Contemporary

Health Issues

Eric W. Banister
Murray Allen
Samia Fadl
Gordon Bhakthan
Dawn Howard

ST. PHILIP'S COLLEGE LIBRARY

JONES AND BARTLETT PUBLISHERS

BOSTON   PORTOLA VALLEY

Copyright © 1988 by Jones and Bartlett Publishers, Inc. All rights reserved. No part of the material protected by this copyright notice may be reproduced or utilized in any form, electronic or mechanical, including photocopying, recording, or by any information storage and retrieval system, without written permission from the copyright owner.

Editorial, Sales, and Customer Service Offices:
Jones and Bartlett Publishers
20 Park Plaza
Boston, MA 02116

Printed in the United States of America
10 9 8 7 6 5 4 3 2 1

Library of Congress Cataloging-in-Publication Data

Contemporary health issues.

    Includes index.
    1. Public health. 2. Medicine, Preventive.
1. Banister, Eric. [DNLM: 1. Delivery of Health Care.
2. Occupational Diseases--prevention & control.
3. Stress--prevention & control. 4. World Health.
WA 540.1 C761]
RA425.C774 1988   362.1   86-27766
ISBN 0-86720-077-4 (pbk.)

ISBN 0-86720-077-4

REPRODUCED FROM CAMERA-READY COPY
SUPPLIED BY THE AUTHORS.

Acknowledgements

The authors would like to thank the many people who contributed to this text. First there are those authors and publishers who allowed our use of material previously published. Early typescripts of the authors' often illegible offerings were made by Laurie Klak and Thelma Ashton of the School of Kinesiology's office staff.

That the text is so superbly illustrated is due to the efforts of several artists in the Instructional Media Center of Simon Fraser University, principally Jacquie Campbell and Connie Bell. The meticulous detective work of Deanne Mackie, permissions clerk, in tracing even the most obscure primary reference source was invaluable. To all the students on whom early iterations of the text were tested and who noted both minor and major errors needing correction, we are grateful. The criticisms whether harsh, constructive or congratulatory, from a wide selection of reviewers improved the final product and encouraged us to think that indeed we had raised some vital concerns relevant to contemporary health care. We are particularly indebted to Kathleen Roe for continued support, suggestions and encouragement.

In the countless revisions the text has undergone in the two year history of its writing, the patient, cheerful, unflagging effort of Patricia Good has been invaluable. Her developing expertness in desktop publishing and deftness of touch in layout are evident throughout the text.

We are especially indebited to Dr. J.C. Yerbury, Director of Distance Education, at Simon Fraser University for his continuing logistic and financial support during the book's preparation.

February, 1988

Introduction

Welcome to Contemporary Health Issues. This dynamic subject cannot help but raise some questions and issues of interest to you, since your life is affected so directly by your health and happiness. These two factors to the exclusion of almost all else uniquely determine the quality of one's life. The very fact of being healthy and happy in one's general and immediate environment implies that the surrounding society is a caring one. To achieve success in this the society must be continuously mindful of its responsibility to provide a sufficient measure of employment, shelter, services, culture, sport, medical care, safety at work and play, and peace and protection. At the same time it must remain flexible and innovative in adapting positively to evolving patterns of change both within itself and relative to others.

It will become obvious to you that societies all over the world face important and complex challenges in their immediate and distant future in maintaining their present, or aspiring to a better, quality of life.

Many of these areas of challenge are discussed at an elementary level in this book. We, the authors, hope that they will stimulate you to dig deeper into the issues brought up and to formulate your own strategies for living which will enrich your society and thus further enhance your own quality of life.

SCOPE AND ORGANIZATION

As you will see from a glance at the Table of Contents this book covers a broad range of topics. The topics are diverse by reason of the fact that it was produced by a team of five authors, all of whom naturally bring differing views and styles to the task. As a group we offer you variations in perspective on the issues dealt with, and a broader knowledge base from which to work than any one of us alone could have provided. We have attempted to keep expressions of individual bias to a minimum, and at least to make them as explicit as possible wherever they are included. Overall, our aim is to present you with current information on each of the health concerns addressed, and we encourage you also to assess the issues objectively and intelligently for yourself. In many cases material on several sides of an issue is presented. This is important not only because the field of health is changing so rapidly, but also because it provides a broader framework for understanding and evaluating concepts and viewpoints at local, national or international levels as they will appear in the future.

The book consists of 16 chapters grouped into four sections, or Parts. **Part One** introduces you to current social issues and national and world concerns relating to health. This part is referred to as **The Global Perspective.** **Part Two,** called **Hazards to Health,** includes pollution, health and the workplace, stress, and disease. Then in **Part Three, Fitness and Health in the 80s,** we address modern developments and trends in areas such as nutrition, sports medicine, drugs (particularly their use in sports), and bioengineering. Finally, (lest we forget!) we return to the "basics" of our lives and our life cycles, to explore the topics of sexuality, reproduction, aging and family violence. These chapters make up **Part Four, The Human Condition.**

OBJECTIVES

When you have completed this book you should be able to:

- **Distinguish** between definitions of health which focus upon avoidance of illness, injury or dying, and those which center around wellness, development and movement toward a fuller, more complete life.
- **Outline** the complex interaction of fundamental forces which control the quality of life, and hence the health, of all people.
- **Describe** the kinds and magnitude of problems facing modern society, and the ways in which these problems dictate the workings and planning for any health care system.
- **List and describe** major contributors to pollution in North America, and discuss the real and potential health effects of each.
- **Explain** the role of work and the workplace in the lives of modern people, and pinpoint at least three aspects of occupational health which are crucial to all workers.
- **Describe** the factors which contribute to one's susceptibility to illness, including diet, lifestyle factors, ergonomics, and exposure to infections and toxins.
- **Discuss** the importance of fitness and sport in modern living, and outline the ways in which participating at all levels may be safely enhanced for optimal benefit (including prevention and care of sports injuries, effective integration of physical activities into daily life, and avoidance of drug misuse/abuse).

- **Outline** modern thoughts on human sexuality and some of the scientific developments which have changed or are changing reproductive practices in our society.
- **Define** bioengineering and describe its possible present and future contributions to the health care system.
- **Describe and discuss** the effects of aging in physiological, psychological and social terms. Outline how these effects may be dealt with in positive ways by the elderly, their families, and society.
- **Describe** the myths associated with family violence in our society and understand the cyclical nature of the problem.

More specific objectives are provided at the beginning of each chapter. Reading them over before you begin to study the chapter will help you prepare mentally for what is to come.

STUDY QUESTIONS

At the end of each chapter you will find Study Questions. They are included to assist you in reviewing the material you have read, and to guide your study of some of the main points. We suggest that you jot down your answers to these questions, particularly those which you find difficult or complex. You may find that this helps you to remember things more easily. This also is a good way to determine exactly where your problems of understanding are, if any.

About the Authors

Murray Allen

Is a graduate of the University of Alberta Medical School in Edmonton. In 1964, Dr. Allen pursued extra training in surgery and orthopaedics before beginning a general practice in North Vancouver, Canada. This gradually extended into a referral practice for the management of pain, and later still into Sports Medicine. In earlier years he used hypnosis as an adjunct to therapy. Starting in 1968, he was one of the first physicians in North America to research and practice acupuncture.

He now has an appointment as Associate Professor in Kinesiology at Simon Fraser University in conjunction with his consulting clinical practice in Sports Medicine and pain management. His research interests extend into the role of endorphins in pain, acupuncture, and sports, and its physical and mental effects upon the body.

Eric W. Banister

Dr. Banister was born in England. He received his undergraduate education in England (B.Sc. Manchester Univ., 1953; Diploma (PE), Loughborough College, 1954). Continuing his studies in North America, he obtained a Master's degree in Physical Education from U.B.C. in 1962, followed by his Ph.D. in 1964 from the University of Illinois.

Dr. Banister joined University of British Columbia as Assistant Professor of Physical Education in 1964, and then came to Simon Fraser University as an Assistant Professor in the Department of Physical Development Studies in 1967. When this department was re-organized in 1970, he became an Associate Professor in the Kinesiology Department and its first chairman. A position he held until 1975 and then again from 1977-82.

As Director of the Institute for Human Performance since 1980, President of Western Fitness Consultants Ltd. (Vancouver) from 1972-75, and an active member of numerous associations involved with Human Factors, engineering, fitness and sports sciences, Dr. Banister contributes a great deal to the academic and professional community. He has authored 3 books, more than 60 articles in scientific journals, several book chapters and reviews, and was Editor of the Canadian Journal of Applied Sports Sciences from 1980-83. Currently, he is on the Editorial Boards of Undersea Medical Research and the Journal of Physiological Anthropology (Japan).

N.M. Gordon Bhakthan

Dr. Gordon Bhakthan received his M.Sc. and Ph.D. degrees in animal physiology from M.S. University in Baroda, India, in 1958 and 1961, respectively. With more than 40 publications in scientific journals and proceedings, Dr. Bhakthan has been a professor in the Kinesiology Department at Simon Fraser University since 1970. His research interests include cellular adaptations to environmental stress and drugs, and the biology of aging.

Currently Dr. Bhakthan serves as Chairman of the Undergraduate Curriculum Committee in the Kinesiology Department, and was Academic Advisor for the Faculty of Interdisciplinary Studies.

Samia Fadl

Dr. Samia Fadl obtained both her B.Sc. (1965) and M.Sc. (1968) in Chemical Engineering from the University of Alexandria, Egypt. In 1978, she obtained her Ph.D. in Engineering from the University of British Columbia, Canada. Prior to coming to Canada, she worked for 8 years as a project engineer in Alexandria. In Vancouver, she worked for two years as scientific project engineer in the pulp and paper industry. At that time she also was working as sessional lecturer in The Department of Bioresource Engineering at U.B.C.

In 1980, Dr. Fadl joined the Department of Kinesiology at Simon Fraser University as Assistant Professor and in 1983 she was appointed by the new Faculty of Engineering Science as Assistant Professor. She held a joint appointment, dividing her time between these two areas. Her field of teaching and research involves Environmental Engineering and Control, and Occupational Health and Safety. She has now left the School of Kinesiology, as it is now, to devote full time to her own high-tech international company specializing in waste effluent purification systems which she has designed and engineered.

Dawn Howard

Since 1982 Dawn Howard has been Academic Coordinator for distance education programs in Education and Kinesiology at Simon Fraser University. She is also currently Editor of the Journal of Distance Education.

Prior to her graduate work in Education, she trained and worked as a Child Care Worker in Ontario. She now serves on the Board of Directors of the North Shore Crisis Services Society (North Vancouver, B.C.), which operates a transition house for battered women and their children.

Contents

Part I

The Global Perspective

CHAPTER 1
Introduction to Health

CHAPTER 2
World Health

CHAPTER 3
Health Care Delivery

ST. PHILIP'S COLLEGE LIBRARY

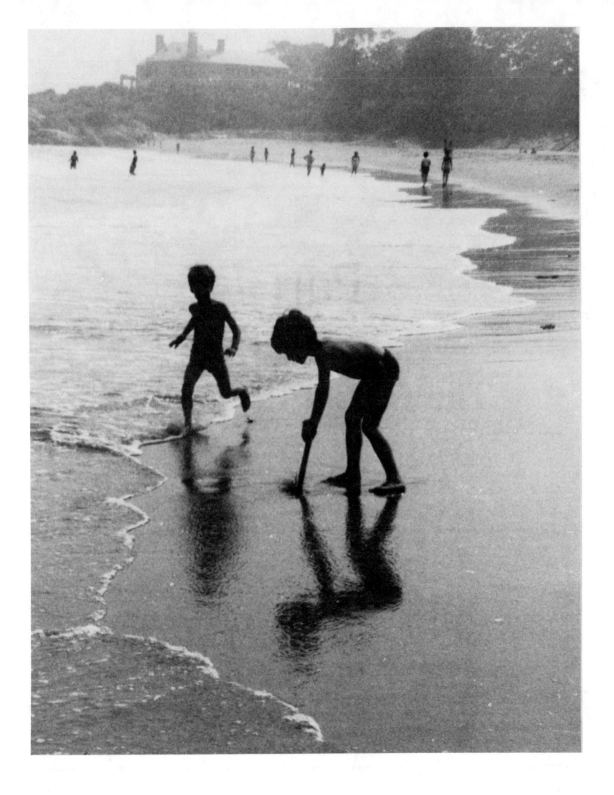

1

Introduction to Health

Health is likely to be our
most valuable possession throughout life.

OBJECTIVES
When you have completed this chapter, you should be able to:
- Recognize that health and disease form a continuum, ranging from high-level health to death, with many intermediate stages in between.
- Compare and contrast the underlying philosophies of allopathic versus holistic health care.
- Briefly outline the relationship between body and mind in determining one's state of health.

KEY TERMS
allopathic health care	lifestyle disease
disease	placebo
health	psychosomatic illness
"holistic" health care	wellness
homeostasis	

1.0 INTRODUCTION
As the title suggests, this book is an introduction to contemporary health issues—issues that should interest us all, from an academic standpoint and personally as well. Since health is likely to be our most valuable possession throughout life, we are well advised to find out as much as possible about what it is and how to maintain and promote it. Society's perception of health has changed dramatically over the past several years and continues to do so as new information is discovered about the human potential and the effect of various environmental influences upon it.

In modern societies it is becoming increasingly evident that traditional medicine is only one of many factors influencing personal health. As society continues to increase in complexity, we are beginning to recognize the impact on health, not only of infectious organisms, but of such diverse influences as industrialization and technology, environmental pollution, pyschological anxiety and dietary concerns. Previously health was thought to be a static condition characterized by the absence of disease or infirmity, and a matter of concern only to medical practitioners who specialized in treating and controlling disease-causing organisms or trauma. However, it is becoming increasingly recognized that health is a dynamic process involving body, mind, and spirit, and that individuals can play an active role in maintaining their own well-being.

This new awareness of the complexity and interrelationships of various health issues has not only had an impact on the traditional health-care delivery system, but on the teaching of health as well. While it once focused primarily on anatomy and hygiene, health education today encompasses a great number of critical contemporary issues. These range from the influence of diet and exercise on longevity, to the burgeoning costs of traditional health-care delivery, environmental pollution, and world population, economics and political systems.

This chapter outlines how the traditional perception of health is evolving into a more contemporary, **holistic view** emphasizing disease prevention rather than cure. It will provide an introduction to preventive health care, which will be a major emphasis throughout the remainder of the book.

1.1 DEFINITIONS OF HEALTH

Before proceeding any further, it is important to clarify the definition of health that will be adhered to throughout this book. The reason for this is that the way in which you define health determines to some extent how you behave. For example, if you define health as the absence of disease and disability, then you are probably a person who has regular medical check-ups, drives with caution and gets enough sleep. If you define health as deriving satisfaction from life, then you may be a person who is willing to risk your physical health to achieve this satisfaction. You may, for example, sky-dive, drive fast or ski for excitement even though these activities pose some threat to your physical health. For most of us, both aspects of health, i.e. quality and quantity, are important; therefore in deciding how to behave in each situation, we must weigh the satisfaction or benefit of each individual risk against its potential danger. As stated above, it is becoming increasingly evident that health is not merely the absence of disease or discomfort. Rather, it is a complete state of physical, mental, social and spiritual well-being that each of us can experience, and which many of us do experience, even if only for short periods of time. Health also is a process of continuous change or adaptation throughout the life cycle. Because there are a variety of influences, both favorable and unfavorable, that confront us throughout life, our health is constantly changing. It is a process not a condition. Being a healthy person does not mean you are never sick. Rather, it means that you possess the resources to cope effectively with a variety of situations and changes, and to respond or adapt to these within the broader context of your well-being.

Health, like love or happiness, is a quality of life that is difficult to define and virtually impossible to measure. For years, health specialists have been unable to agree unanimously upon such a definition. The World Health Organization (WHO) defines health as a

"complete state of physical, mental and social well-being and not merely the absence of disease or infirmity".

This definition is so broad that some critics regard it as meaningless, but its universality can also be seen as its strongest point. You might like to develop your own definition of health. Try writing down one which is meaningful to you, and then look at it again at the end of this book, to see whether there has been a change in your views. Here is a slightly different definition:

Health is a relative state of ability to mobilize one's resources to respond effectively with one's environment to the stresses that come one's way.

(Eisenberg and Eisenberg, 1979).

As you can see, this definition implies, as mentioned earlier, that health is a process. It also states clearly that people can influence their own state of health by using the resources they already possess. The definition goes on to suggest that our state of health occurs in relationship with (not in opposition to) our environment. Finally, it also includes the state of your mind, which is undoubtedly one of the most important influences on your health. In order to mobilize your internal resources, you must first make a conscious decision to do so.

1.2 THE WELLNESS MODEL

Considering health as the totality of a person's existence is a holistic view of health. This approach recognizes the contribution and interrelatedness of physical, psychological, emotional, spiritual and environmental factors to the overall quality of a person's life. Unfortunately, the word holistic has often been misunderstood and maligned in recent years. Since it may include alternative therapies such as biofeedback, naturopathy and acupuncture, it has mistakenly been associated with a whole array of less scientific, or as yet unproven, approaches to health care. However, the philosophy of holistic health is not based on all or anyone of these therapies. Nor is the philosophy incompatible with the ideas of conventional medicine. Rather, a holistic philosophy of health emphasizes a view that has gained wide acceptance among members of the medical community: that each person has the capacity and the responsibility for optimizing his or her sense of well-being and for creating conditions and feelings that can help prevent disease.

To illustrate, consider whether you would regard a diabetic as being healthy. If your definition of health is merely the absence of disease, you probably wouldn't. However, if a diabetic has adjusted his or her life to be happy and self-fulfilled, we probably would say that he/she has developed a quite adequate **wellness**. Wellness as defined here, concerns the quality of life. It means being in control of your life while at

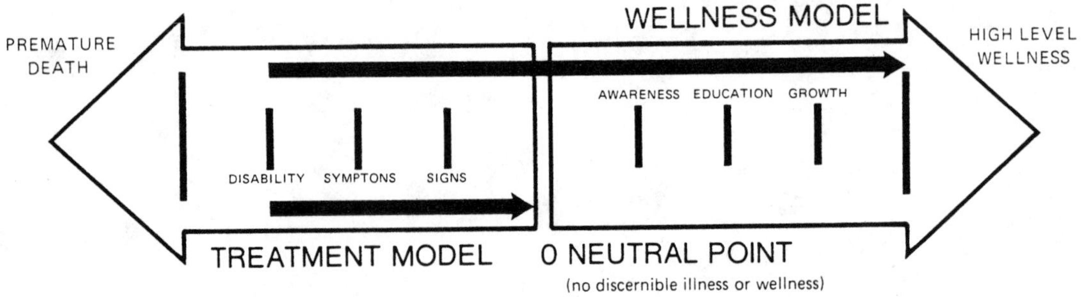

Figure 1.1. The Wellness Model versus the Treatment Model. Reproduced with permission from Travis, 1977.

the same time recognizing that you cannot control everything affecting you. It means living your life so that it is rewarding and satisfying. Thus, with this definition, it is possible to be **physically healthy** but to not have **wellness**, and it also is possible to have wellness without being completely healthy physically.

Wellness may be said to begin when a person sees him/herself as a growing, changing person (Carroll and Miller, p. 6, 1986). High level wellness (Figure 1.1), means giving care to the physical self, using the mind constructively, channeling stress energies positively, expressing emotions effectively, becoming creatively involved with others, and staying in touch with the environment (Travis, 1977).

Figure 1.1 illustrates the distinction between the **Wellness Model** and the **Treatment Model** which it overlaps. Moving to the right of centre in the diagram indicates

"increasing levels of health and well-being. The treatment model can bring you from varying states of disease to the neutral point, where symptoms have been alleviated. The wellness model, which can be utilized at any point, directs you beyond neutral, and encourages you to move as far to the right as possible. It is not meant to replace the treatment model on the left side of the continuum, but to work in harmony with it." (Travis, facing p.1, 1977).

1.3 RESPONSIBILITY FOR HEALTH AND WELLNESS

There are a great many facets of life over which we have no immediate or direct control. Some of these, such as unemployment, poverty, political power struggles and nuclear warfare, environmental pollution and the rising cost of medical care, seem to be such massive problems that we, as individuals, are left feeling powerless to effect change. Ultimately, we all want the world to be a better place in which to live, but how can we, as individuals, possibly influence issues of such magnitude? How can we help bring an end to world malnutrition, hunger and starvation when food and material goods are sometimes used by wealthy nations to barter for influence in less fortunate nations? What can you do to solve the problem of decreasing funds for old-age security and medical care for increasing numbers of senior citizens? How can one protect one's own lungs from deteriorating while living in a city constantly exposed to automobile exhaust and other people's cigarette smoke? Unfortunately, many times the response to these questions is to throw one's hands in the air in frustration and do nothing.

Change, however, begins with the individual. As demonstrated so frequently over the past several years, whether this be in the types of food available on supermarket shelves or (optimistically) the number of nuclear warheads readied for a devastating war, cumulative personal action can have an effect. There undoubtedly are a number of things which we all still can do to improve our own (and, indirectly, the world's) health. Hopefully, this book will help you identify some of the positive actions you can take in your own life.

Fortunately, achieving a healthy lifestyle is possible, and is not terribly expensive or difficult. It is not always necessary to lobby a government, participate in demonstrations or convince some large organization to change its rules. Moreover, one need not rely completely upon assurances from a third party (i.e. medical insurance) to guarantee care or protection against the inevitability of illness or the need for tonics, vitamin supplements or drugs. While it is comforting to know that such help is available, planning to use it to a minimum is desirable. The majority of today's health problems are more likely to be self-inflicted perils than ills over which we have no control. Diseases such as heart disease, cancer and hypertension, which today account for the largest loss of life in people over forty, may be preventable through self-directed healthful living. (This will be discussed in Chapter 7).

To achieve a healthy life, simply live healthfully. Apply some of the principles of health science, coupled with an understanding of how your mind, body and emotions interrelate. Set some health goals for yourself, and follow through in achieving these goals. The first step in achieving a healthy lifestyle is to take responsibility for your own health and well-being. Take **responsibility** (not blame or guilt) for your feelings, your relationships, your diet, your level of physical activity, your drug-taking behavior (including smoking cigarettes and drinking alcohol) and your social environment. **Social environment** means where you live, work or go to school, and the stresses that may result from them. All these factors, to a certain extent lie within your power to control, change, or accept, depending on what you want out of life.

Once you take responsibility for your health and well-being, you will begin to feel more powerful and confident. People usually find that it feels better to take care of themselves than to abuse themselves—to engage in nurturing rather than self-destructive behaviors.

1.4 DISEASE

If one accepts a holistic concept of health, what does this imply for the definition of disease? Most people in our society take health for granted, paying little attention to their physical condition until pain or discomfort signals that something has gone wrong. Our reaction is usually that of surprise, frustration or anger at such an unwarranted intrusion, accompanied by anxiety and a sense of helplessness. Often we are uncertain of what has gone wrong, why it has happened, or how to make it better. The solution is a trip to the family physician for some medication and a cure. Disease is thought of as being caused by an external invader attacking a previously healthy body. The blame goes to defective genes, bad luck, last night's meal, or something in the air. Most of all, one just wants to feel better.

In contrast, the holistic concept of disease views it as a failure to respond appropriately to challenge. Remember that we are constantly being exposed to both favourable and unfavourable influences. Failure to respond effectively to unfavourable challenges, whether these be viruses, poor diet or stress, results in disease. Disease is not a static event, or an alien presence within us. Rather, it is a conflict of opposing forces of different strengths which can be expressed on different levels: physical, psychological, social or spiritual.

1.4.1 Homeostasis

Threats to health are resisted and reacted to by the body's struggle to preserve **homeostasis**. Homeostasis is the tendency for the body systems to interact and to be regulated in such a way as to maintain a relatively constant physiological state. For example, homeostatic mechanisms maintain internal body temperature near 37°C, heart rate between 60 and 90 beats per minute, and blood glucose (sugar) levels around 80 mg per 100 ml of blood. Opposing forces to increase or decrease these values function harmoniously to maintain homeostasis, a phenomenon referred to by physiologist Walter B. Canon as the **wisdom of the body**. A weakening of some of the opposing forces results in disruption of homeostasis, and maybe the onset of disease.

Those of you familiar with Eastern philosophy may recognize similarities between the concept of homeostatis and the idea of mind-body harmony, Yin and Yang. Yin and Yang are viewed as two opposite but complimentary types of natural forces or energies. Yin is characterized by darkness, receptiveness and quiet. Yang, on the other hand, symbolizes light, creativity and movement. When Yin and Yang forces are in balance in an individual, a state of internal harmony (homeostasis) exists and the person experiences health and well-being. If, however, either Yin or Yang forces predominate in a person, a state of disharmony or disease may result.

Disease therefore can serve as a valuable source of feedback regarding one's inner harmony and one's relationship with the environment.

At this point, however, it is important to distinguish between a disease and its symptoms. For example, increased blood pressure is a symptom, not a disease. It is a symptom of an underlying disorder or imbalance, which may have originated from unknown causes or from a long history of poor eating habits, lack of exercise and poor reaction to stress. No single element in this system is, by itself, the disease; the symptom results from dynamic interaction between various stresses and the body's attempt to compensate. Treating high blood pressure with anti-hypertensive drugs will not provide a complete cure especially if the absolute cause of it remains unknown, although it may relieve the symptom. Also, if the underlying imbalances which have been allied to hypertensive symptoms, are not corrected through improved diet, exercise and stress management, then as soon as the drugs are withdrawn, the symptoms will return. Elevated blood pressure is the feedback signal that lets us know there is an underlying problem.

A similar distinction should be made between illness and disease. The former refers to a general feeling of ill-health, while the latter refers to various structural or functional disorders of tissues and organs. A person may feel ill without an actual disease being evident or diagnosed, a condition sometimes referred to as **psychosomatic**. While the term **psychosomatic illness** was used previously to refer to the imaginary ailments of the hypochondriac, it is now recognized that such disturbances are just as real and damaging as infectious organisms or toxic chemicals. People can affect their physical health by what they think and feel, and a distinctive feature of psychosomatic illness is that psychological, social and environmental influences can contribute to actual physical disorders. Stress-related illnesses all are classified as psychosomatic (see Chapter 6). On the other hand, a person can suffer from a diagnosed disease without feeling ill, as in the case of the diabetic described earlier. In other words, experiencing good health does not imply that one never feels ill or experiences disease. Again there are many causes of illness and disease, and one's attitude towards health to a large degree determines the outcome of both.

1.5 REFERENCES

Carroll, C. and Miller, D. Health: **The Science of Human Adapatation, (4th ed.).** Dubuque, Iowa: Wm. C. Brown, 1986.

Eisenberg, A. and Eisenberg, H. **Alive and Well: Decisions in Health.** New York: McGraw-Hill, 1979.

Travis, J.W. **Wellness Inventory.** Mill Valley, California: Wellness Resource Centre, 1977.

1.6 STUDY QUESTIONS

1. Explain how a positive attitude toward health and well-being can function as a placebo effect. Can you cite examples from your own personal experience that demonstrate the power of the mind to affect health and disease? (Perhaps you've felt ill on the morning of a big exam.)
2. Briefly explain, in biological terms, the relationship between thoughts, feelings and physiology.
3. What is the relationship between homeostasis, illness and disease?

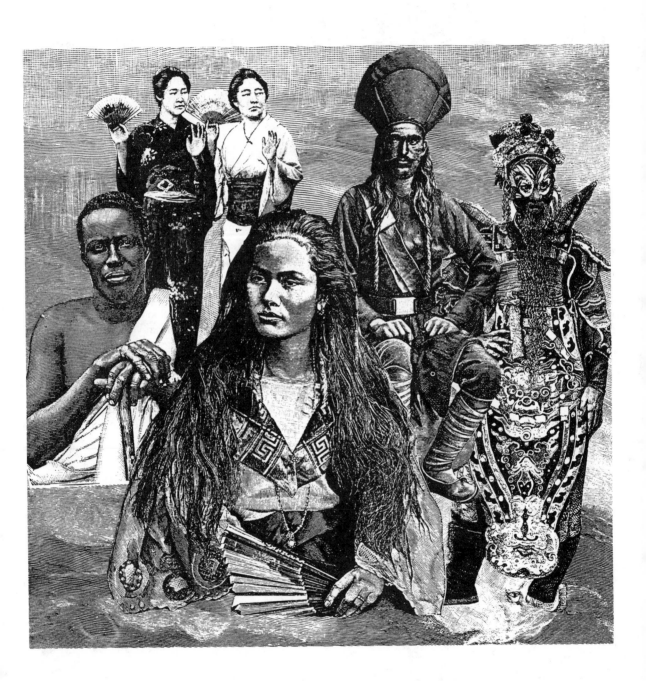

2

World Health

Health is a vital aspect of daily living and must be
a prime consideration in any society's welfare concerns.

OBJECTIVES

When you have completed this chapter, you should be able to:

- **Integrate** and **discuss** divergent reports in the media on local or global health care issues, or the quality of life.
- **Draw up** simple models of the underlying forces which interact to cause observable changes in personal, community, national or international health care.
- **Understand** the forces that lead to excess population growth and **describe** the strain that an uncontrolled rise in population puts upon any society's resources and ability to care for the health and welfare of its people.
- **Outline** trends in world living habits in the future, predictable through the analysis of past events.
- **Understand** the nature of the simple growth curves of any attribute, particularly one in which the attribute grows out of control, and another in which the attribute is controlled by feedback effects so that it grows to a steady state or equilibrium value.
- **Distinguish** between morbidity and mortality and life expectancy and longevity.
- **Discuss** the issues raised, for life in the 21st century, by the model of interactive world forces proposed by Meadows and Meadows in Limits to Growth (1972), and the weaknesses of that model raised by studies like Simon's and his group in **Global Report—Revised.**
- **Outline** the changing pattern of morbidity and mortality in developed countries and the increased interest in disease prevention and health promotion in them.
- **Outline** the changing nature of health care delivery in developed countries from one emphasizing sick care only to one emphasizing, equally, if not more, self-care, self-responsibility and the provision of systems within the society to train and sustain the body in a healthy state for as long as possible.

• **Describe** the imminent onset of a more leisured society and the ramifications this has for living and work habits and the fabric of future society in industrialized nations.

KEY TERMS

asymptote   population expansion
global modeling   systems model interactions and feedback
morbidity   replacement fertility
mortality

2.0 INTRODUCTION

Later chapters of this book deal with health concerns of individuals. In order to give you a wider perspective, this chapter and the next deal with issues that affect **all** the world's people, issues that involve important social and economic trends in the late twentieth century.

Health is a vital aspect of daily living and must be a prime consideration in any society's welfare concerns. Changes in our own western society have been accomplished, are being introduced, or are being planned in such areas as:

• Population control
• Abortion
• Euthanasia
• Management of criminals
• Preservation and enhancement of the environment
• Treatment of drug addiction and alcoholism
• Protecting the food supply from contamination
• Changing lifestyle patterns incorporating recreation, exercise, nutritional concerns.
• Provision of health care for all.

Table 2.1. Comparison of age structures in developed and developing countries, 1980. Reproduced with permission from **World Development Report, World Bank**, 1984.

Country Group	Age distribution (percent)					Total fertility rate
	0-4	5-14	15-64	over 65	all ages	
All developed countries	7.6	15.5	65.6	11.3	100.0	1.9[a]
Japan	7.3	16.1	67.7	8.9	100.0	1.8
United States	7.9	15.0	66.3	10.7	100.0	1.9
Hungary	8.0	13.7	64.9	15.9	100.0	2.1
All developing countries	13.6	25.5	57.0	4.0	100.0	4.2[a]
Korea, Republic of	10.6	22.7	62.7	4.0	100.0	3.0
Colombia	14.0	25.4	57.1	3.5	100.0	3.8
Bangladesh	17.9	24.9	54.6	2.6	100.0	6.3
Kenya	22.4	28.6	46.1	2.9	100.0	8.0

[a.] Weighted average

There are many other areas of concern and you can probably list some yourself. Any Government's Department of Health carries responsibility for all or most of these issues.

2.0.1 Health, Happiness and Quality of Life

Health is a major determinant of happiness. The capability of a society's systems to look after its people depends to a large extent on the sheer number of people needing care. Other important factors are the quality of the population, the physical and intellectual vigor of a people, their developed technology, environmental surroundings, and general affluence. These all bear upon the quality of life within a society and consequently, upon any individual's health within that society. Methods have been adopted in the so-called developed (industrialized) countries to influence substantially both the quantity of the population and its quality of life. These methods are, as yet, unexplored in the less well developed or emergent nations. Some of the methods themselves provoke debate, even violence, and include such issues as:

• Population control, either by contraception or planned abortion
• Prolongation of life by modern medical technology and chronic care of the elderly
• Diagnosis of genetic deficiency and control of propagation in genetically deficient adults
• Adoption and rearing of children born of surrogate mothers
• Environmental protection and occupational health and safety
• The cost of health care
• Eradication of prejudice and racism

You may be able to list some other important issues from your own knowledge. Do this for yourself.

Inevitably the conclusion remains that both the **Quantity and Quality** of a society's population determine its ability to care for the health and happiness of the people within it.

Table 2.2. Rural and urban population growth, 1950-2000. Reproduced with permission from *World Development Report*, World Bank, 1984.

Country group	Percentage urban population			Average annual percentage growth			
				1950-1980		1980-2000	
	1950	1980	2000	Urban	Rural	Urban	Rural
All developing countries	18.9	28.7	-	3.4	1.7	-	-
Excluding China	22.2	35.4	43.3	3.8	1.7	3.5	1.1
Low-income							
Asia	10.7	19.5	31.3	4.4	2.0	4.2	0.9
China	11.2	13.2[a]	-	2.5	1.8	-	-
India	16.8	23.3	35.5	3.2	1.8	4.2	1.1
Africa	5.7	19.2	34.9	7.0	2.5	5.8	1.5
Middle-income							
East Asia and Pacific	19.6	31.9	41.9	4.1	1.8	3.1	0.9
Middle East & North Africa	27.7	46.8	59.9	4.4	1.6	4.3	1.6
Sub-Saharan Africa	33.7	49.4	55.2	3.1	1.0	2.9	1.7
Latin America & Caribbean	41.4	65.3	75.4	4.1	0.8	2.9	0.4
Southern Europe	24.7	47.1	62.3	3.8	0.5	2.9	-0.2
Industrial countries[b]	61.3	77.0	83.7	1.8	-0.7	1.0	-1.1

a. Government estimate for 1979.　b. Excludes East European nonmarket economies.

2.1 TRENDS IN LIVING HABITS, MORTALITY, MORBIDITY AND HEALTH CARE EXPENDITURE

2.1.1 Living Habits in 2000 AD

Table 2.1 shows some recent demographic trends. The population probably will continue to expand at an annual percentage rate of 0.8 to 1.0 in industrialized nations and from 1.8 to 2.4 in the rest of the world. The proportion of people over 65 will also increase dramatically to some 15-20% of the population in developed nations (see Chapter 14). This will impose an increasingly heavy economic burden, as many of these older people become non-working, infirm and suffer increasingly from degenerative diseases.

The pace of urbanization will be greatest in developing countries. Even now over 2/5 of the world's 5 billion people live in cities. In the Western world 4 out of 5 people already do. Figure 2.1 shows the aggregation of people in world cities (urban areas of greater than 10 million inhabitants) projected to the year 2000. Soon some of the former great cities of the west may no longer rank as such by population count and the majority of world cities will be in developing countries. The problems attendant upon the aggregation of such numbers for societies with insufficient resources to care for them are immense.

Urbanization will continue to increase (Table 2.2) until 80-85% of the population of industrialized countries live within urban concentrations. With this will come all the attendant nervous and physical strain on individuals from traffic, the hustle of daily life, pollution, noise, etc.

High technology computer-integrated manufacturing (CIM) increasingly will invade the work place replacing **people intensive** processes. This may be visualized as a move from the **smokestack** to the **robot** (Figure 2.2). General Motors spent no less than $40 Billion over the last 5 years (1981-86) on CIM factories of the future. In such factories Information Technology (IT) and computer control slash waste

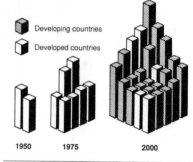

Urban agglomerations with more than 10 million inhabitants: 1950, 1975, and 2000

Developing countries

Developed countries

1950　1975　2000

1950	(millions)		(millions)
New York, northeast New Jersey	12.2	London	10.4

1975			
New York, northeast New Jersey	19.8	London	10.4
Mexico City	11.9	Tokyo, Yokohama	17.7
Los Angeles		Shanghai	11.6
Long Beach	10.8	Sao Paulo	10.7

2000			
Mexico City	31.10	Sao Paulo	25.8
Tokyo, Yokohama	24.2	New York, northeast	
Shanghai	22.7	New Jersey	22.8
Beijing	19.9	Rio de Janeiro	19.0
Greater Bombay	17.1	Calcutta	16.7
Jakarta	16.6	Seoul	14.2
Los Angeles		Cairo, Giza, Imbaba	13.1
Long Beach	14.2	Manila	12.3
Madras	12.9	Bangkok, Thonburi	11.9
Greater Buenos Aires	12.1	Delhi	11.7
Karachi	11.8	Paris	11.3
Bagota	11.7	Istanbul	11.2
Tehran	11.3	Osaka, Kobe	11.1
Baghdad	11.1		

Source: United Nations, 1980

Figure 2.1. Shows urban agglomerations with more than 10 million inhabitants: 1950, 1975 and 2000. Reproduced with permission from **World Development Report**, World Bank, 1984.

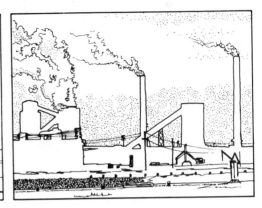

Figure 2.2. From smokestack to robots. Reproduced with permission from **Macleans**, p. 18 and 28, March 20, 1987.

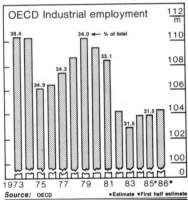

Fewer on the factory floor

Figure 2.3. Decline in jobs in the six largest countries.... the organization for economic co-operation and development (OECD) in the last 8 years. Reproduced with permission from **The Economist**, Dec. 20, p. 94, 1986.

Table 2.3. Growth in participation in games and sports in Canada from 1972-1976. Reproduced with permission from **The 1976 Fitness and Sport Survey**, Dec. 1977.

Activity	Number in 1972 1,000's	Number in 1976 1,000's	Growth (%)
Tennis	732	2,175	197
Skiing	1,000	2,534	153
Jogging	1,039	2,575	148
Golf	1,100	1,911	74
Swimming	4,191	7,117	70
Skating	2,155	2,930	36
Bicycling	1,743	2,225	28
Curling	643	826	28
Hockey	1,191	1,459	23
Walking	6,167	6,984	13

through information on: machine wear, minimal inventory needs, pricing, overhead, handling and management costs. Benefits from this, if indeed they may be viewed as such, will include a reduction in working hours and a decrease in amounts of physical effort needed from the worker.

This change will not be without its attendent problems **particularly** for established societies, **especially** the inflexible economies. Unfortunately, the post World War II boom in the economies of developed nations, fuelled by labor intensive methods, promoted and encouraged a rise in the wages and expectations of millions of blue collar workers (and white collars too). These expectations are now being crushed by the increasing technology of modern manufacturing, leaving people at every level suddenly unneeded (Figure 2.3). More seriously, the minimum level of competence needed to do a modern job is often greater than the qualifications of many aspiring applicants without their undertaking retraining, and then further retraining, as even their new skills/knowledge become quickly outmoded in the accelerating pace of technological change. This is a daunting task indeed for the average person and an unwanted stress and daily worry threatening the happiness and health of many.

Leisure time will increase significantly for most people, as a result of shorter working hours, earlier retirement from conventional jobs, increased robotization and efficiency in producing material goods.

The amount of leisure time spent by Canadians in physical activity is shown in Table 2.3. These data are somewhat unreliable since the defined time and frequency of participation by many were really not high enough to classify them as true participants. Nevertheless, the promotion of physical activity as a national goal will probably lessen the incidence of costly degenerative diseases in a society in the future. The increasing availability of leisure time for people to do this must certainly then be considered as a factor. The United States has been more realistic

Table 2.5. Principal causes of death in industrial countries expressed as a percent of all deaths in the years between 1960 and 1984.

Cause of Death	1960	1965	1984
Cardiovascular diseases	36	32	33
Cancer	22	19	38
Apoplexy (cerebrovascular accidents)	10.5	13	6
Accidents	6.7	5	6.6
Influenza/pulmonary infections	3.1	3.3	2.1

in counting its physically active participants. One survey made recently showed that although 42% of adults over 18 years exercised or played sports, only 10-20% did so with sufficient frequency and intensity to produce increased cardiorespiratory fitness. In another survey of 22 states, 1/2 of them reported 50% of their citizenry sedentary, defined by the criterion of their not taking physical activity of some form for 20 minutes at least 3 times per week (Table 2.4). Participation in all other forms of leisue activity e.g. education, the arts and sciences is probably no less than this.

2.1.2 Disease and Mortality

Table 2.5 shows principal causes of death in industrialized countries, between 1960 and 1984. These categories and proportions have not altered materially in the last 20 years except for cancer. Table 2.6 shows principal causes of death in the U.S. in 1984. Check for yourself that the leading causes are similar. Is modern medicine failing here? The main cause of death is degenerative disease; infectious diseases are essentially conquered. Deaths in underdeveloped nations, however, still occur mainly from infections, both bacterial and viral, and from hunger. Infant mortality is particularly high and high mortality rates continue throughout childhood in those nations. Infant mortality is also high in some industrial nations in some disadvantaged groups. Thus, in the American non-white population, infant mortality is 2-3 times greater than in the white population.

New diseases continually advance throughout the world, to take the place of those already eradicated, and in their turn threaten life. For example, no cure is presently known for Acquired Immune Deficiency Syndrome (AIDS). Life expectancy has been increased in developed countries for some sections of the population (principally those financially better off) by the virtual elimination of infant and childhood mortality. But even if a cure for degenerative diseases, heart disease, cancer and stroke were found, little more than 12 years would be added to life beyond the allotted 3 score and 10 (70 years).

Table 2.4. Percentage of sedentary adults in various states. Reproduced with permission from Simmons, K. **The Physician and Sports Medicine**, 15(1): 190-195, January, 1987.

Idaho	44.2
Montana	45.0
Arizona	46.1
Utah	47.5
Florida	51.5
New York	51.5
Illinois	52.4
Connecticut	52.8
California	53.5
Wisconsin	53.5
North Dakota	54.6
District of Columbia	54.9
Minnesota	55.7
North Carolina	57.7
Ohio	61.3
Kentucky	61.4
West Virginia	61.7
Georgia	63.8
Indiana	64.5
South Carolina	64.5
Rhode Island	65.1
Tennessee	67.8

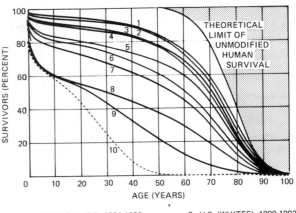

Figure 2.4. Historical changes in the human survival curve.

1. NEW ZEALAND, 1934-1938
2. U.S. (WHITES), 1939-1941
3. U.S. (WHITES), 1929-1931
4. ENGLAND AND WALES, 1930-1932
5. ITALY, 1930-1932
6. U.S. (WHITES), 1900-1902
7. JAPAN, 1926-1930
8. MEXICO, 1930
9. BRITISH INDIA, 1921-1930
10. STONE AGE MAN

Table 2.6. Causes of deaths in the United States in 1984. Modified and reproduced with permission from **Centers for Disease Control,** 35: 1986.

Cause of death	deaths per 100,000	(rank)
All causes (total)	866.7	
Unintentional injuries	40.1	(4)
Malignant neoplasms	191.6	(2)
Heart diseases	324.4	(1)
Suicide, homicide	20.6	(7)
Congenital anomalies	5.6	(10)
Prematurity	3.5	(11)
Sudden infant death syndrome	2.4	(12)
Cerebrovascular diseases	65.6	(3)
Chronic liver diseases and cirrhosis	11.3	(9)
Pneumonia and influenza	25.0	(6)
Chronic obstructive pulmonary diseases	29.8	(5)
Diabetes mellitus	15.6	(8)

Table 2.7. Principal causes of disablement morbidity in France (%) from 1950 to 1968.

Causes of disablement	1950	1958	1965	1968
Psychoses	6.25	9.53	15.00	20.17
Arthritis and rheumatism	5.72	9.08	10.61	10.24
Tuberculosis	26.60	22.92	9.04	5.72
Cerebrovascular injuries	2.30	3.84	6.39	7.59
Arteriosclerotic and degenerative diseases of the heart	7.19	7.74	9.03	8.55
Tumours	3.44	3.88	4.26	5.51
Accidents	1.75	3.12	2.97	3.04

Figure 2.4 shows the principal way in which modern medicine has increased life expectancy in industrialized nations, compared with under-developed countries. This has been achieved by protecting the infant. There has been a steady increase in life expectancy: from 40 years in 1870 to 68-77 years in 1970 (this varies according to sex and country). In fact, the sexagenarian of today can hope to live another 18 years beyond this, compared with the 12 years he or she could have expected 150 years ago. However, further progress in achieving greater life expectancy would necessitate a decline in mortality not among young children, but among older people. Perhaps you can estimate from your own research, and draw in for yourself, on the graph in Figure 2.4, the approximate curve for America's non-white population as it exists today.

2.1.3 Disease and Morbidity

Morbidity, or incapacity due to chronic disease states, is probably more to be feared than death. A decreasing ability for locomotion and social interaction must inevitably decrease the quality of life to a point where even the strongest spirit is daunted. Table 2.7 shows some principal causes of disability through recent decades in an industrialized nation. It may be seen in Chapter 8 that morbidity today is still due to these causes. Some of these causes are also common to the principal causes of death. You should review all 3 tables, 2.5, 2.6, and 2.7 to find these common causes.

2.1.4 The Cost of Health Care

Table 2.8 shows how accessibility to health care, either direct (medical, nursing) or indirect (public sanitation) is much higher in developed countries. Notice in column 10, the gross discrepancy in the number of people sharing one physician between a low income country (37,000 people) and an industrialized nation (860). Analyse some of the other statistics in the table for yourself.

In developed countries the increasing costs of medical care are of grave concern, as they assume ever increasing proportions of the Gross

Table 2.8. Changes in statistics related to improved health care in the different economies between 1960 and 1980. Reproduced with permission from **World Development reports 1978 and 1984**, The World Bank.

	Life Expectancy at birth			Mortality per 1,000						Population per						% with access to safe water supply
				0-1 year			1-4 year			Physician			Nurse			
	1960	1975	1982	1960	1975	1982	1960	1975	1982	1960	1974	1980	1960	1974	1980	1975
Low income	36	44	59	144	122	87	27	-	11	37,000	21,185	15,931	4,515	6,710	4,564	25
Middle income	49	58	65	101	46	32	15	5	6	3,050	2,430	2,021	2,235	1,570	2,018	52
Industrialized	70	72	75	25	15	20	1	1	0.1	860	650	554	390	230	180	-
Oil Exporting	45	53	63	175	110	96	44	30	13	5,800	1,140	1,355	4996	1500	836	87
Centrally Planned (communist)	66	70	73	38	30	21	3	2	1	830	480	349	358	245	131	-

National Product (GNP) and National Budget. Table 2.9 shows the rise in health care costs in some developed countries from 1953-1983, and Figure 2.5 shows graphically the trends in Canada and the USA. The costs of Health Care in the USA in 1986 reached a staggering total of $365 billion. Good health, however, is regarded as a right in most industrialized nations and its provision is seen as a virtual necessity, regardless of cost. And, as with many social issues, the bourgeoning costs of health care, even in the wealthier countries, are likely to be ignored by many of us until it becomes such a problem that we must act. By then, unfortunately, we may not have any money left to act with, even prudently!

2.2 POPULATION

Until 1700 the world population grew at less than .002% per year. Overall the world population is now near 5.2 billion people with an overall annual growth at 2%. Population expansion in industrialized nations now is 0.8% and probably will continue at an annual rate of 0.8 to 1.0 in these countries, and at higher rates up to 2.5 in underdeveloped countries. Thus, it is clear that the distribution of population between rich and poor countries is anomalous, and is becoming increasingly so (see Table 2.10).

2.2.1 The Pressures Resulting from Large Populations

An increasing population in a society compounds all its social and welfare problems. The central problem of feeding the population either from its own resources or through international trade becomes critical for a nation. When provision is no longer adequate, malnutrition, even famine, disease, and death ensue. In industrialized nations, even though food is adequate, over-population has already resulted in overcrowding, noise, pollution, crime and violence, and these bring different threats to the quality of life. Experiments with animal colonies show that in crowded conditions: (a) Mothers become unable to suckle their young; and (b) Anger and violence increase dramatically.

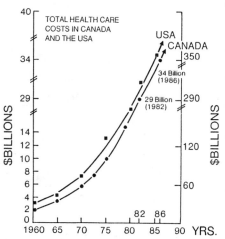

Figure 2.5. Exponential rising costs of health care in Canada and the U.S.A. Data reproduced with permission from **World Development Reports 1978 and 1984**, The World Bank.

Table 2.9. Rising expenditures on personal Health Care as a % GNP in developed countries between 1958 and 1983. Data from Reville, P. **Sport for All**; Maxwell, P.J. **Health and Wealth**, 1981 and **World Development Bank Report, 1984**, World Bank, 1984. Reproduced with permission.

	1953	1965	1977	1983
West Germany	3.0	6.0	9.2	17
USA	2.3	6.1	8.9	15
Sweden	3.4	5.6	9.8	-
Netherlands	4.0	5.3	8.2	-
Framce	3.4	5.8	7.9	-
Australia	3.0	5.2	7.7	12
Canada	4.1	6.1	7.1	17
Switzerland	-	-	6.9	-
United Kingom	3.5	3.9	5.2	10

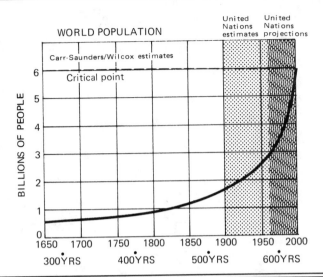

Figure 2.6. World population growth. Reproduced with permission from Bogue, D.J. Principles of Demography, New York: John Wiley and Sons, 1969.

Table 2.10. Distribution of population versus percentage total world population in rich and poor countires.

Year	Rich*	Poor**
1974	30	70
1984	20	80
Predicted 2000	10	90

*   Gross National Product (GNP), per capita US dollars 6200. Average Annual Growth in GNP 3.4

** GNP per capita US dollars   100 Average Annual Growth in GNP 0.5

Table 2.11. Nature of exponential growth with a doubling period of 50 years.

Year	Millions People	Year	Millions People
0	1	250	32
50	2	300	64
100	4	600	4,096
150	8	650	8,192
200	16	700	16,384

2.2.2 Uncontrolled Population Growth

The dangers of a rising human population have been hidden from us for a long time. We seem to be suddenly confronted with a world population growing out of control. However, this is the very nature of growth. For a long time it seems quite slow and steady. However, this is only because the original numbers were small. In effect, growing populations double their number in defined periods of time (e.g. about 50 years, Table 2.11). Thus, a population of one million people at year zero becomes 2 million fifty years later. In another fifty years the population is 4 million. Not too much later it is 4 billion and in the next 50 years it becomes 8 billion. Thus, after a Critical Point (shown on the part of the curve after 1950 in Figure 2.6) the consequences of a doubling population every 50 years is immensely important for health, happiness and survival.

The kind of graph the data in Table 2.11 produces is seen in Figure 2.6 and in alternative ways in the box enclosure on page 25. The world population since 1650 has been growing exponentially and now the population increase is on the steep part of the graph (out of control). In early years the increase per 50 years didn't seem too much. Now it is frighteningly rapid and poses a serious threat to the economies of many nations. The present world population growth rate is about 2.1% per year, corresponding to a doubling time of 33 years. In 1986 the world population was 5 billion people.

The mathematical expression of the curve shown in Figure 2.6 is:

$$Y = ae^{bx} \text{ or } P = ae^{bx}$$

where Y = Population (P)

a = a constant

b = velocity constant

x = years

Three views of population change

The charts in this box provide three different perspectives on past and present population growth. Although each looks different, all are based on the same facts.

The top chart shows the change in the absolute size of world population from about 9000 B.C. (the beginning of the agricultural age) to the end of the present century. The middle chart shows population growth rates from A.D. 1750 to 2000. The bottom chart, like the top one, shows change in the size of the human population, but over a longer period—back to 1 million B.C.— and on a logarithmic scale.

The three charts suggest strikingly different impressions of population growth. The top one conveys the impression of an enormous population explosion beginning sometime after 1750 (the beginning of the industrial age). It points upward at the year 2000 with no apparent limit. The middle chart indicates that these recent dramatic increases have been produced by relatively small, though accelerating growth rates. Annual growth was about 0.4 percent between 1750 and 1800, crept up steadily until it reached 0.8 percent in 1900-50, and then rose sharply to 1.7 percent between 1950 and 1975. The line for growth rates points upward, but shows a recent dip, and is therefore not as dramatically threatening as that in the top chart.

The bottom chart shows that population has growth from somewhat less than 10 million on the eve of the agricultural age. In the first rise in the curve, population expanded gradually toward the limit supportable by hunting and gathering. With the adoption of arming and animal husbandry, a second burst of population growth began.

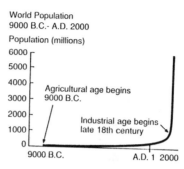

World Population
9000 B.C.- A.D. 2000
Population (millions)

Agricultural age begins 9000 B.C.

Industrial age begins late 18th century

9000 B.C.　　　　　A.D. 1 2000

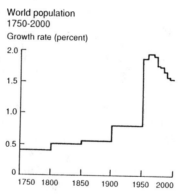

World population
1750-2000
Growth rate (percent)

1750 1800　1850　1900　1950 2000

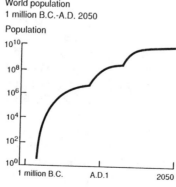

World population
1 million B.C.-A.D. 2050
Population

1 million B.C.　　A.D.1　　　2050

Eventually—though much more quickly than in the first case—the technological limits were again reached, and population stabilized at around 300 million in the first millenium A.D. From the late eighteenth century the industrial age triggered a third burst of population growth. It began from a much higher base and has covered a much shorter period, but on a logarithmic scale it appears no more rapid or unusual than earlier growth spurts.

Which chart best portrays the past and the prospects for the future? The top one emphasizes the special character of recent population growth, setting current experience apart from thousands of years of earlier history. It conveys a sense of crisis. The middle chart highlights the substantial acceleration in growth rates, especially in the past quarter century, that produced this expansion, and the current downward trend in those rates. It suggests that managing population growth is possible. The bottom figure underlines the likelihood of an eventual equilibrium between population and resources, achieved either by a decline in birth rates or an unwelcome rise in death rates. It calls attention to the need to achieve equilibrium by a decline in birth rates.

Reproduced with permission from **World Development Report 1984,** World Bank 1984.

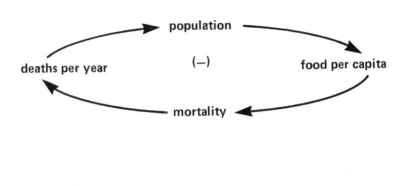

Figure 2.8. Typical feedback loop. Reproduced with permission from **The Limits to Growth: A report for The Club of Rome's Project on the Predicament of Mankind** by Donella H. Meadows, Dennis L. Meadows, Jørgen Randers, William W. Behrens, III. A Potomac Associates book published by Universe Books N.Y., 1972. Graphics by Potomac Associates.

This equation enables us to predict that, without some control, a population explosion will eventually smother the earth. Can you think of other instances of population explosions (besides human)? Perhaps you can suggest methods that either have been, or else could be, used to control them.

2.2.3 Controlled Growth

Controlled growth results from feedback of some controlling factor or factors to retard growth. Controlled growth curves appear like those in Figure 2.7, where there is some upper limit to the growth function (height, weight, life expectancy, whatever it may be). This upper limit is called the **asymptote**, or steady state. As the asymptote is approached very small increases in the growth variable take place, even for very large changes in the factor producing the growth.

Examine Figure 2.7 and suggest why (since life expectancy seems to depend on adequate nutrition), despite very high nutritional levels, life expectancy levels off. Can you think of any other natural growth phenomenon which has this general shape?

The ability to describe and even predict the cause of an event by a mathematical equation has led to the development of a technique called Systems Modeling or Forecasting. This technique was used first in engineering science. Here there is a set of events interacting with and influencing one another (feedback). A complex computer systems model of those interactions may be developed. If a reasonable estimate of begining levels of each component of a system and their rate of change into another (e.g. the change of raw materials manufactured into a motor vehicle) may be made, then the model may be allowed to run for a fixed period to forecast where the model will be (i.e. what its wealth is from capital investment, how much pollution from manufacturing has occurred, or what stimulus to increased population, and wealth it has produced, etc.) at a defined point in the future.

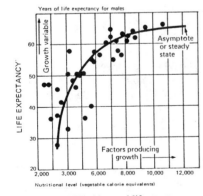

Figure 2.7. Nutrition and life expectancy. Modified and reproduced with permission from **The Limits to Growth: A report for The Club of Rome's Project on the Predicament of Mankind** by Donella H. Meadows, Dennis L. Meadows, Jørgen Randers, William W. Behrens, III. A Potomac Associates book published by Universe Books N.Y., 1972. Graphics by Potomac Associates.

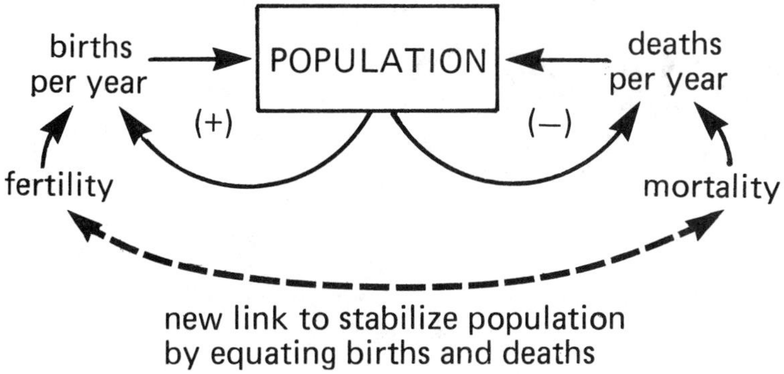

Figure 2.9. Excess population deaths feedback positively on a population total. Reproduced with permission from Meadows & Meadows, **Limits to Growth**, 1972.

This is how a group of scientists led by D.H. Meadows, D.L. Meadows, and J.W. Forester formulated the First Global Model of world forces for the Club of Rome Organization in the 1960's. It resulted in publication of the book Limits to Growth in 1972. Now even more powerful Global Models have been developed by Strategic Planners for the American Joint Chiefs of Staff (JCS) in order to estimate the consequences of patterns of action taken by governments. Recently the model "Forecasts" (1983) replaced a previous World Integrated Model (WIM) being used by the JCS (Science, Nov. 11, 1983). The National Research Council of America also recently completed a report in 1986 on Global issues entitled Population Growth and Economic Development: Policy Questions. In addition, many governments are developing agencies similar to the American Office of Technological Assessment (OTA) to advise policymakers on the future consequences of technological innovation. Germany, Holland and Great Britain all are forming agencies and France has had its Office for the Evaluation of Scientific and Technological Choices since 1983 (Economist, Sept. 13, 1986).

A typical feedback loop negatively affecting population growth is shown in Figure 2.8. According to this figure, as population increases less food is available to feed the increasing population and famine and deaths ensue. This exerts a negative or controlling effect on further population growth. Similarly, excess population deaths from other causes feed-back positively on a population total, making more resources available to those left, encouraging births, until again the number of births balances deaths (Figure 2.9).

2.2.4 The Approach to Stability
Table 2.12 shows that in both so-called developed countries (industrialized) and underdeveloped countries (so-called Third World) the fertility level is dropping, although fertility rates in less developed nations are still twice as high as in developed nations they have decreased remarkably in the last decade.

Table 2.12. Demographic indicators of approaching stabilization in population growth. Reproduced with permission from **World Development Report 1984**, World Bank, 1984.

	Crude Birth Rate per 1,000 pop. CBR			Crude Death Rate per 1,000 pop. CDR			% change CBR	CDR	Total Fertility Rate	
	1960	1975	1982	1960	1975	1982	1960-82	1960-82	1982	2000
Low income	48	47	30	26	20	11	-34.2	-54.7	4.1	3.2
Middle income	45	40	31	17	12	8	-23.2	-36.4	4.2	3.1
Industrialized	18	16	14	10	10	9	-31.4	-5.4	1.7	2.0
Oil exporting	48	46	42	19	14	11	-12.9	-49.8	6.9	5.8
Centrally planned	24	18	18	10	9	10	-20.5	+34.4	2.3	2.1

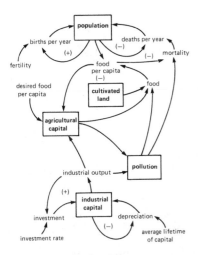

Figure 2.10. Feedback loops of population, capital, agriculture and population. Reproduced with permission from **The Limits to Growth: A report for The Club of Rome's Project on the Predicament of Mankind** by Donella H. Meadows, Dennis L. Meadows, Jørgen Randers, William W. Behrens, III. A Potomac Associates book published by Universe Books N.Y., 1972. Graphics by Potomac Associates.

If **replacement fertility** is achieved, that is if deaths are paralleled exactly by live births, the world population will tend to stabilize. The exact level at which this occurs depends on when replacement fertility is achieved. Table 2.13 shows the population forecast for this case. By now you will realize that in any system there are many interacting factors exerting both positive (uncontrolled, destabilising) and negative (controlling) feedback effects (loops) upon each other in any system. These factors influence the achievement of a stable world system in many ways besides population control. They are most easily recognizable in developed countries, where industrialization, agricultural development, exploitation of natural resources, social services, available investment capital, and pollution have all reached a high level and have a direct and important effect upon the general quality of life, health, and happiness of the individual (Figures 2.10 and 2.11).

Similarly, a concomitant lack of resources and services contribute to the poor quality of life generally experienced in underdeveloped countries, where people naturally aspire to the same quality of life as their more fortunate fellow human beings in developed countries.

Examine some of the interconnections between population and industrial capital and you'll find they operate through agricultural capital, cultivated land, and pollution. Each arrow indicates a causal relationship, which may be immediate or delayed, large or small, positive or negative, depending on the assumptions included in each model run.

It seems logical that the expectations of people in developed countries for continuing improvement in their quality of life must be damped somewhat, if the world is to reach a state of equilibrium and approach equality.

Let's take one turn around Figure 2.11 and then you can take a different one for yourself, assuming a different primary premise. Let us assume times are good. The investment rate is high, capital investment is large and these forces promote a great deal of industrial activity and

Table 2.13. Momentum for World Population Growth. Reproduced with permission from **The Limits to Growth: A report for The Club of Rome's Project on the Predicament of Mankind** by Donella H. Meadows, Dennis L. Meadows, Jørgen Randers, William W. Behrens, III. A Potomac Associates book published by Universe Books N.Y., 1972. Graphics by Potomac Associates.

If world attains replacement fertility* in	Current World Population will be (billions)	Stable World Population will reach (billions)
2000-2005	5.9	8.5
2020-2025	8.0	10.7
2040-2045	10.8	13.5

* 2.1-2.5 live births per woman.

products (see all the arrows leading to industrial output). Now follow the arrows straight up. This product has to be sold, a successful product attracts a sales force, wholesalers, retailers, transport workers etc., and service capital is attracted. All these people and companies pay taxes and social services grow (e.g. health services, family planning etc.). Health services help decrease mortality so that death rate (DR) goes down; family planning education should control the population, but times are good; and industrial output per capita is high, so everyone can afford children. The balance of these effects determines fertility and thus the birth rate (BR). If BR rises, there are more people to die and thus population feeds back on (DR). There also are more people to marry and so this feeds back on the BR. Times are good, the population on balance rises. Now, what if our non-renewable resources begin to be depleted? Say oil reserves begin to get low. What happens to the system? Analyze Figure 2.10 similarly.

2.3 STUDYING INTERACTIVE WORLD FORCES

The following issues are raised by the study of how world forces interact in "Limits to Growth". Most of us do not tend to think about these issues a lot, because we are generally concerned with our own day-to-day life issues. The issues are:

1. Industrialization may be a more fundamentally disruptive force than population increase. Population increases may result from feedback pressure of industrialization and increased availability of goods, unless this factor is consciously appreciated and controlled.

2. In the next century it seems that we face a choice in maintaining our well-being by:
   a. controlling the development of the modern industrial society
   b. allowing decline in world population from diseases caused by pollution
   c. limiting the world population by famine
   d. limiting the world population by other means (and what are these "other means"?)

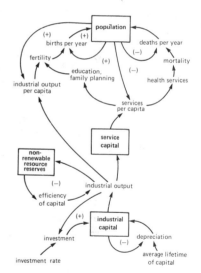

Figure 2.11. Population and industrial capital are also influenced by the levels of service capital (such as health and education services) and of non-renewable resource reserves e.g. oil, coal and minerals. Reproduced with permission from **The Limits to Growth: A report for The Club of Rome's Project on the Predicament of Mankind** by Donella H. Meadows, Dennis L. Meadows, Jørgen Randers, William W. Behrens, III. A Potomac Associates book published by Universe Books N.Y., 1972. Graphics by Potomac Associates.

3. We face the collapse of the social order within smaller societies (riots, crime) or between nations (war) because of physical and psychological overcrowding.
4. Strategies directed at population control alone may be self-defeating. (Can you suggest why this is so?)
5. We must face the fact that the underdeveloped nations may catch up to the developed nations, and solve the present problems affecting world stability. However the population of underdeveloped nations is 4 times greater than that of developed nations. Thus, if the underdeveloped countries reached a similar level of development to that of the developed countries, the subsequent load on the world's available resources, pollution control and dissipation systems would become intolerable. The quality of life, and hence health, would have to decline somewhat in developed countries to accommodate this change.
6. Highly industrialized countries may be self extinguishing as pollution increases and natural resources are used up or contaminated. After reading the list try convincing yourself that these problems will disappear without people's concern (e.g. our concern!).

2.3.1 Existing in the 21st Century: Problems and Challenges

We must acknowledge that forces could interact to threaten human life on this planet. We need endurance, self discipline and optimism to sustain these pressures and maintain the best mode of living for ourselves.

Industrial societies, which have previously encouraged and rewarded growth, may have to change their assumptions radically. Characteristic of the change from growth into equilibrium is stress. Forces of supression must rise far enough so that forces now sustaining growth are depressed or we must find ways to continue evolving without the accompanying disruptive forces on society. The world thus faces pressures to:

• Stop population increases
• Stop industrialization increasing

• Stop increases in the standard of living in developed countries but work to maintain present standards and make them more equal throughout the society.

Social stresses, connected with shortages of land, housing, and unemployment will increase. All of these factors will accompany transition from urban growth to equilibrium. People will move into new coherent cities rather than aggravating existing urban sprawl. Governments will have incentives to improve transit services, port facilities, industrial control. Adaptation to Information Technology and Robotized manufacturing industry will occur. Leisure for learning, sport and individual enterprise will occur.

2.4 THE FUTURE ORGANIZATION OF MEDICAL CARE IN DEVELOPED COUNTRIES

Even within developed nations the provision of medical care is often haphazard; funds for its operation often are ill-directed and the real goal of maintaining good health by self discipline, education and provision of relevant health maintaining services is still little appreciated.

Only a small part of the chapter has dealt with medical health care delivery, since this will be covered in Chapter 3. We have taken a **systems model approach** because it is felt that this method of analysis offers you the best comprehensive picture of a good, all-embracing societal health care system. Such a system should be flexible and responsive to the varying feedback demands placed on it by an evolving, complicated, society.

Figure 2.12 models the development of the health care expectations of a person living in an industrialized nation between the years 1900 to 1970. Medical care has become more complex in this century and as it has become more effective, the entry mix of people has changed significantly. Yet the entry point is still the doctor's appointment. Before 1900 (Figure 2.12, left) medicine had little to offer and only sick people entered medical care. By 1935, as medicine began to have more to offer, as insurance plans appeared, some "early sick" people were entering the

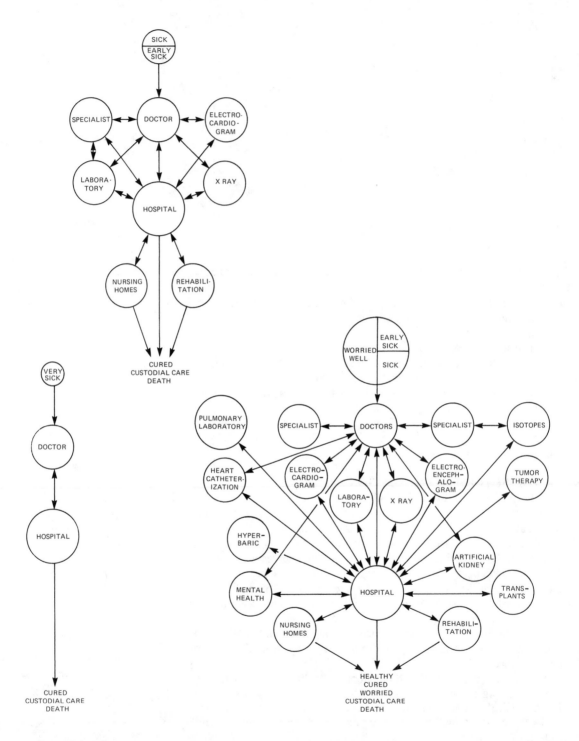

Figure 2.12. The complex nature of modern medical care. Reproduced with permission from Garfield, Sidney R. The Delivery of Medical Care. Copyright © April 1970, **Scientific American, Inc.** All rights reserved.

system (Figure 2.12, top). Since World War II medical technology has proliferated as indicated by the display of treatment components (Figure 2.12, right), and well people enter the system, largely because of prepayment, insurance plans, or Medicare and Medicaid in the U.S.A.

Figure 2.13 shows a model of a future health care delivery system. The new system would be more interactive with the community group it serves, taking responsibility for providing: preventive health care information and service, practical health care experiences (e.g., exercise, diet clinics, self measurement of fitness etc.), and conventionally understood diagnosis of illness, sick care, and extended care services. The infrastructure of the new system could very well use many of the agencies already existing in a community. They would now be linked by an information system (computer centre) allowing rationalization, co-ordination, and increasing efficiency.

2.5 SUMMARY

This chapter stresses important factors which will determine the future health and happiness of the people of the world. While it is impossible to predict outcomes with any certainty, the issues raised here have been of concern to some perceptive demographers, social scientists, anthropologists, physical scientists, engineers, and physicians for at least the last two decades. During this period we have moved inexorably and, more recently, somewhat precipitously toward some of the predictions made by their interactive model system. (Thus the world population was 4.09 billion people in 1983, and 5.0 billion in 1986.)

The conservation of our health and happiness, for an adequate period of time, and compatible with an amount a society can afford to pay, is a global as well as a national ideal. Its attainment depends only fractionally upon developing health care technology: It depends primarily upon our management of the interactive world forces abroad today, and this gives us an entirely new perspective from which to view contemporary health care issues.

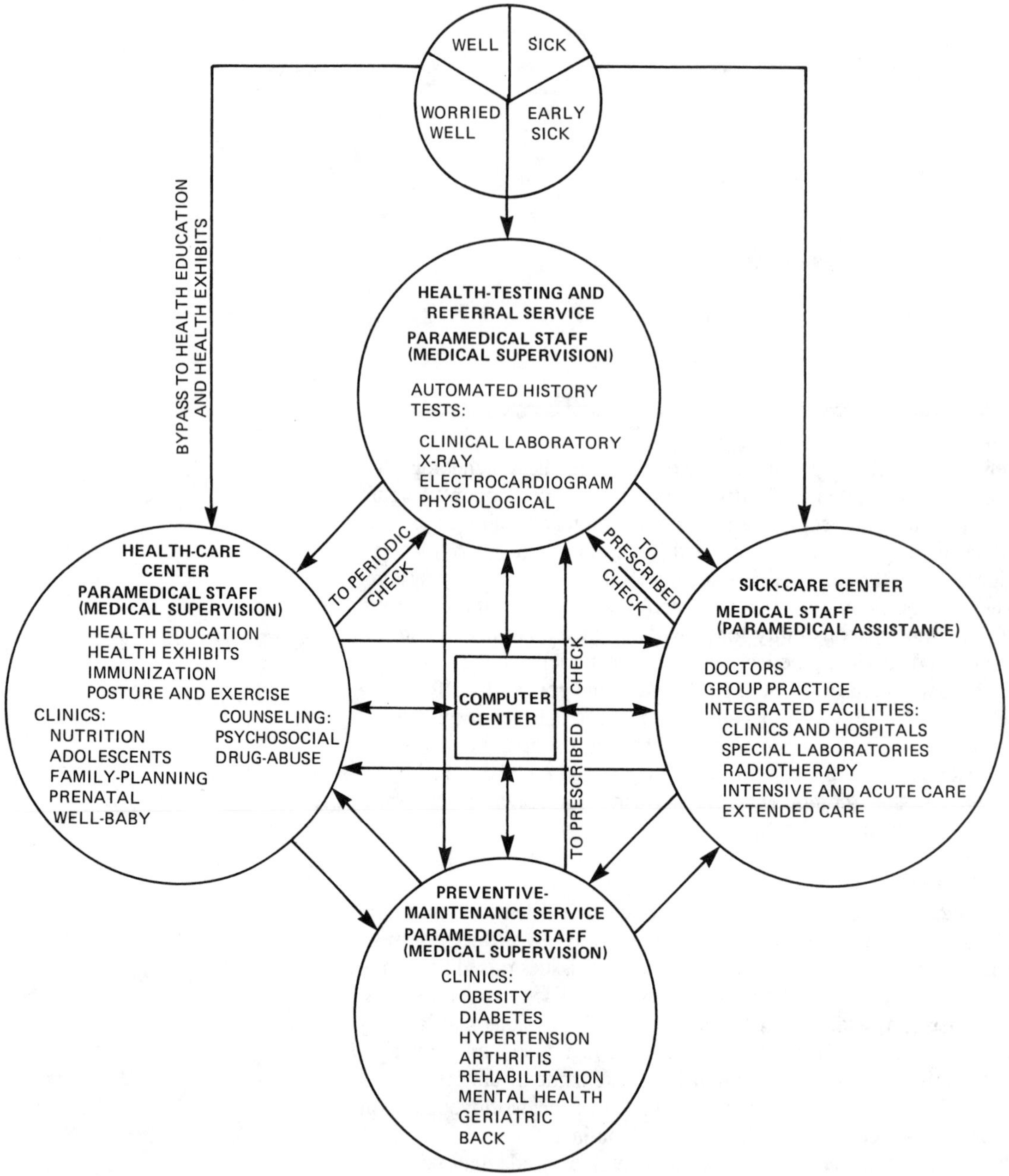

Figure 2.13. Separating the sick from the well is the basis of a new health care delivery system.
Reproduced with permission from Garfield, Sidney R. The Delivery of Medical Care. Copyright © April 1970,
Scientific American, Inc. All rights reserved.

2.6 REFERENCES

Allison, A.C., Natural Checks and Balances in Man, **Proceedings of Royal Society in Medicine, 66**, 1973.

Bannister, R., Sport, Physical Recreation, and the National Health, **British Medical Journal, 4:** 711-715, 1972.

Bauer, P. and Yarney, B. Why We Should Close Our Purse to the Third World, **The Times (London)**, April 11, page 10, 1983.

Bogue, D.J. Principles of Demography, New York: John Wiley and Sons, 1969.

Centers for Disease Control. **Morbidity, Mortality Weekly, Report, 31:**109, 1982.

Centers for Disease Control. **Morbidity, Mortality Weekly Report, 35:**457, 1986.

Durrand, J.D. Historical Estimates of World Population: An Evaluation. **Population and Development Review 3**, 3: 253-296, 1977.

Forrester, J.W., **World Dynamics**, Cambridge, Mass., Wright-Allen Press, 1971.

Garfield, S.R., The Delivery of Medical Care, **Scientific American, 222:** April, 1970.

Getting Smart: The Retooling of America. **The Economist, Aug. 23:** 14-16, 1986.

Ginzberg, E. and Vojta, G. Beyond Human Scale: The Large Corporation at Risk. **Basic Books**, p. 255, 1986.

Glass, R.I. **Science**, 234: 1986.

Hayes, H. A Conversation with Garret Hardin: A Controversial View that Feeding Starving Countries Will Ultimately Harm Them. **The Atlantic Monthly**, 66-70, 1981.

Holden, Constance. World Model for Joint Chiefs. **Science**, 11th Nov., 1983.

Lalonde, M. **A New Persective on the Health of Canadians**, Government of Canada, Ottawa, 1974.

Letters to Editor, Bad News Is It True? **Science, 210:** pp.1296-1308, 1980.

McDermott, W. Pharmaceuticals: Their Role in Developing Societies, **Science 29**: 240-245, 1980.

Meadows, D.H. and Meadows, D.L. **The Limits to Growth**, Signet, The New American Library Inc., New York, 1972.

Population Growth and Economic Development: Policy Questions, The National Research Council (U.S.A.). Reviewed by Holden, C. **Science, 231**, 28 March, 1493-4, 1986.

Reville, P. **Sport For All: Physical Activity and Prevention of Disease**, Council for Cultural Cooperation, Council of Europe, Strasbourg, 1970.

Robertson, G. **Future Work**, Gower/Temple Smith - Universe Books, 238, 1986.

Science and Technology. When decision makers turn to the experts. **The Economist**, Sept. 13, 1986.

Simmons, Kathryn. The Federal Government: Keeping Tabs on the Nation's Fitness. **The Physician and Sports Medicine 15(1):** 190-195, January, 1987.

Simon, J.L. Resources, Population Environment An Oversupply of False Bad News, **Science, 208**: 1431-1437, 1980.

Simon, J.L. World Population Growth, **The Atlantic Monthly**, August, pp.70-76, 1981.

Simon, J.L. and Kahn, H. **Global 2000** (Revised 1983), Annual Meeting of American Advancement for Science.

World Development Report 1984. New York, Oxford University Press, Oxford, v. 27 cm. annual, published for the World Bank.

Training for Work. **The Economist,** 93-101, Dec. 20, 1986.

2.7 STUDY QUESTIONS

1. Compare the state of malnutrition in the world today with that of the past, taking into account the symptoms, numbers of people involved,   and the problems encountered in evaluating the situation.
2. What are the implications of a rising world population to the quality of life and health in the world?
3. Define the concept of ergonomics and outline the contribution it can make to quality of life.
4. Draw a simple diagram showing interactions among the forces of population, natural resources, capital investment, pollution, and the quality of life.

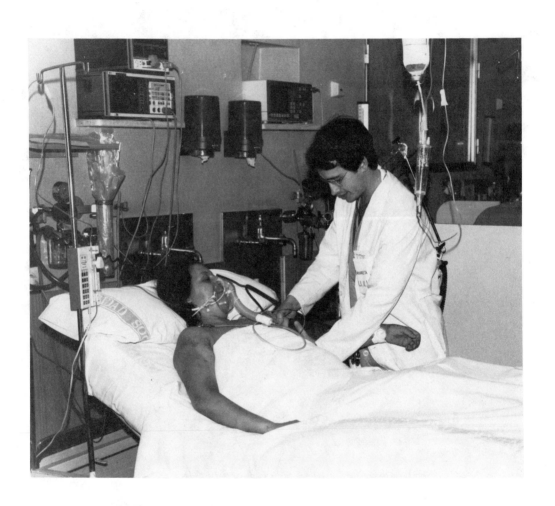

3

Health Care Delivery

No single model of health care delivery will operate
with the same effectiveness in all nations.

OBJECTIVES

When you have completed this chapter, you should be able to:
- **Distinguish** between the major characteristics of health care delivery systems in five political economies.
- **Outline** some of the major factors contributing to the rising cost of health care in many countries.
- **Propose** ways in which individuals can use their society's health care system most efficiently and effectively.
- **Discuss** the underlying factors contributing to fraudulent health care practices, and outline ways of discriminating between these and more legitimate approaches to health care.
- **Outline** procedures for selecting and using the services of a physician or related health professional.

KEY TERMS

Catastrophic Health Care
Fee-for-service
For-profit Hospitals
Free enterprise system of health care delivery
Health Maintenance Organization
Iatrogenic disease
Pathogenic theory of disease
Placebo Effect
Preventive Health Care
Socialist system of health care delivery
Transitional system of health care delivery
Underdeveloped system of health care delivery
Welfare state system of health care delivery

3.0 INTRODUCTION

The state of a nation's health, to some degree, reflects the effectiveness of its health care delivery system. Because of diverse historical backgrounds, socio-economic conditions, political ideologies and other cul-

*The state of a nation's health,
to some degree, reflects the effectiveness
of its health care delivery system.*

tural factors, no two countries are exactly alike in their health care systems. Also, because of these diversities, no single model of health care delivery will operate with the same effectiveness in all nations.

The nature and effectiveness of any health care delivery system is determined predominantly by the prevailing economic health of the society. While **Welfare State** systems (total care provided by the State) may be regarded as the ideal, combining abundant resources with freedom of access to all, their burgeoning costs threaten major budgetary crises even in relatively affluent nations. Policymakers thus are having to face serious strategic choices in the use of health care monies. If one considers the eradication of disease as the ideal criterion, on the **pathogenic model**, most sophisticated health care systems have been experiencing ever-diminishing health returns from the increasingly large sums of money invested. Most evidence indicates that an adequate return in curing opportunistic disease states and trauma in the majority of the population has been achieved. The major causes of morbidity and mortality in modern society are now related to lifestyle and age, but the potential impact of preventive health care is still drastically unexploited.

This chapter will examine health care delivery from an international perspective, and examine some of the current problems facing several systems. It will present the pros and cons of some proposed solutions, and discuss the implications of today's **systems-in-transition** for the health consumer.

3.1 HEALTH CARE DELIVERY SYSTEMS

For purposes of comparison, it is useful to consider the predominant characteristics of health care delivery systems in five different political economies. These will be referred to as **free enterprise, welfare, underdeveloped, transitional,** and **socialist** economies. One must keep in mind that the health care systems in many countries categorized under each of these headings are in continual flux, and that a component of any one country's system may be common to others.

"Today the country as a whole tends to be a little more commercial in its attitude to health care than it was in the sixties for example. Maybe medicine is viewed a little less ecclesiastically and a little more pragmatically."

W.J. McNernly

3.1.1 Free Enterprise Systems

The closest example of a health care delivery system based on free enterprise is that of the United States. Here, more than anywhere else in the world, the provision of health services is influenced by an open economic market, even though one may observe increasing intervention in that market. Evidence of such free enterprise is that in 1975 only 6% (378) of hospitals in the country were run by investor-owned corporations. In 1984 the number was 878, a jump to 13% of the total. Hospital Corporation of America (HCA), by far the biggest chain, owned more than 440 hospitals.

Prophetically W.J. McNernly, former chairman of Blue Cross and Chairman of the National Academy Institute of Medicine's report (1981) on **For-Profit Enterprises in Health Care**, remarked, "Today the country as a whole tends to be a little more commercial in its attitude to health care than it was in the sixties for example. Maybe medicine is viewed a little less ecclesiastically and a little more pragmatically."

The essential characteristics of the free enterprise system are:
- development and use of health care resources in a predominantly open consumer market
- minimum intervention by government, or other mechanisms of control, over demand or price
- health services are bought and sold like any other commodity
- since societal intervention is at a minimum, the distribution of services is dependent mainly on individual purchasing power
- efforts to modify this process arise through private or local initiative, hence a multiplicity of programs may arise to organize, finance and deliver services for **special needs**. This results in a pluralism of organized sub-systems, dependent upon local strength, creativity and wealth. Differentials in money and power result in great discrepancies in access to health care.

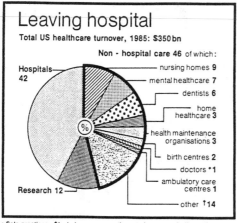

Leaving hospital

Total US healthcare turnover, 1985: $350 bn

Non - hospital care 46 of which:

- nursing homes 9
- mental healthcare 7
- dentists 6
- home healthcare 3
- health maintenance organisations 3
- birth centres 2
- doctors *1
- ambulatory care centres 1
- other †14

Hospitals 42

Research 12

* Solo practices †Includes group practices, pain centres & diagnosis centres
Source: Health Industry Manufacturers Association

Figure 3.1. Distribution of $350 billion Health Care Resources in the USA in 1985.

In the past few decades, political pressures to change this system in the United States have been generated by the inequities inherent in any free enterprise system. Several organized health programs have arisen to interrupt the free flow of economic market forces and local political autonomies. Yet vestiges of earlier conditions remain. Hospitals and doctors alike remain predominantly private agents, receiving fees (until recently relatively unconstrained) for each service rendered, charging what the market will bear.

Of the total monies spent on health in 1975 (about $150 billion) in the U.S., 43% came from government agencies, 25% from voluntary health insurance agencies, 27% from purely private payments, and the balance of 5% from charity and industry (Roemer, 1977). In 1986 the cost of health care in the USA had risen to an enormous $365 billion whose distribution among health care institutions is shown in Figure 3.1 for 1985. In 1986, however, a rising degree of accountability in the operation of the entire health care system is being demanded by both government and medical insurers. Both Medicare (care of the over 65 group) and Medicaid (care of the indigenous younger-than-65 group), which pay for 30% of all hospital admissions, now limit the number of total in-patient days covered and individual lengths of stay. Whether the quality of care in American society has gone down in the process of this cutback is undetermined. Medicare and Medicaid also now pay on a fixed schedule for some 470 types of illnesses as opposed to actual costs as previously. Large employers and other insurers have also instituted stricter policies and require higher contributions toward medical expenses by employees. Regulation has also been introduced through licensing of hospitals and health personnel, certification of medical specialties by professional bodies, increased hospital discipline over medical staff, and expanded peer review procedures. The pharmaceutical industry, which is entirely private, has been subjected to expanding controls over the production, marketing, and distribution of its products, and patients

*The usual indices of comparing health status among
different countries are
life expectancy and infant mortality.*

are exercising increasing influence on the performance of health care workers through court actions for malpractice and through a movement for consumer participation in health-related policy decisions. An omnibus Health Bill, recently signed into law (1986), eliminated some of the former federal support for Health Maintenance Organizations (HMOs), which prospectively contract to provide for the health needs of an individual for a fixed sum. Although this action may be seen as negatively affecting a key unit of the Nation's health care system, other actions of the bill are positive. They are: (1) to take action against the 18,000 incompetent doctors in the system; (2) to provide money to train physicians in geriatric medicine; (3) to provide for increased research and education on Alzheimer's disease; (4) to improve mental Health Services; (5) to study Infant Mortality; and (6) to allow distribution abroad of pharmaceutical products not yet licensed internally by the Food and Drug agency.

3.1.2 Health Care in Canada*
Interposed between the essentially free enterprise health care system of the U.S.A. and the Welfare State System of Britain and the Scandanavian countries is that of Canada, whose experience crystallizes the problems set for the modern developed state by a burgeoning industry trained primarily to consider only the cure and not the cost.

The usual indices of comparing health status among different countries are life expectancy and infant mortality. In 1971 Canada ranked eighth among 21 nations in a composite ranking of the seven most widely used measures of premature death. In life expectancy, Canadian men ranked seventh (69.9 yrs.) while women were second only to their Swedish counterparts (76.9 yrs.). Of those countries who fared better (e.g., the Scandinavian countries, the Netherlands and Switzerland), health analysts note that most are geographically small and have relatively small populations, making the job of providing high quality health care easier.

*Adapted in part from a series of six articles by Bennett and Krasny on Health Care in Canada. **The Financial Post**, March 26-May 7, 1977.

The high level of health enjoyed by the majority of Canadians is typical of western industrialized nations, particularly when compared with less-developed countries, where life expectancy may be in the low 40's and infant mortality three to four times as great (see chapter 2). Two important influences on these favourable health indices are abundant health care resources and an extensive health care insurance system.

HEALTH CARE RESOURCES
In purely quantitative terms, the Canadian system is impressive. Close to 40,000 physicians and 350,000 other health-care workers serve 1,400 hospitals. Compared with other countries, Canada now ranks fourth in number of physicians per 10,000 population and third in number of nurses. Table 3.1 shows the comparative distribution of physicians in some industrialized and developing nations of the world between 1960 and 1980.

MEDICAL INSURANCE
More than 99% of Canadians have comprehensive, prepaid protection against the costs of medical services from physicians and surgeons, hospital inpatient treatment, and a wide range of outpatient and extended care services. Such extensive coverage, exceeded only by Britain and the Scandinavian countries, makes access to health services a right of all rather than a privilege of those who can pay. This is in contrast to the U.S., where public funds pay only 40% of the nation's health care bill, and where prolonged or catastrophic episodes of illness often result in personal bankruptcy. However, President Reagan recently (1987) proposed provisions for the elderly under a Catastrophic Health Insurance. These provisions would ensure hospital care after an elderly patient's out-of-pocket costs reached $2,000. An extra $4.92 on the current $17.50 per month Medicare Part B premium would help pay for this. For those under 65 the plan asks individual states to consider mandating catastrophic insurance through employers. Currently however, millions of people in the U.S., are not covered by any plan.

Table 3.1. Comparative physician distribution in industrialized societies and some developing nations.

Country	Population per physician			Physician per* 100,00 people
	1960	1965	1980	1980
Germany	670	630	450	222
USA	750	670	520	192
Sweden	1,050	910	490	204
Netherlands	900	860	540	185
France	930	810	580	172
Australia	750	720	560	178
Italy	640	590	340	294
Canada	910	770	550	182
Switzerland	740	750	410	244
United King.	940	860	650	154
Zair	79,620	39,050	13940	7
Nicaragua	2,690	2,490	1,800	55
India	4,850	4,860	3,690	27

* WHO ideal is 150 per 100,000 population. Reproduced with permission **World Development Reports**, 1984, World Bank, 1984.

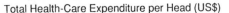
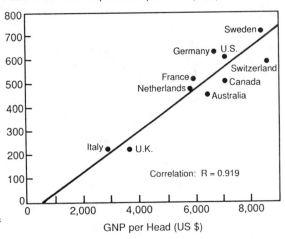

Total Health-Care Expenditure per Head (US$)

Correlation: R = 0.919

GNP per Head (US $)

Figure 3.3. Total health-care expenditures and GNP, 1975.

Cost of health care per person

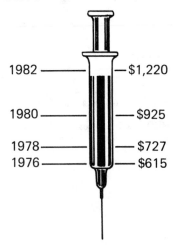

1982 — $1,220

1980 — $925

1978 — $727
1976 — $615

Figure 3.2. Health care costs, in Canada in terms of individual consumers, has doubled since 1976. Reproduced with permission from **Financial Post**, Aug. 6, 1983.

It must be emphasized that the increasing cost of an extensive prepaid system is not sustainable. Canada now spends proportionately more on health care than any country except the U.S., possibly Sweden, and the Netherlands. In Canada the total of public and private per capita expenditure on health care experienced an annual growth rate of 9% during the 60s, 10% in the early 70s, and 15% in the late 70s, reaching approximately $615 per capita in 1976. Since 1976 the per capita cost of health care has doubled, reaching an astonishing $1,220 [a total Federal cost of $25 billion] in 1982 (Figure 3.2). In the same period, consumer prices climbed 75%. However, more notable than the growth in per capita spending is the change expressed as a proportion of Gross National Product (GNP). Whereas health care expenditures were 5.5% of GNP in 1960, they had risen to 7.3% in 1975 and 8.5 % in 1982. Comparable figures in the U.S. for 1976 were 8.3% of GNP or $615 per capita ($124 billion). In contrast, Britain's $160 per capita expenditure in 1976 was one-third of Canada's, and its 5.4% of GNP was three-quarters of the Canadian figure.Comparative positions held by industrialized nations in 1975 is shown in Figure 3.3 from (Maxwell, 1981). Expenditure on health care seems inexorably tied to the growing affluence of a society (reflected in its Gross National Product or GNP). Figure 3.4 clearly shows this relationship. Since 1975 a veritable explosion in health care costs has occured in the U.S.A. reached $365 billion and in Canada topped $34 billion (Figure 3.4).

Predictions of future health care costs suggest that they will continue to rise, largely as a result of two major trends in society. The first of these is the aging of the population. People over 65 years old need nearly eight times as many hospital beds as those under the age of 45. By 1996 there will be 3.2 million Canadians over 65, compared with today's 2 million. America will have 29 million elderly compared with the 26 million of today. Canada therefore will have over 1 million more elderly people, who will not only need more medical care, but will be in a political position to demand it. The second major trend is that medi-

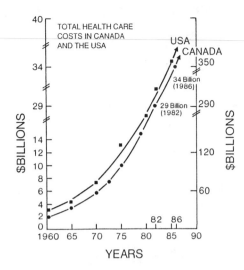

Figure 3.4. Exponential growth of Health Care Costs in the U.S.A. and Canada typical of the growth in cost of many industrialized societies.

cal and dental skills required to treat the chronic and degenerative diseases affecting elderly people will have to be added to the training of primary care physicians.

Increasing competition for support for Health Care from scarce dollar resources will increase social tension. In Canada several provincial ministries have already decided to close hospitals or charge additional user fees to prevent health care siphoning off resources from other urgent priorities. In the U.S. too, dollar expenditures on 470 types of illness have been capped at certain levels (see earlier). Of course, such political strategies have met with considerable resistance, particularly by those who feel that a decrease in size of current health care allocations will result in a diminished state of health.

But is this true? Many health specialists agree that as optimal a state of health as may reasonably be expected in Canadians has now been achieved. Instead, many argue that further significant improvements will not accrue through applying more of today's hi-tech medical science, but rather by the population practicing restraint and discipline in lifestyle. In common with other western nations, Canada has been experiencing ever-diminishing returns in indices of the Nation's health from the large sums of money invested in the system in recent years.

In the three decades from 1931 to 1961, Canada increased its spending on health care by approximately 1-3/4 percentage points of GNP and life expectancy (at birth) increased by nearly eight years. In the following decade, when the proportion of GNP devoted to health care also grew by 1-3/4 percentage points, life expectancy rose by only one year. After a certain point in the economic development of a society and the evolution of its health care system, there appears to be no correlation between resources supplied and health status. In both developed and less-developed countries, life expectancy shows a marked correlation with the number of physicians up to 100 per 100,000 population; after that point there is no apparent relationship. Table 3.2 emphasises the point that more spending is not necssssarily effective in preserving health. By

Table 3.2. Health care expenditures related to mortality statistics in some industrialized nations, 1975.

Country	% *	Rank	Index	Rank
West Germany	9.4	1	1.23	10
United States	8.6	2	1.18	9
Sweden	8.5	3	0.76	1
Netherlands	8.1	4	0.80	2
France	7.9	5	1.11	8
Australia	7.3	6	1.01	5
Italy	7.1	7	1.04	6
Canada	7.1	7	1.08	7
Switzerland	6.9	9	0.86	3
United King.	5.5	10	0.91	4

* % Gross National Product (GNP).

the same token tight fiscal constraint over a long period slows research and development and discoveries potentially able to effect large cost saving in the future. Levels of service are also substantially reduced.

PHYSICIAN SUPPLY

Among western developed nations, Canada is fourth in physician supply (175/100,000 people), exceeded by only West Germany, Scotland and the U.S., and considerably richer than the World Health Organization's (WHO) optimal level of 150 doctors for every 100,000 people. This was not always the case, however. In the early 60s it was believed that Canada had too few doctors, with a physician-to-population ratio of 127 per 100,000. In 1964 the Royal Commission on Health Services recommended a major effort to increase the physician supply, aiming to have 175 doctors per 100,000 by 1990. By doubling the output of graduates through the creation of four new medical schools, expanding existing programs and doubling immigration of foreign medical graduates, the objective of 175 physicians per 100,000 was achieved in 1976—14 years ahead of schedule and the developed system continues the spate of medical graduates.

Physicians undoubtedly also hold the keys to success of the health care system; prescribing a patient's care and in large measure determining its quality. They may also provide the human element in what seems to be an otherwise impersonal system, and for many people they become trusted advisors on family problems as well as health.

Less obvious is the enormous impact that doctors have on health care costs. Although their fees are a highly visible portion, they only represent about 1/5 of total health care expenditures. More significant, is how their decisions determine the costs of treating individual patients. Consider, for instance, the impact of such a decision of whether a patient goes to hospital or stays at home (the difference being approximately $100 a day); the number and type of diagnostic tests which will

*...it is a costly luxury to have an
over-abundance, even an abundance of doctors,
and cost effectiveness must, increasingly, be
a prime consideration.*

be performed; or the amount and type of medication prescribed. Physicians are trained to focus on the quality of care, on what is best for the patient, almost without regard for cost, and the advent of medicare in 1968 in Canada removed even the constraint posed by what the patient could afford. An attitude is taken that if there is any chance at all that an expensive treatment might help a patient, why not try it? And after all, doing everything possible, regardless of cost, may prevent malpractice suits.

Studies have shown that the presence of additional physicians creates greater usage and overall demand on the system; each single doctor generating annual costs of $500,000. There is also substantial evidence that the incidence of elective surgery is closely correlated with the number of physicians per unit of population. Even though physicians have increased in numbers proportionately faster than the population, their incomes continue to rise, suggesting either that the number of medical incidents has truly increased, or, more likely, that an increased number of incidents have been diagnosed by the increasing number of physicians in the field.

This state of affairs is not entirely negative. Some people get far more frequent treatment than was the case in earlier years, which alleviates pain and provides security. Others have more ready access to doctors, which in some instances can literally be life-saving. Nonetheless, it is a costly luxury to have an over-abundance, perhaps even an abundance of doctors, and cost effectiveness must, increasingly, be a prime consideration.

HOSPITAL COSTS

One out of every six Canadians is admitted to a hospital each year, the highest rate in the western world. In addition, it is estimated that non-emergency outpatient visits to hospitals are as high as 10 million a year, or one for every two Canadians. Not surprisingly, hospitals contribute most to health-care spending, representing almost 1/2 of total

*Projections of future health costs, based on the
growing proportion of elderly and the increased
specialization required to treat the diseases
with which they are affected,
predict that there simply will not be enough
public money available to maintain the
current system in developed countries.*

health care costs. Hospital costs are also the fastest growing component of health expenditures. In some provinces the latter increase at annual rates of up to 20 percent. Moreover, hospital spending is bound to increase as the number of people over 65 years (who already account for over a third of all hospital inpatient days) continue to increase.

While 3/4 of the growth in hospital costs over the past ten years has been caused by wage increases for hospital employees (excluding fee-for-service physicians), it is likely that many patients are being admitted to hospitals who should not be, for minor ailments such as warts, for example. Patients may also be staying longer in the hospital than necessary. At a cost of over $100 per day, unnecessary time in the hospital is very expensive. In the opinion of some critics, it is also medically dangerous, as an often quoted **rule of thumb** is that 15 percent of all disease is **iatrogenic**, that is contracted during treatment.

COST CONTAINMENT
The rapidly rising health care costs in Canada represents a universally common problem in developed nations, one that must be immediately addressed before it gets any worse. Projections of future health costs, based on the growing proportion of elderly and the increased specialization required to treat the diseases with which they are affected, predict that there simply will not be enough public money available to maintain the current system in developed countries.

In attempting to reduce spiralling costs, policy-makers have proposed a number of alternatives, such as:
• Reduce the number of entrants to and/or graduates from medical schools.
• Reduce the fee schedules for physicians and other health professionals.
• Limit the number of physicians who can receive remuneration from medicare.
• Include cost-effectiveness training in medical school curricula.
• Strengthen peer review by physicians of the appropriateness of hospital admissions and length of patient stay in institutions.
• Introduce salaries for physicians, independent of the volume of work.

None of these proposals are without drawbacks. Simply limiting the number of medical graduates may create a shortage of physicians in rural areas, since most doctors prefer to locate in urban centers with close access to sophisticated support services. Holding down the fee schedules may encourage physicians to recall patients more often for follow-up visits, lengthen their work week, or shift their practice toward more lucrative services. In addition, provincial regulation of these practices could mean that control over the day-to-day work of the medical profession would pass from its practitioners to the government. Restricting the income of health professionals, particularly physicians, could also mean declining morale, a reduced quality of care, and a mass exodus of top quality doctors to other countries.

Making physicians managers of cost would divert their attention from what should be their overriding concern: the quality of care received by the patient. Peer review, which is already carried out by at least one committee of physicians in each hospital, is cumbersome and time consuming, and increasing its stringency may cost more than it saves in reducing admissions or length of stay.

Limiting the number of physicians who can receive remuneration from government will encourage some physicians to practice independently of government assistance, and to bill their patients directly. The result would be a two-tiered system of health care delivery: one for those can afford to pay, and another for those who cannot.

The idea of salaries for physicians has been implemented **de facto** in Health Maintenance Organizations (HMO), now in use in parts of the U.S. In an HMO, patients prepay all their health care from physicians in a group practice. Regular monthly payments constitute a prepayment for all services required on a per-person basis (rather than **fee-for-service**). Physicians are salaried and have an incentive to treat patients as economically as possible, since they retain any revenue in excess of operating costs. Conversely, they have to pay shortfalls themselves, and there is therefore a heavy emphasis on preventive health care.

Hospital admission rates for HMO's, such as Kaiser Permanente in California, have been shown to be 60% below the Canadian average, but such data may be distorted since HMO's have been accused of preferentially selecting only young and healthy clients.

Nonetheless, it has increasingly been recognized over the past several years that the potential impact of preventive health care has been drastically underexploited. Whereas the major health problems 50 years ago could be effectively treated by physicians at minimal cost, the major illnesses of today are chronic and degenerative in nature. Many of these illnesses have no effective cure, but more importantly, most are related to lifestyle and therefore are preventible. Smoking-induced disease alone kills close to 250 Canadians a day, but neither smoking-induced disease nor other lifestyle related maladies can be ameliorated by spending more money on our traditional health care system. Indeed, as Marc Lalonde, then Canada's Minister of Health, wrote in **New Perspective on the Health of Canadians** (1974),

"the organized health care system can do little more than serve as a catchment net for the victims ... measures other than medicine have to be put to work in order to insure better health for everyone."

This New Perspective radically challenged many of the traditional assumptions of medical care and set the stage more than a decade ago for the current interest in prevention.

3.1.3 The Welfare State

When the government assumes responsibility for assuring health services to most of the population in accordance with their needs, the resulting system can be described as that of a welfare state. Even though access to health services has been equalized through collectivized insurance, much of the delivery system remains in private hands, with a variety of measures applied by the government to control quality and cost.

Social visibility of these costs, and their escalation with advanced technology and utilization rates create political pressure to increase the scope of controls.

The welfare state system most closely approximates that which exists in western Europe, and to a large extent, Canada, where a great percentage of health services is financed through collective channels. If we use Sweden as an example, approximately 8-10% of its gross national product (GNP) is devoted to health. Social insurance for almost complete medical care covers 100% of the population. Outside of hospital care, for which the individual pays nothing, physician care and drugs require a 80% cost-sharing by the patient on the first three visits, but not on continuing treatment for chronic illness. Publicly financed dental services are highly developed for school children of all income levels, although adults must pay privately. Altogether, it may be estimated that about 92% of health costs in Sweden are borne by social insurance and government revenues. Of the remaining 8%, a small amount comes from charity and industry (Roemer, 1977; Maxwell, 1981).

The Swedish supply of physicians is about the same as that in the U.S., but there are fewer specialists and more general practitioners. Being in relatively greater supply than in the U.S., the general practitioner plays a much greater role in general patient care and has few, if any, ties to a hospital. Practically all in-hospital service is provided by salaried specialists. A patient requiring specialist care or hospitalization is referred to a hospital doctor, and returns to the care of the general practitioner after discharge. Although the rate of hospital admissions is lower in Sweden than in the U.S., the average length of stay is longer, so that the total hospital days per 1000 population is greater.

Administratively, the authority of local government in general, and central government in particular, is much greater in the Swedish welfare state than in the U.S. Hospitals are overwhelmingly owned and operated by units of government, and because elected officials already control the health care delivery system, competition for the consumer dollar is not as prominent. Satisfaction with the system is generally very high, and litigation for malpractice is rare.

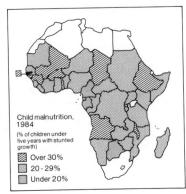

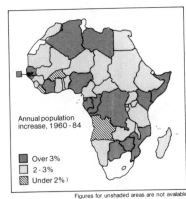

Source: UNICEF

Figure 3.5. Primary indices of health shown for some African countries. Figures for unshaded areas are not available. Reproduced with permission from **The Economist**, p. 91, May 31, 1986.

3.1.4 Underdeveloped Country Systems

In the poorest of countries, such as those in Africa and much of Asia, resources for modern health services are extremely deficient. Being only slightly industrialized, the population is predominantly rural, illiterate and impoverished, with all the concomitants of malnutrition and disease. Some primary indices of health in such countries are shown in Figure 3.5 for the countries of Africa.

The country of Ghana, located on the northwest coast of Africa, provides a typical example of such a system. Ghana invests only a small proportion (1.8%) of its GNP in health services. A significant part of even this small amount comes from international donations, either through foreign governmental aid or religious missions. While the doctor-to-population ratio improved from 1:18,000 in 1961 to 1:12,700 in 1970, it is the number of physicians practising in the urban rather than the rural sector that has increased. More than 50% of doctors in Ghana are in and around the capital of Accra, where less than 10% of the population live. The balance of doctors must serve the remaining 90% of the population, meaning that for the majority of the population the supply of physicians is **very low** (Roemer, 1977).

The large majority of people therefore depend for most of their health care on primitive traditional healers located in the villages. Most minor illnesses go untreated, and the more severe disorders are typically brought to the attention of village healers, who may prescribe a variety of empirical or mystical techniques to effect a cure. Insofar as modern medical science is applied, it is by central government authorities.

Since only a small proportion of the population earns a regular wage, there are neither social insurance nor voluntary insurance programs for medical care. Occasionally a large corporation may operate a closed system of health services for its workers and their families, and in some rural areas there may be religious missions offering semi-charitable medical care for small payments by the people.

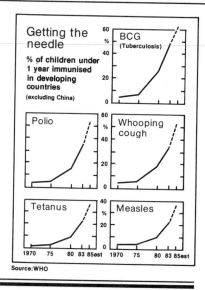

Getting the needle

% of children under 1 year immunised in developing countries (excluding China)

Source: WHO

Figure 3.6. Shows the percentage of children under 1 year immunized in developing countries (excluding China). Reproduced with permission from **The Economist**, p. 92, May 31, 1986.

In 1978 the World Health Organization (WHO) set a goal of **Health for All by the year 2,000**, proposing a low-technology packet of primary health care in poor countries designed to prevent disease. Primary tenets were to provide clean water, vaccination (see Figure 3.6), contraception, mother and child medical treatment, and essential drugs (200 of them) for all. The WHO considered that if poor countries would provide only 10% of their GNP to health the goal was possible. To date, 35 to 40 countries have, to varying degrees, adopted these policies. Between 1980 and 1983 15 million more rural people were served with good water. Eighty developing countries adopted the essential drug list and worldwide the demand for vaccines is at 3 times its 1983 level. The first 5 year phase of the WHO initiative has recently been studied in some African countries. In Gambia there were fewer deaths among very small babies and fewer deaths from malaria. Overall though infant mortality had not changed. Nonetheless, since 1980 Gambia had installed pump wells in 700 of its 2,000 villages, immunized 70% of its children, and improved access of villages with greater than 400 population to trained health care workers.

In Kenya, the number of modest health centres and dispensaries serving other than the large cities more than doubled, to 1600 by 1986 from their late 1970's level. Kenya also decreased infant mortality to 100 per 1,000 live births from a high of 140 in the 1960s while doubling its spending on health care.

Poverty and lack of prenatal and infant care, similar reasons to those causing the problem in underdeveloped nations, even caused the U.S. record of infant deaths to reach 10.8/1000 births in 1984. That was good for last place in a ranking of 20 industrial nations. The majority of these deaths were recorded among the impoverished black and hispanic American populations.

3.1.5 Transitional Systems

Many predominantly agricultural and rural countries, such as those in Latin America and the Middle East, have made great progress in developing their health care systems. Although the majority of the population still lives under very poor conditions, a modest structure of organized health services has been developed. Although traditional healers still treat patients, they are noticeably being replaced by more modern resources. For the affluent, a substantial private medical sector still functions and the distribution of doctors typically remains uneven, with the concentration living in the largest cities.

As an example, health services in Peru reflect several different historical influences. The original Indian culture gave rise to traditional healing practices that are still widely found in rural areas. The presence of the Catholic Church of Spain gave rise to many charitable hospitals for the care of the urban poor. North American influence has promoted public health programs, especially through environmental sanitation and mass campaigns against infectious disease. Finally, modern Europe disseminated the social security idea which gave rise to a special subsystem of health services for insured workers. At the same time, a class of wealthy families developed, mainly in the large cities, and a private medical care sector took shape.

Thus, the economic support for health services in Peru is quite diversified. The total percentage of GNP devoted to health is nearly 3%, with 50% of this going toward the care of only 10% of the population.

3.1.6 Socialist Systems

SOVIET UNION

Since the Russian Revolution of 1917 a markedly different type of health care system has arisen in the Soviet Union, with health care essentially a public service, and with almost all personnel employed as

*In the Soviet Union every new doctor was required to serve
three years at a rural post, in order to repay the state for
their (all-expenses-paid) medical training.*

civil servants and all facilities owned and operated by the government.
Health service has become, theoretically, a right of citizenship.

In the first twenty years or so after the Russian Revolution, a high
priority was assigned to health, especially for workers and for children.
Remarkably large numbers of doctors and other health professionals
were rapidly trained. These graduates then were employed, on state salaries, in newly built hospitals, clinics, and health centres. While it has
not disappeared entirely, private medical and dental practice gradually
declined as the public system was developed.

The Soviets managed the problem of rural health care more effectively than did many other countries. First of all, every new doctor (and
most are female) was required to serve three years at a rural post, in
order to repay the state for their (all-expenses-paid) medical training.
Should a doctor choose to stay longer than the three years, she/he would
be paid a higher salary than that paid in urban centres. As more and
more health personnel graduated, the job market began to dictate where
they would go for employment, and often this meant working in rural
areas because city positions were filled. The large supply of auxiliary
health workers in the Soviet Union, coupled with the strategy described
above, has meant greater equity between urban and rural services than
most other nations enjoy. Generally speaking, the Soviet model of
health care delivery is one which emphasizes quantity rather than quality. In other words, it is seen as more important to provide modestly
adequate services to most of the population (which is greatly spread out,
geographically) than technologically superior service to only a few. Preventive services also are emphasized, and higher priority is given to
children and industrial workers (Roemer, 1977).

Approximately 4% of total Soviet GNP is spent on health services.
Health workers account for 5-6% of the total workforce, about the same
as that in the U.S., but the American system absorbs more than double
the percent of the U.S. GNP. While the Soviet health system would
seem rigid in many ways compared with free enterprise standards, it pro-

In China thousands of peasants have been trained as "barefoot doctors" in order to offer at least minimal health care to everyone.

vides all citizens with virtually free medical services, and the level of consumer satisfaction seemed to be high. In the period of Gladnost or openness characterizing the Gorbachev regime however widespread degenerative disease, alcoholism, smoking and sedentarinism is now acknowledged. It is repported that life expectancy of Russian males is no more than 67 years.

CHINA

China's health care system changed from the Soviet model when it broke away politically in 1960. Even more drastic changes were incorporated by 1970, following the Proletarian Cultural Revolution. The bureaucratic hierarchy of the Soviet model did not prove useful in China, where the population was so much larger, and after 20 years, rural areas still lacked adequate services (Sidel, 1982).

The present system is much more decentralized, and thousands of peasants have been trained as "barefoot doctors" in order to offer at least minimal health care to everyone (Roemer, 1977). The result is economical, with the use of traditional methods, low-cost facilities, and an incentive system for health workers based on social rather than economic motivation. Although regular health care is not paid for by the state, the costs (which are minimal) are paid under cooperative plans or by factory or commune donations. The government covers most specialist costs.

Modern China's health care delivery system is a remarkable accomplishment. In a single generation, China changed from a starving, ignorant disease-laden and elitist society to one that is healthy, productive, literate and characterized by mass participation. Because China's social, economic, political and cultural circumstances are so unique, it is often difficult to apply her experience to other nations in any useful way. However, some important lessons may be learned from her methods, such as the value of local self-sufficiency, of brief, goal-oriented training and well-organized but part-time use of local workers, and of preventive health care (Roemer, 1977). An even more important lesson, and one more difficult to learn, is the need for society's basic attitudes toward health and health care to change fundamentally, in order for all to benefit. Specifically, it should be a primary goal in any society that health services, as well as other resources, be distributed equitably. Moreover, the very opportunity to be of help to others ought to be a prime motivator to individuals and groups working in health services (Roemer, 1977).

3.1.7 An Overall Analysis

Each of the five principal types of health care systems described above is distinguishable from the others, even though each has variations within its own type. Over time, changes occur in all systems. If one considers all the systems currently displayed by different countries, as part of a continuum, it is understandable that any given system may eventually merge into another type. For example, Australia has recently begun moving from the free enterprise to the welfare state pattern; Egypt appears to be moving from the underdeveloped to the transitional type of system; Costa Rica seems to be evolving into the welfare state pattern from a transitional one; and Great Britain in many ways is moving from a welfare state to a socialist system (Roemer, 1977).

While the classification of health care systems offered here may be considered theoretical or somewhat arbitrary in terms of how divisions are made among categories, it should serve to place each in an international perspective.

3.2 CURRENT THEORIES
AND FUTURE DEVELOPMENTS

3.2.1 Pathogenic Theory Versus Holism

Throughout history, medical science has attempted to explain the cause of disease. In primitive times, disease was thought to be a punishment inflicted by unseen gods for offences committed against them. Later, the environment was considered to be a cause of illness; unsanitary conditions or swamp air were linked to disease. Finally, when the pathogenic theory, or germ theory, was proposed, it was thought that the ultimate answer had been found. Diseases that never before had been understood were clarified and indeed, viewing germs as the cause of infec-

"More than 90% of modern medicine could disappear
from the face of the earth—doctors, hospitals,
drugs and equipment—and the health of the nation
would immediately and drastically be improved".
........*Robert Mendelsohn*

tious disease truly was a breakthrough in bringing about prevention and treatment. But as medical science has become more sophisticated, it has been found that disease rarely has a singular cause. Even the germ theory never completely explains a disease's cause.

Relying exclusively on the pathogenic theory made it difficult to determine why some people who obviously had contact with a germ were not infected, while others with the same exposure did get sick. It also makes it virtually impossible to address some of the major health problems we face today, since these are generally not the result of infectious microorganisms. As indicated in Chapter 1, traditional, or allopathic, medical practice has been criticized for relying too heavily upon the germ theory of disease. That is, practitioners of the traditional medical model are criticized for assuming that disease is avoidable and undesirable, and that every disease is caused by a pathological lesion which can be treated and cured by external manipulation. Critics of this approach point to excessive use of drugs, invasive techniques, and dehumanized treatment as evidence that today's medical system is not so much concerned with health promotion as with disease treatment. Some medical heretics, such as Robert Mendelsohn in his book **Male Practice** (1982), go so far as to say that *"More than 90% of modern medicine could disappear from the face of the earth—doctors, hospitals, drugs and equipment—and the health of the nation would immediately and drastically be improved"*. Ivan Illich, in his controversial book, **Medical Nemesis**, states that *"the medical establishment has become a major threat to health"*, and that *"a society which can reduce professional intervention to a minimum will provide the best conditions of health"*.

While such harsh criticisms may be partially justified, they are undoubtedly over-generalizations and do not apply carte blanche to the entire medical profession, which continues to make invaluable contributions to our health care system. Where the medical system leaves itself open to criticism, however, is in its continuing inability to deal with the major causes of death and debility in society today. Examples of these are accidents and suicide in youth, and chronic degenerative disease among adults.

The current practice of holistic health care, defined in Chapter 1, arose out of such criticism and provides an alternative philosophy to allopathic medical practice. Rather than viewing any disease in isolation, to be destroyed as quickly as possible, holistic medicine considers disease to be feedback about the state of harmony arising between an individual and his/her environment. It recognizes that there is no single cause of disease, that mind and body are inseparably linked, and hence regards **psychosomatic disease** as being very real (rather than a figment of one's imagination). Note that the concept of holism is not an alternative health care delivery system. Rather, it is a philosophy whose basic premises are not dissimilar to those prescribed in the Hippocratic Oath taken by all medical school graduates. In other words, holistic health care is not new. It is as old as medical science itself.

3.2.2 The Changing Medical Paradigm

There is little doubt that our health care system, including traditional medical practice, is undergoing a transition in response to rising costs, professional criticism, consumer demand, and the changing patterns of morbidity and mortality. The final outcome has yet to be determined, but, as is the case with most other institutions currently undergoing transition, it will likely be more responsive to human needs.

The shift in philosophy from allopathic to holistic health care has not and will not take place without its own set of difficulties. One of greatest concern to the health consumer is the growing number of alternative therapists, prescriptions and modalities which have arisen to meet the rising demand for **anything other than traditional medicine**. Many of these alternatives may be useful complements to a good physician-patient relationship. In fact, preventive/holistic health centers may include nutritionists, psychologists and acupuncturists on their staff as well as a physician. Physicians also refer their patients to naturopaths, physiotherapists, chiropractors, massage- or hypno-therapists. Unfortunately, many adjunct health services are not covered by medical insurance, and prolonged therapy may incur a substantial cost to the individual, especially if he/she is not referred to it by a physician.

Some unfortunate people, who have experienced frustration with their traditional allopathic doctors, have set out on their own, visiting one anti-establishment practitioner after another, searching for a miraculous cure for a disease for which modern medicine has no answer to offer (arthritis and terminal cancer are two examples). Personal testimonies of successful treatment often lure them to far-away clinics at great personal expense, only to meet finally, once again, with disappointment and failure.

3.2.3 Placebo Effects

A phenomenon which often makes it difficult to determine whether a particular therapy or medication is itself effective is the placebo effect. Traditionally, the term placebo has been used to describe an imitation medicine for placating imaginary illnesses. A hypochondriac, or person who repeatedly appears in the doctor's office complaining of pain for which there is no apparent cause may be given a sugar pill to satisfy his/her apparent need for treatment. Another traditional use for placebos, or inert medications, is in the testing of new drugs. In this case, one group of subjects is given the active drug and another the placebo to determine the physical effect of the new drug (i.e., without any possiblity of the observed effect being psychological only). A peculiar observation in this type of testing is that approximately one-third of people taking placebo medication actually experience the anticipated drug effects. In other words, their belief that the pill they are taking will affect their health is enough to create an effect in such varying conditions as seasickness, ulcers, warts, and the healing of post-operative wounds.

The placebo effect, while still not completely understood, has been

A peculiar observation.... is that approximately one-third
of people taking placebo medication
actually experience the anticipated drug effect.

central to medical practice for hundreds of years across all cultures.
Much of the success of witch doctors and their concoctions of lizard's
blood, animal dung and frog sperm may be attributed to the belief their
patients have in their ability to cure. Even today, the placebo plays an
important role in the physician-patient relationship. Lack of faith in a
doctor's ability to cure illness of course will undoubtedly affect the
outcome of treatment.

should find a physician who shares your philosophy and is willing to

3.2.4 Health Quackery

Quackery is a term referring to the use of misrepresented, questionable,
ineffective or dangerous treatments, often involving very high fees.
Stereotyped images of **quacks** probably include the shifty-eyed sales-
man who travels door-to-door with miraculous products claiming to be
a panacea for all that ails you. But quackery of a sort also may originate
from qualified persons who, in an honest attempt to provide answers to
difficult questions, misinterpret available information or extrapolate beyond what is currently known about a particular issue or phenomenon.
Our concept of quackery also changes with time. When William Withering began prescribing digitalis, a derivative of the fox-glove plant, for
heart patients in England in 1775, he was labelled a quack. So was
Ignaz Semmelweis, when he declared in 1848 that deadly childbed fever
could be prevented by physicians washing their hands before delivering
a baby.

Both Withering and Semmelweis eventually became medical heroes,
and their discoveries became recognized as major contributions to medical science. The differences between quack treatments and monumental
discoveries are not always immediately clear. Sometimes a truly well-
intentioned physician, or even a entire medical community, can use a
treatment that later proves as dangerous, or more so, than that of a
quack. X-rays, for example, were used very freely until it was discovered that heavy use could cause cancer.

A belief in quack therapy however may result in a beneficial outcome even though the treatment by itself may be totally ineffective.

Although some forms of health quackery may be essentially harmless, and even provide a placebo effect which aids the body's own healing process, others may have a deleterious effect. In most situations they are expensive, and may delay or discourage a person from seeking needed medical attention. Although efforts are made by government to control fraudulent health practices, they nonetheless abound—particularly when so many people are looking for alternative therapies for incurable diseases. Until we have completed the transition to a preventive health care system, this trend is likely to continue.

As mentioned earlier, fraudulent health practices are often difficult to detect, and some forms of **quackery** eventually become incorporated into acceptable procedures once additional information becomes available. During an era of transition, such as we are presently experiencing, it is often difficult for the health consumer to make decisions about the variety of options that are available. The American Medical Association offers the following guidelines to assist the individual in identifying phony products of medical quacks:

- The quack often claims that a special or **secret formula** or machine can cure disease.
- The quack promises or implies a quick or easy cure or offers to solve a variety of seemingly unrelated problems.
- Quacks often use case histories and testimonials from patients to impress people.
- Quacks are usually very critical of traditional medical methods and may claim personal persecution by the medical establishment.
- Reported "scientific" evidence for a quack's method is usually not from reliable sources.

3.3 PERSONAL STRATEGIES: HEALTH CONSUMERISM

Today's marketplace of health provides a vast array of options for the consumer, ranging from traditional medical care to alternative therapies, unorthodox services and sometimes questionable products. Medical services have long been regarded as somewhat mysterious to the average person, who has preferred to entrust health care management to a physician, especially during periods of crisis. But the purchase of health care services should be similar to the purchase of any other commodity in terms of consumer approach. In order to make appropriate choices, the health consumer must identify reliable sources of information, develop a personal health strategy, replace fears and superstitions with objectivity in health-related matters, and avoid fraudulent health practices by insisting on explanation and evidence.

Central to accomplishing this is selection of a physician whom you trust and can communicate with. This is by no means an easy task. While general reputation and recommendation by a reliable friend may be appropriate starting points, someone else's criteria for a good doctor may be different from your own. Some people prefer an authority figure, someone who effectively will tell them what to do when things go wrong. However, if you are interested in becoming more responsible for your own health and preventing disease as much as possible, you should

3.4 REFERENCES

Bennett, J.E. and Krasny, K. Health Care in Canada. **The Financial Post**, March 26-May 7, 1977.

Benson, H. **The Relaxation Response**. New York: Avon, 1975.

Capital Line. 30 Million May Find Health Care Relief. **U.S.A. Today**, Feb. 13, 1987.

Capital Line. Elderly: Reagan Health Plan Falls Short. **U.S.A. Today**, Feb. 18, 1987.

Culliton, B.J. Omnibus Health Bill: Vaccines, Drug Exports, Physicians Peer Review. **Science 234**: 1313, 1986.

Culliton, B.J. For-Profit Hospitals Loom Large on the Health Care Scene. **Science 233**: 928, 1986.

Healy, M. U.S.A. Failing to Save Babies' Lives. **U.S.A. Today**, Feb. 4, 1987.

Health care costs in Canada. The **Financial Post**, Aug. 6, 1983.

Illich, I. **Medical Nemesis: The Expropriation of Health**. New York: Pantheon, 1976.

Maxwell, R.J. **Health and Wealth**. Massachusetts, Toronto. Lexington Books, D.C. Heath and Company, 1981.

McNemly, W.J. For-Profit Enterprise in Health Care. **Science, 233**: 928, 1986.

Mendelsohn, R. **Male Practice**. Chicago: Contemporary Books, 1982.

National Academy Institute of Medicine. **For-Profit Enterprise in Health Care**, Washington, National Academy Press (2101 Constitution Ave., N.W. Washington, D.C. 20418). 1986.

Roemer, M.J. **Comparative National Policies on Health Care**. New York: Marcel Dekker, 1977.

Science and Technology. Health Care is Not Curing Africa's Ills. **The Economist,** May 31, 91-92, 1986.

Sidel, Ruth and Sidel, Victor. **The Health of China**. Beacon: Boston, 1982.

Standard and Poor's Market Month, Hospital Market Stocks Poised for Recovery, 3, Dec. 1986.

World Bank, **World Development Report, 1984**. New York. Oxford University Press, 1984.

World Bank, **World Development Report, 1985**. New York. Oxford University Press, 1985.

3.5 STUDY QUESTIONS

1. Compare and contrast the major characteristics of free enterprise, welfare state, and socialist health care delivery systems.
2. Outline several reasons why people are dissatisfied with medical care in developed countries today. What sort of changes would increase public satisfaction with the medical care received?
3. Cite several examples of medical or surgical procedures that may be carried out in unwarranted numbers.
4. Describe several ways by which a person can increase his or her satisfaction with the results of a visit to a physician's office or stay in a hospital.
5. Explain why a search for the appropriate healing methods is so complicated.

Part II

Hazards to Health

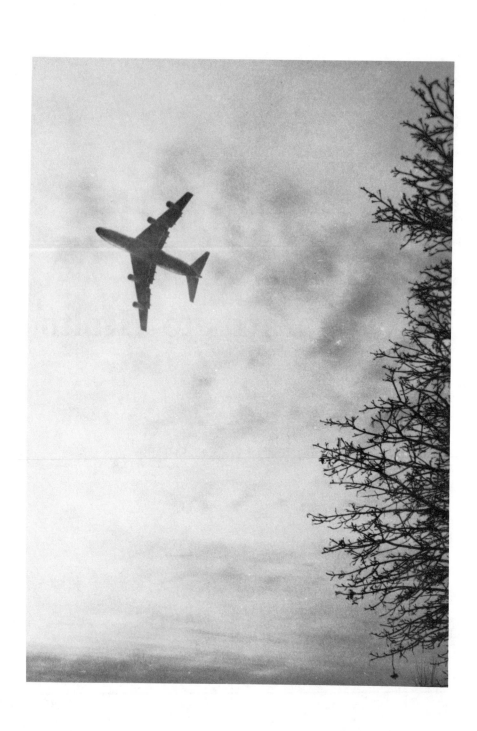

4

Environmental Stressors

The central truth of the human-environment relation today:
we are still part of nature, not masters of nature.

OBJECTIVES

When you have completed this unit, you should be able to:

- **Define** the terms "pollution," "pollutants," and "toxic agents," and the concept of a healthful environment.
- **Identify** the different types and sources of air pollution and their effects on human health.
- **Explain** the concepts of temperature inversion, green-house effect, cooling effect.
- **Describe** the process leading to photochemical smog.
- **Identify** the major sources and harmful effects of water pollution.
- **Explain** some effects of unsafe chemical waste disposal.
- **Evaluate** the use of pesticides in light of their known hazardous effects.
- **Outline** the major contributors to noise pollution, and their effects.
- **List** major sources of exposure to radiation and its adverse health effects.
- **Explain** the role of politics and the role of the individual in preserving the environmental quality.
- **Describe** some effective steps to controlling air, water, and land pollution.

KEY TERMS

ambient air	eutrophication	P.C.B.
asbestos	heavy metals	pesticides
biodegradable	hydrocarbons	pollutant
Canada Water Act	ionizing radiation	ozone (O_3)
carcinogens	leach	rad
Clean Air Act	mutagens	smog
CO	NO_x	SO_x
decibel (dB)	particulates	temperature inversion
Environmental Protection Agency (EPA)		UFFI
Environmental Protection Service (EPS)		

The environment is the unique skin of soil, water,
gaseous atmosphere, mineral nutrients,
and organisms that covers this planet.

4.0 INTRODUCTION

In both World and Individual Health, one vital operating factor is the relationship between human beings and the environment. This chapter considers some of the most important features of this relationship.

The **environment** is the unique skin of soil, water, gaseous atmosphere (air), mineral nutrients, and organisms that covers this planet. For thousands of centuries, humans have learned to modify and exploit the environment to their advantage: to clear, to plant, to mine, to dam, to dredge, to domesticate animals, to breed varieties of plants and animals suitable to their needs, and to increase the yields of crops, fish, and fiber extracted from the natural system of the planet. Yet, in the last third of the twentieth century, we still cannot claim either full understanding or control of the environmental systems that support our growing population. This is the central truth of the human-environment relation today: **we are still part of nature, not masters of nature.**

The problem with our human-environment relationship, though, is that we are systematically diminishing the capacity of the natural environment to perform waste disposal, nutrient cycling, and other vital roles. At the same time, our growing population and rising affluence are imposing larger and larger demands on these natural processes. Any encompassing concept of the environment must also include social and cultural conditions contributing to it, not just physical conditions. The entire environment is, therefore, a dynamic system, reacting to every abuse and social value.

4.0.1 Healthy Environment

A **healthy environment** is essential to the maintenance of everyone's physical and mental health. If we let the environment deteriorate too far, all our other efforts at achieving good health will be in vain.

The concept of a healthy environment must not only emphasize the absence of harmful substances, but it also must include positive qual-

LAND POLLUTION

Erosion
Agricultural manure
Chemicals in soil
  and food
Junk cars
Septic tanks
Chemical wastes
Power plants
Ashes and residue

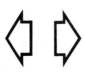

AIR POLLUTION

Open dumps
Dust
Odors
Pesticide sprays
Vehicle exhaust
Sewage odors
Radiation and smoke
Industrial gases
Incineration-smoke
  and fly ash
Smoke and odors

WATER POLLUTION

Silt in water
Nutrients in runoff
Chemicals in water
Contaminated rainfall
Contaminated water supply
Thermal pollution
Chemical wastes and oil
Process water wastes
Drainage to surface waters

Figure 4.1. Major Environmental pollutants and their interrelationships.

ities such as scenic beauty, pleasant communities, recreational facilities, adequate housing, educational and economic opportunities, a choice of various life-styles, and a social and technological environment lying within human adaptive capacities.

4.0.2 Pollution - Pollutant

A **pollutant** may be a single chemical element such as lead or mercury, a chemical compound such as DDT or carbon monoxide, or a more complicated combination of materials such as silt or sewage. Pollutants may also include various forms of energy such as noise, radiation, and heat. Pollution, simply defined, is a condition in which a substance(s) has so contaminated, dirtied, or corrupted the environment that it becomes unfit to support life in a healthy way. The major environmental pollutants in air, water, and land and their interrelatedness are summarized in Figure 4.1.

The production of pollutants has increased due to the following:
• **increased population,**
• **increased technology:** each year hundreds of new chemicals are produced and their long term health effects on human beings are largely unknown.

It is important to realize that a human environment can never be absolutely clean because, by definition, it includes at least one contaminant source, a person. An environment passes from a clean to a contaminated state when the source of contamination, relative to its rate of elimination, is sufficiently large, or where there are enough sources whose aggregate output is sufficiently large, to exceed some sensory or physical concentration limit for living organisms. Almost everything an individual in an industralized society does affects the environment. Without careful planning, good controls, and the cooperation between groups and individuals, the impact will be all bad and an unhealthy environment will be created.

Because there are many kinds of pollutants, there are many different sorts of harm produced by them. It is useful to divide these into four categories:

1. Direct assaults on human health (for example, lead poisoning or aggravation of lung disease by air pollution),
2. Damage to goods and services that society provides for itself (for example, the corrosive effects of air pollution on buildings and crops),
3. Other direct effects on what one perceives as the "quality of life" (i.e. congestion and litter), and
4. Indirect effects on society through interference with the ecological balance in fish production and effects on vegetation or other forms of life.

4.0.3 Political Aspects

The pollution problem has been growing since the onset of the Industrial Revolution in the late eighteenth and early nineteenth centuries, but the situation has lately become much worse and much more urgent. During the early sixties great political efforts in both the United States and Canada were made to control air, water, and land pollution. Governments tried to regulate discharge of any hazardous substances from motor vehicles and industrial emissions. The political fervor of the late 1960s and early 1970s over environmental quality has suffered several setbacks in recent years, becoming a secondary political issue as national economic problems (such as scarce and expensive energy, unemployment, inflation, and taxes) became more urgent.

The first Clean Air Act in the U.S.A., passed in 1963, provided federal support for pollution control activities. The second Clean Air Act, passed in 1970, required each state to submit to the Environmental Protection Agency (EPA) a plan to achieve the air quality standards specified in the act. These standards were to be met by 1975. Complications in achieving these standards have resulted in several extensions of the time period before their inception. Similarly, discussions between countries, such as Canada and the U.S.A., on the elimination of contam-

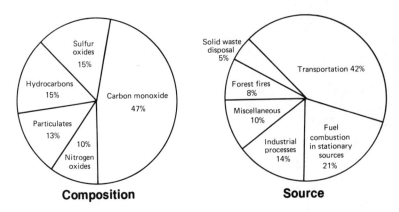

Composition   **Source**

Figure 4.2. Composition and sources of air pollution in the United States. (Data from the National Air Pollution Control Administration, Dept. of Health and Human Services, 1982.)

ination of each other's water and air space has dragged in protracted negotiations, while contamination continues unabated.

4.1 AIR POLLUTION

Normal air consists of nitrogen, oxygen, carbon dioxide, and several other lesser known gases. Approximately 21% of the air we breathe is oxygen; this is necessary for the maintenance of life. But our air supply is limited. Exhaled air contains only 17-18% oxygen, and its content must be continually refurbished by oxygen generated by our green vegetation (photosynthesis in plants).

For many years people have been treating the atmosphere as if it were a sewer, letting different kinds of waste products escape into it—gases, dusts, fumes, vapors and smoke. However, only in the past thirty years or so has serious concern been expressed regarding the deteriorating quality of the air we breathe and its effect upon the well being of people. While we can adapt to subtle and ongoing changes in the air quality, we cannot continue to function in polluted air if we wish to be healthy.

4.1.1 Sources of Air Pollution

The composition and sources of air pollution are summarized in Table 4.1 and represented by Figure 4.2, above.

TRANSPORTATION

By far the greatest source of air pollution in North America is the motor vehicle, which expels millions of tons of pollutants into our air each year, virtually all of which are by-products of combustion (Figure 4.2). Pollution from burned gasoline emitted from gas tanks, exhaust pipes, crankcases, and carburetors increases every year and accounts for more than half of all man-made pollutants. The internal combustion engine is not very efficient; it does not completely burn the fuel it uses: nearly 15% non-combusted gases escape into the air in the form of poisons. However, the main by-products of gasoline combustion are carbon monoxide and hydrocarbons. A comparison between the pollutant emission from three different transportation sources (automobiles, diesel engines, and aircraft) is summarized in Table 4.2.

Table 4.1. Sources and concentrations of atmospheric trace gases.

Contaminant	Main Anthropogenic Source	Natural Source	Estimated Global Emissions (tons·yr^{-1}) Anthropogenic	Natural	Atmospheric Background Concentration	Remarks
Sulfur dioxide (SO$_2$)	combustion of coal and oil	volcanoes	146 x 10^6	no estimate	0.2 ppb$_v$	-
Hydrogen sulfide (H$_2$S)	chemical processes sewage treatment	volcanoes, biological action in swamps	3 x 10^6	100 x 10^6	0.2 ppb$_v$	background concentration based on only 1 set of data
Carbon monoxide (CO)	auto exhaust, other combustion	forest fires, oceans terpene reactions	304 x 10^6	33 x 10^6	0.1 ppm$_v$	ocean contribution to natural source; very small
Nitric oxide (NO); Nitrogen dioxide (NO$_2$)	combustion	bacterial action in soil (?)	53 x 10^6	NO: 430 x 10^6 NO2: 658 x 10^6	NO: 0.2-2 ppb$_v$ NO2: 0.5 - 4 ppb$_v$	little data on natural sources
Ammonia (NH$_3$)	waste treatment	biological decay	4 x 10^6	1160 x 10^6	6-20 ppb$_v$	-
Nitrous oxide (N$_2$O)	none	bact. action in soil	-	590 x 10^6	0.25 ppm$_v$	-
Hydrocarbons	combustion, chemical processes	biological processes	88 x 10^6	CH$_4$: 1.6 x 10^9 terpene: 200 x 10^6	CH$_4$: 1.5 ppm$_v$ non-CH$_4$: <1 ppb$_v$	"reactive" hydrocarbon emissions from anthropogenic sources = 27 x 10^6 tons·year^{-1}
Carbon dioxide (CO$_2$)	combustion	biological decay, release from ocean	1.4 x 10^{10}	10^{12}	330 ppm$_v$	atmospheric concentration increasing yearly

Adapted and reproduced with permission from John Wiley and Sons, Inc. Robinson and Robbins. Emissions, Concentrations and Fate of Gaseous Atmospheric Pollutants, pages 1-93. In Air Pollution Control, Part II, W. Strauss (ed.). New York: Wiley-Interscience, ©1972.

Table 4.2. Emission factors from transportation sources. Emission factor is a parameter commonly used to indicate how much of a contaminant is released for a given amount of fuel consumed.

	SOURCE		
	Automobiles mean emission rate in pounds per 1,000 gallons of fuel consumed	**Diesel Engines**	**Jet Aircraft** emission rate in pounds per flight at altitude of 35,000 ft
Contaminant			
Carbon monoxide	2,300	60	20.6
Nitrogen oxides	113	222	23
Sulfur oxides (as SO$_2$)	9	40	-
Aldehydes (as HCHO)	4	10	4
Hydrocarbons	200	136	19
Organic acids (acetic)	4	31	-
Particulates	12	110	34

Compiled from: Office of Air Programs, EPA. Compilation of Air Pollutant Emission Factors. Publication No. AP-42, U.S. EPA, Research Triangle Park, N.D., 1972.

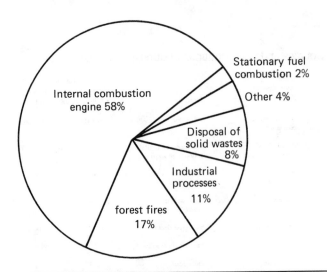

Figure 4.3. Sources of carbon monoxide emissions into the air. (Source: U.S. Department of Health, Education and Welfare, DHEW Publication, 1982.)

INDUSTRIAL PROCESSES AND POWER PLANTS
Industrial installations such as iron and steel mills, chemical plants, oil refineries, smelters, phosphate plants, and pulp and paper mills generate about 35% of air pollutants each year, particularly sulfur and nitrogen gases produced by burning heavy fuel oil and coal for low-cost industrial power and heat. As fuel consumption increases over the coming decades, this source of emission may produce dangerously high levels of harmful materials.

SOLID WASTE DISPOSAL
Belching incinerators annually process about 1800 lbs. of refuse for each person and produce 25 lbs. of airborne waste (mainly carbon monoxide) for each ton of garbage burned. Smoldering city dumps and municipal facilities also contribute foul odors and smoke to the air, as does the private burning of garbage in backyards.

4.1.2 Types of Air Pollutants
Five types of substances, known as primary pollutants, account for more than 90% of the worldwide air pollution problem. These are listed below:
- Carbon monoxide (CO),
- Nitrogen oxides (NO_x),
- Sulfur oxides (SO_x),
- Particulates (part.),
- Hydrocarbons (HC).

Refer again to Figure 4.2 to see the elements and composition of air pollution in terms of these five contaminants.

CARBON MONOXIDE (CO)
Carbon monoxide is the most abundant and widely distributed air pollutant found in the lower atmosphere. Approximately half of all air pollutant emissions are carbon monoxide, with the internal combustion en-

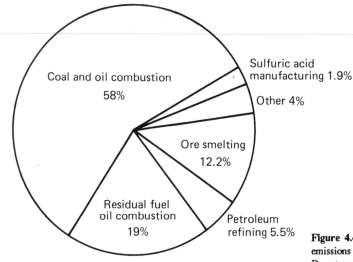

Figure 4.4. Sources of sulfur dioxide emissions into the air. (Source: U.S. Department of Health, Education and Welfare, DHEW, 1982.)

gine of the automobile the principal source. Figure 4.3 shows the various sources of carbon monoxide and indicates the percentage of the carbon monoxide in the air that is emitted by each.

CO is a colorless, odorless, and highly poisonous gas. It is produced through imperfect gasoline combustion in automobiles. Carbon monoxide poses a threat to health because of its ability to react with hemoglobin in blood and reduce the ability of the blood to transport oxygen, causing death by asphyxiation. For this reason it is extremely dangerous in heavy traffic, tunnels, and garages where concentrations can build up. In small quantities CO can cause dizziness, headache, and tiredness.

NITROGEN OXIDES (NO_x)

Two of the various nitrogen oxide compounds present a serious threat to air quality: nitrogen dioxide (NO_2) and, to some extent, nitric oxide (NO). Nitrogen dioxide is a foul smelling, brown gas produced when engine heat breaks up nitrogen molecules and combines them with oxygen. It is attributed mostly to motor vehicle emissions and chemical manufacturing processes. These gases can irritate the nose and eyes, cause plant damage, shut out sunlight, and reduce visibility. Nitrogen oxides constitute 8% of all air pollutants.

SULFUR OXIDES (SO_x)

The sulfur oxide emitted into the atmosphere in the largest quantities is sulfur dioxide (SO_2) accompanied by a small amount of sulfur trioxide (SO_3). SO_2 accounts for 15% of all air pollution. Its major source is the combustion of fuel and oil in homes and factories (see Figure 4.4). SO_2 is a colorless gas with an unpleasant odor that irritates the lungs and cardiovascular system. It combines with water vapour in the air in falling rain to form sulfuric acid (Acid Rain), which corrodes metal, stone, and fabric, and threatens plant life. Sulfuric acid formed by sulfur dioxide has been the primary cause of sickness and death in every major air pollution disaster.

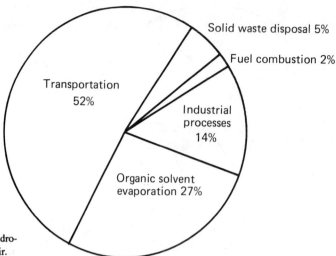

Figure 4.5. Sources of hydrocarbon emissions into the air. (Source: U.S. Department of Health, Education and Welfare, DHEW, 1982.)

PARTICULATES

Particulates are found in fly ash, smoke, and dust produced mainly combustion. Particulates account for 14% of air contamination, and are often found in smog conditions. Particles and the gases that adhere to them (e.g., SO_2) are not easily filtered by the upper respiratory tract and thus can be carried deep into the lungs. Particulates damage vegetation by forming hard crusts on leaves, killing plant tissue. High levels of particulates in the air are chiefly responsible for the visibility problems experienced in and around major industrial areas.

HYDROCARBONS

Hydrocarbons are mainly found in automobile exhaust as shown in Figure 4.5. These organic chemicals account for 15% of airborne pollutants. Suspected of being a cancer-producing agent, hydrocarbons are most dangerous when combined with other pollutants to produce smog.

THERMAL (OR TEMPERATURE) INVERSION

The problem of air pollution is complicated by the existence of inversion layers over many of the world's major cities. Normally the temperature of the atmosphere decreases steadily with increased altitude; but during an inversion, a layer of warm air overlying cooler air below severely limits vertical mixing of the atmosphere, and pollutants accumulate in the layer of air trapped near the earth's surface (see Figure 4.6).

When the pollutants contained by the cool air are unable to rise through the warm air, pollutants that would normally disperse through an atmosphere 12 miles deep are concentrated a few hundred feet off the ground and create what is called "killer smog." Inversions usually occur in areas surrounded by mountains and along seacoasts. The Los Angeles basin, for example, can have inversions for as many as 340 days per year, which produce dangerous pollutant concentrations. The Meuse Valley, an industrial section of Belgium, is another such area. In 1930, 63 people died there and another 6,000 were taken ill as a result of an inversion that held factory smoke close to the ground for several days.

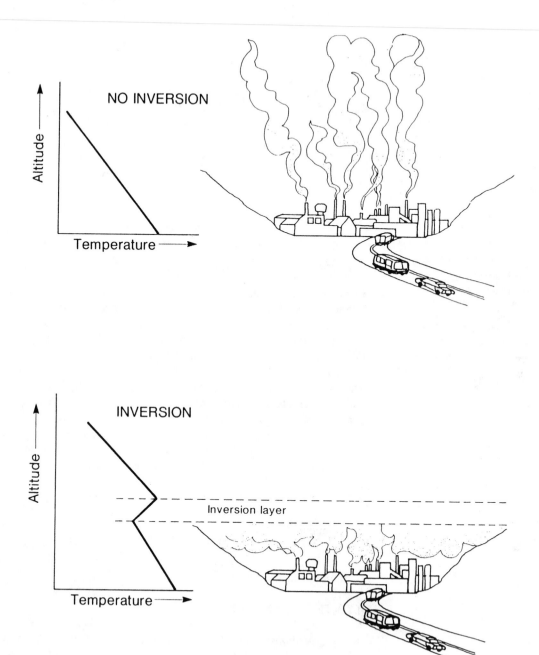

Figure 4.6. Temperature inversion, in which a layer of warm air overlies a layer of cooler air, trapping air pollution close to the ground. Redrawn and reproduced with permission from **ECOSCIENCE: Population, Resources, Environment** by Paul R. Ehrlich et al. Copright © 1970, 1972, 1977 W.H. Freeman and Co.

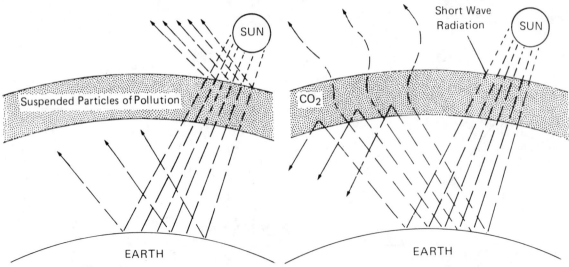

Figure 4.7. Which do you feel is more likely to occur? A cooling trend in the world—"Ice Age" development, left, or a warming trend in the world—"greenhouse effect," right? (Adapted and reproduced with permission from Miller, C.D. "Health, The Science of Human Adaptation".)

PHOTOCHEMICAL SMOG

The word smog is a contracted form of s̲mo̲ke and f̲o̲g. Smog is a common phenomenon in many metropolitan areas, especially those along seacoasts. Photochemical smog is a result of a series of chemical reactions in the atmosphere, when air pollutants trapped under an inversion layer are changed to more harmful chemicals by the action of sunlight. The basic ingredients of photochemical smog include nitrogen dioxide and incompletely burned hydrocarbons from auto exhausts. When nitrogen dioxide absorbs energy from sunlight, it forms nitric oxide (NO) and atomic oxygen (O). The atomic oxygen then unites with oxygen in the atmosphere (O_2) to form ozone (O_3). Ozone is an irritant to the lungs, eyes, and throat, causing headache, cough, and shortness of breath. It is therefore used as a key indicator of air pollution levels in areas where photochemical smog occurs. Ozone reacts with other air pollutants, especially hydrocarbons, to form hundreds of undesirable compounds. Among the worst offenders in producing photochemical smog are PAN (peroxyacetyl nitrate) and various aldehydes. Both compounds are highly irritating to the eyes and the respiratory tract and are harmful to vegetation as well.

4.1.3 The Greenhouse Effect

Much publicity has been given to a problem that has become known as the **greenhouse effect**. It involves the concept that increased concentrations of carbon dioxide (CO_2) in the atmosphere, as the result of human activities, can cause climatic changes by affecting the surface temperature of the earth. The greenhouse effect results from an interaction between the increasing amounts of atmospheric CO_2 and radiation leaving the earth. In this case CO_2 is behaving as a one-way filter, allowing visible light to pass through in one direction, but preventing the light in a longer wavelength form from passing in the opposite direction. This behavior is represented in Figure 4.7.

Recently scientists have predicted that a surface temperature increase of 0.8 to 2.9° C would result from a doubling of atmospheric CO_2 levels. It has been suggested that average temperature increases of this magnitude could lead to increased melting of ice caps and glaciers. The actual decrease in the average worldwide temperature seems to be more consistent with the increasing concentration of atmospheric particles that has been observed. The decrease in the earth temperature has been attributed to increased cloud cover and increased atmospheric particulate concentrations, creating a potential for a new "Ice Age." Obviously, a number of variables are involved in all of these conflicting predictions and much remains to be learned about these phenomena.

4.1.4 Indoor Pollution

Many people spend large amounts of each day indoors. In many cases, 80-90% of one's time is spent in a house, an automobile, a waiting room, an office or other workplace, or a confined space accessible to the general public, such as a store or a restaurant.

In keeping with the notion that wherever people spend a lot of time pollution tends to grow, indoor pollution cannot be ignored or underestimated. Increases in energy prices have encouraged individuals to seek alternative fuels and to reduce energy consumption. Therefore, efforts have been made to reduce energy use in the residential and commercial sectors by adding more insulation, reducing air-exchange rates, and switching fuels. Increased use of wood and coal-burning stoves and kerosene heaters leads to increased emissions of toxic and carcinogenic particles and gas. Reduced air-exchange rates in the presence of emissions from building materials and consumer products may adversely affect human health, welfare, and comfort. Urea formaldehyde foam insulation (UFFI), for example, has been shown to be a significant source of formaldehyde in the air. Complaints, symptoms, and illnesses have been reported by occupants of buildings with UFFI, and its use has been abandoned in Canada.

It has been shown that indoor exposure to environmental pollutants may be substantial, although there is little epidemiologic evidence of the health effects of indoor pollutants. Indoor concentrations of some pollutants (for which primary ambient air quality standards have been determined) often exceed quoted standards.

Indoor pollution in residences, public buildings, and offices is created by their occupants' activities and the use of appliances, power equipment, and chemicals (i.e. organic vapours, gases such as CO, NO_2, and SO_2); by wear and tear and outgassing of some structural or decorative materials (formaldehyde and asbestos fibers); by thermal factors (combustion byproducts), and by the intrusion of outdoor pollutants (i.e. SO_2). Some other pollutant sources such as cigarette smoking have been recognized as a major source of indoor pollution. Table 4.3 summarizes some typical indoor pollutants, their sources, and possible indoor concentrations as compared to outdoor levels.

Side-stream tobacco smoke, Radon, and Radon decay products (natural background radiation existing in construction materials and ground water), asbestos fibers, fiberglass, formaldehyde combustion by-products (such as polycyclic aromatic hydrocarbons, nitrogen dioxide, carbon monoxide, hydrogen cyanide, and sulfur dioxide), aeropathogens (disease-causing microorganisms), and allergens are all associated with a range of problems from mild irritation of nasal and mucous membranes, to irreversible toxic and carcinogenic effects. Reductions in damage to health from exposure to indoor contaminants may be attained simply by reducing exposure to those contaminants. Effective control strategies must be based on understanding several factors, such as contaminant characteristics (including concentrations, reactivity, physical state and particle size) and emission source configurations.

Indoor pollution control methods fall into five categories. These are ventilation, source removal or substitution, source modification, air purification, and behavioral adjustments to reduce exposures. Combinations of these can be used in certain cases (e.g. ventilation, source removal, and behavioral changes to reduce involuntary exposure to tobacco smoke). Table 4.4 summarizes the applicability of control methods to important indoor air contaminants.

Table 4.3. Sources, possible concentrations, and indoor-to-outdoor concentration ratios of some indoor pollutants.

Pollutant	Sources of Indoor Pollution	Possible Indoor Concentration[a]	I/O Concentration Ratio	Location
Carbon monoxide	Combustion equipment, engines, faulty heating system	100 ppm	>>1	Skating rinks, offices, homes, cars, shops
Respirable particles	Stoves, fireplaces, cigarettes, condensation of volatiles, aerosol sprays, resuspension, cooking	100-500 $\mu g \cdot m^{-3}$	>>1	Homes, offices, cars, public facilities, bars, restaurants
Organic vapors	Combustion, solvents, resin products, pesticides, aerosol sprays	NA	>1	Homes, restaurants, public facilities, offices, hospitals
Nitrogen dioxide	Combustion, gas stoves, water heaters, dryers, cigarettes, engines	200-1,000 $\mu g \cdot m^{-3}$	>>1	Homes, skating rinks
Sulfur dioxide	Heating system	20 $\mu g \cdot m^{-3}$	<1	Removal inside
Total suspended particles without smoking	Combustion, resuspension, heating system	100 $\mu g \cdot m^{-3}$	1	Homes, offices, transportation, restaurants
Sulfate	Matches, gas stoves	5 $\mu g \cdot m^{-3}$	<1	Removal inside
Formaldehyde	Insulation, product binders, particleboard	0.05-1.0 ppm	>1	Homes, offices
Radon and progeny	Building materials, groundwater, soil	0.1-30 $nCi \cdot m^{-3}$	>>1	Homes, buildings
Asbestos	Fireproofing	<1 $fiber \cdot cc^{-1}$	1	Home, school, office
Mineral and synthetic fibers	Products, cloth, rugs, wallboard	NA	-	Homes, schools, offices
Carbon dioxide	Combustion, humans, pets	3,000 ppm	>>1	Homes, schools, offices
Viable organisms	Humans, pets, rodents, insects, plants, fungi, humidifiers, air conditioners	NA	>1	Homes, hospitals, schools, offices, public facilities
Ozone	Electric arcing, UV light sources	20 ppb 200 ppb	<1 >1	Airplanes Offices

[a]Concentrations listed are only illustrative of those reported indoors. Both higher and lower concentrations have been measured. No averaging times are given. NA=not appropriate to list a concentration.

Table 4.4. Control strategies for indoor pollution.

Type of Control	Specific Strategies
Ventilation	a) general ventilation b) spot (zone or localized) ventilation c) infiltration
Control by source removal	a) material or product substitution b) restrictions on source use, sales, and activities by type of indoor facilities
Control by source modification	a) change in combustion design b) material substitution c) reduction in emission rates by intervention of barriers
Control by air-cleaning (pollutant removal)	a) particle filtering b) gas and vapor removal c) passive scavenging or absorption
Education	a) consumer information on products and materials b) public information on health, soiling, productivity, and nuisance effects c) resolution of legal rights and liabilities of consumer, tenant, manufacturer, etc., related to indoor quality

Adapted from: **Indoor Pollutants**. Committee on Indoor Pollutants, Board of Toxicology and Environmental Health Hazards, Assembly of Life Sciences, New York. National Academy Press, p. IX-40, 1981.

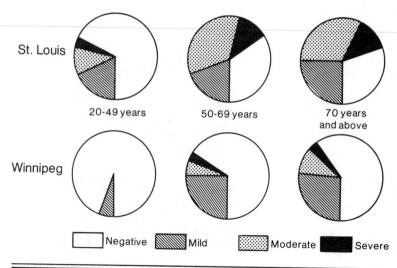

St. Louis

20-49 years   50-69 years   70 years and above

Winnipeg

☐ Negative   ▨ Mild   ▩ Moderate   ■ Severe

Figure 4.8. Prevalence and extent of emphysema in St. Louis, Missouri and Winnipeg, Canada. (Redrawn and reproduced from data of Williamson, S.J., **Air Pollution**, 1973.)

4.1.5 Health Effects of Air Pollution

Polluted air has a significant impact on the health of human beings and is responsible for a significant number of deaths and illnesses daily. According to Dr. Herbert Schimmel, biophysicist of Albert Einstein College of Medicine, air pollution triggered approximately 28 deaths daily from 1963 to 1972 in New York City alone. The severe effects of air contaminants upon health were brought to general attention following several acute air pollution crises, known as "episodes." Some of the major air pollution episodes are presented in Table 4.5. In addition to these major ones, many minor air pollution episodes occur regularly in the United States and other areas of the world (Figure 4.8).

Accurate analysis of effects of low levels of air contaminants (e.g. chronic exposure) are very difficult to establish. The available **epidemiological** evidence suggests that concentrations of air pollutants in the atmosphere contribute to certain chronic diseases in urban populations. The diseases most often associated with general air contamination involve the respiratory tract (i.e., **chronic bronchitis, pulmonary emphysema**) and, perhaps, lung cancer.

Air pollution levels also have been connected to some incidences of heart disease. Air pollution seems to be particularly harmful to infants, the elderly, pregnant women, and those suffering from chronic respiratory disorders. Some observed relations between contaminant levels and health effects are summarized in Tables 4.6, 4.7, and 4.8.

There is enough definite evidence of harmful effects of air pollution for many public health authorities now to recommend that people curtail vigorous outdoor activities while intense smog is in the area. In southern California, ozone levels are monitored daily as indicators of photochemical smog levels. Schools there are advised to keep pupils indoors during recess and lunch periods when ozone levels exceed 0.35 parts per million, a level reached on several days each year.

Table 4.5. Major air pollution episodes.

Location	Date	Topography Meteorological	Chemical Agents Involved
Meuse Valley, Belgium	Dec. 1-5, 1930	River valley; temperature inversion, weak winds, fog	Responsible agents not definitively known; those implicated include SO_2, fluorides, H_2SO_4. Estimated 9.6-38.4 ppm_v SO_2
Donora, Pennsylvania	Oct. 26-31, 1948	River valley; temperature inversion, weak winds, fog	No conclusive proof for health effects from any single agent; combination of SO_2 and particulates implicated. Estimated 0.5-2.0 ppm_v SO_2 4 $mg \cdot m^{-3}$ total particulates
Poza Rica, Mexico	Nov. 24, 1950	Flat terrain; temperature inversion, weak winds, fog	Hydrogen sulfide (H_2S)
London, England	Dec. 5-9, 1952	River plain; temperature inversion, weak winds, fog	Health effects due to any single agent not proven; SO_2, H_2SO_4, particulate levels high; SO_2 max. of 1.34 ppm_v, average 0.7 ppm_v; smoke particles max. 4.46 $mg \cdot m^{-3}$
New York City	Nov. 23-26, 1966	Temperature inversion, weak winds	Believed due to SO_2 and particulates. Max. 24 hr average of hourly SO_2 concentration = 0.51 ppm_v; max hourly SO_2 = 1.02 ppm_v

Table 4.6. Mortality and morbidity due to industrial and domestic sources of air pollution.

Main Sources	Mortality/Morbidity
Industry (steel mills, glass factories, Zn smelters, H_2SO_4 plants)	63 excess deaths; several hundred attributable illnesses; higher mortality in older age groups. Symptoms: respiratory tract irritation, coughing, chest pain, eye irritation.
Industry (steel mills, Zn smelter, H_2SO_4 plant)	20 excess deaths; 5,000-7,000 attributable illnesses; mortality in older age groups. Symptoms: respiratory tract irritation, eye irritation, cough, nausea.
Single industrial plant accidental discharge	22 excess deaths; 320 attributable illnesses. Persons of all age groups affected. Symptoms: respiratory tract irritation and nervous system disorders.
Space heating using coal in homes and factories	3,500-4,000 excess deaths; excess morbidity, but no estimate of numbers made; higher mortality in older age groups. Symptoms: respiratory tract irritation and nervous system disorders.
General urban sources: household and industry	168 excess deaths; unknown number of attributable illnesses; higher mortality in older age groups.

Table 4.7. Effects of air pollution on human health.

Pollutant	Known or suspected effect
Oxides of sulfur	Aggravation of existing respiratory diseases and contribution to their development; impairment of lung function; eye and throat irritation.
Oxides of nitrogen	Eye and throat irritation; contribute to development of photochemical smog.
Ozone	Considerable eye and throat irritation; possible association with asthmatic attacks; possible lung damage (pulmonary fibrosis)
Carbon monoxide	By combining with hemoglobin, reduces oxygen-carrying capacity of blood, deprives tissues of oxygen; low concentrations may cause severe impairment of mental abilities; higher concentrations cause death.
Lead	Intake through air adds to burden through food and water; may result in lead poisoning.
Asbestos	Particles inhaled into lungs remain permanently, irritate lung tissues, cause cancer and other lung diseases (extreme care must be taken to avoid asbestos inhalation).
Beryllium	Causes bronchitis and systemic poisoning; has poisoned people living three-quarters of a mile from a processing plant.

Table 4.8. Some observed relations between contaminant levels and health effects.

Contaminant	Concentration level Producing Adverse Health Effects	Adverse Health Effects
Particulate matter and sulfur oxides	• 80-100 $\mu g \cdot m^{-3}$ particulates (annual geometric mean) • 130 $\mu g \cdot m^{-3}$ (0.046 ppm_v) of SO_2 (annual mean) accompanied by particulate concentrations of 130 $\mu g \cdot m^{-3}$ • 190 $\mu g \cdot m^{-3}$ (0.068 ppm_v) of SO_2 (annual mean) accompanied by particulate concentrations of about 177 $\mu g \cdot m^{-3}$ • 105-265 $\mu g \cdot m^{-3}$ (0.037-0.092 ppm_v) of SO_2 (annual mean) accompanied by particulate concentrations of 185 $\mu g \cdot m^{-3}$ • 140-260 $\mu g \cdot m^{-3}$ (0.05-0.09 ppm_v) of SO_2 (24-hour average) • 300-500 $\mu g \cdot m^{-3}$ (0.11-0.19 ppm_v) of SO_2 (24-hour mean) with low particulate levels • 300 $\mu g \cdot m^{-3}$ particulates for 24 hr mean accompanied by SO_2 concentrations of 630 $\mu g \cdot m^{-3}$ (0.22 ppm_v)	• increased death rates for persons over 50 years of age • increased frequency and severity of respiratory diseases in school children • increased frequency and severity of respiratory diseases in school children • increased frequency of respiratory symptoms and lung disease • increased illness rate of older persons with severe bronchitis • increased hospital admissions for respiratory disease and absenteeism from work of older persons • chronic bronchitis patients suffering acute worsening of symptoms
Carbon monoxide (CO)	• 58 $mg \cdot m^{-3}$ (50 ppm_v) for 90 minutes (similar effects) upon exposure to 10 to 17 $mg \cdot m^{-3}$ (10-15 ppm_v) for 8 or more hours • effects upon equivalent exposure to 35 $mg \cdot m^{-3}$ (30 ppm_v) for 8 or more hours • effects upon equivalent exposure to 35 $mg \cdot m^{-3}$ (30 ppm_v) for 8 or more hours	• impaired time-interval discrimination • impaired performance in psychomotor tests • increase in visual threshold
Photochemical oxidants (O3 and peroxyorganic nitrates)	• in excess of 130 $\mu g \cdot m^{-3}$ (0.07 ppm_v) • 200 $\mu g \cdot m^{-3}$ (0.1 ppm_v) maximum daily value • 490 $\mu g \cdot m^{-3}$ (0.25 ppm_v) maximum daily value. (This value would be expected to be associated with a maximum hourly average concentration as low as 300 $\mu g \cdot m^{-3}$ [0.15 ppm_v])	• impairment of performance by student athletes • eye irritation • aggravation of asthma attacks

Tables 4.5, 4.6, 4.7 and 4.8 are from **Air Pollution and Industry**, R.D. Ross (ed.), Litton Educational Publishing, Inc., 1972. Reprinted by permission of Van Nostrand Reinhold Co.

Key: $\mu g \cdot m^{-3}$ = microgram per cubic meter
$mg \cdot m^{-3}$ = milligram per cubic meter
ppm_v = parts per million (volume basis)

Table 4.9. Pre-1969 ambient air quality standards for carbon monoxide.

Jurisdiction	Concentration mg·m^{-3}	Concentration ppm$_v$	Averaging Time
California	33	30	8 hrs
	132	120	1 hr
Czechoslovakia	1	0.9	24 hrs
	6	5.4	30 min
New York	16.5	15	8 hrs
	66	60	1 hr
Ontario	5.5	5	30 min
Pennsylvania	27.5	25	24 hrs
Poland	0.5	0.45	24 hrs
	3	2.7	20 min
U.S.S.R.	1	0.9	24 hrs
	3	2.7	20 min

Compiled from Stern, S.C. (ed.). **Air Pollution** 2nd Ed. New York: Academic Press, 1968.

4.1.6 Air Quality Standards

Since air contamination is a local problem, standards for contaminant levels usually have been established for local jurisdictions such as cities, countries, and provinces or states. Different jurisdictions, however, often have regulated different air contaminants and have proclaimed varying standards for the same contaminant. The most frequently regulated contaminants are smoke, carbon monoxide, and sulfur dioxide. The extent of variation in regulations for ambient air quality in different countries, and even in different cities in the same country, is illustrated in Table 4.9.

The first **Clean Air Act** was passed in 1963 in the United States. The Act provided federal support for pollution control activities. The second Clean Air Act, passed in 1970, required each state to submit to the Environmental Protection Agency (EPA) a plan to achieve the air quality standards specified in the Act. Table 4.10 shows the federal air quality standards that have been promulgated in the United States. In Canada, The Clean Air Act was officially proclaimed in November 1971. The Act provides the basis for the federal government's air pollution control activities and has three main objectives.

1. To protect the health of the public of Canada from air pollution. Federal regulations are laid down limiting the emission of hazardous pollutants such as lead, mercury, vinyl chloride, asbestos and arsenic from specific industrial sectors.
2. To promote a uniform approach across Canada in the control of other pollutants. The Act enables the issuance of industrial sector guidelines which, if adopted by a province as models for legislation, become enforceable by that province.
3. To provide the mechanisms and institutions needed to ensure that all measures to control air pollution can be taken. Provinces have a direct responsibility in controlling air pollution and cooperative efforts between provincial and federal authorities are required.

Table 4.10. United States Federal Air-quality Standards in $\mu g \cdot m^{-3}$.

	Primary	Secondary
Particulates:		
Annual mean	75	60
24-hour maximum	260	150
Sulfur dioxide:		
Annual mean	80	60
24-hour maximum	365	260
Carbon monoxide:		
8-hour maximum	10,000	10,000
1-hour maximum	40,000	40,000
Photochemical oxidants:		
1-hour maximum	160	160
Hydrocarbons:		
1-hour maximum	160	160
Nitrogen oxides:		
Annual mean	100	100

Source: U.S. Environmental Protection Agency. Health Effects of Environmental Pollution, 1973.

The Clean Air Act is administered within the Department of the Environment by the Environmental Protection Service (EPSW) through five regional offices across Canada located in Dartmouth, Montreal, Toronto, Edmonton, and Vancouver.

In addition to the general objectives above, the Government of Canada has proposed national air quality objectives that set specific limits on levels of pollution in the ambient air. The Clean Air Act refers to three levels of air quality for each major air pollutant: **desirable, acceptable,** and **tolerable.** The objectives proposed to date concern only the first two of these levels. The National Air Quality objectives, in their latest formulation, are given in Table 4.11. A complete formulation of the National Air Quality Objectives as revised appeared in the March 30,1974, and April,1974, editions of the **Canada Gazette.**

National emission guidelines for various industries are now under development with the cooperation of the provinces and industry. Emission Standards for lead from the secondary lead smelting industry, for mercury emissions from chlor-alkali plants, and for asbestos emissions from mining and milling operations were established and published in the Clean Air Act Annual Report, 1976-1977.

MOTOR VEHICLE EMISSION STANDARDS
Federal standards regulating exhaust emissions from new motor vehicles manufactured or imported into Canada are issued and enforced under the Motor Vehicle Safety Act, administered by the Ministry of Transport. They require compliance on a uniform national basis. Emission standards were first enforced on the 1971 model year and became more stringent for following models. Canadian standards are similar to those of the United States, not only because of proximity and the resultant flow of vehicles across the border but also because Canada tends to have similar pollution problems. Table 4.12 indicates the emission standards for different automobile model years, as published by the U.S. EPA.

Table 4.11. National air quality objectives in Canada of concentrations of various air contaminants.

Air Contaminant	Maximum Desirable Level	Maximum Acceptable Level	Maximum Tolerable Level
Sulphur dioxide			
Annual arithmetic mean	30 μg·m^{-3} (0.01 ppm)	60 μg·m^{-3} (0.02 ppm)	
Average over 24 hours	150 μg·m^{-3} (0.06 ppm)	300 μg·m^{-3} (0.11 ppm)	800 μg·m^{-3} (0.31 ppm)*
Average over 1 hour	450 μg·m^{-3} (0.17 ppm)	900 μg·m^{-3} (0.34 ppm)	
Suspended particulate matter			
Annual geometric mean	60 μg·m^{-3}	70 μg·m^{-3}	
Average over 24 hours		120 μg·m^{-3}	400 μg·m^{-3} *
Carbon monoxide			
Average over 8 hours	6 mg·m^{-3} (5 ppm)	15 mg·m^{-3} (13 ppm)	20 mg·m^{-3} (18 ppm)*
Average over 1 hour	15 mg·m^{-3} (13 ppm)	35 mg·m^{-3} (30 ppm)	
Oxidants (ozone)			
Annual arithmetic mean		30 μg·m^{-3} (0.015 ppm)	
Average over 24 hours	30 μg·m^{-3} (0.015 ppm)	50 μg·m^{-3} (0.025 ppm)	
Average over 1 hour	100 μg·m^{-3} (0.05 ppm)	160 μg·m^{-3} (0.08 ppm)	300 μg·m^{-3} (0.15 ppm)*
Nitrogen dioxide			
Annual arithmetic mean	60 μg·m^{-3} (0.033 ppm)	100 μg·m^{-3} (0.055 ppm)	
Average over 24 hours		200 μg·m^{-3} (0.11 ppm)	300 μg·m^{-3} (0.16 ppm)*
Average over 1 hour		400 μg·m^{-3} (0.22 ppm)	1,000 μg·m^{-3} (0.53 ppm)*
Sulphur dioxide times suspended particulate matter			
Average over 24 hours			12,500 (μg·m^{-3})2*
Hydrogen fluoride			
Average over 70 days		0.20 μg·m^{-3} (0.24 ppb)*	
Average over 30 days		0.35 μg·m^{-3} (0.43 ppb)*	
Average over 7 hours	0.20 μg·m^{-3} (0.24 ppb)*	0.55 μg·m^{-3} (0.67 ppb)*	
Average over 24 hours	0.40 μg·m^{-3} (0.49 ppb)*	0.85 μg·m^{-3} (1.05 ppb)*	
Hydrogen sulphide			
Average over 24 hours		5.0 μg·m^{-3} (3.29 ppb)*	
Average over 1 hour	1.0 μg·m^{-3} (0.66 ppb)*	15.0 μg·m^{-3} (9.88 ppb)*	

* Proposed
ppb = parts per billion

Source: "Air Pollution in Canada" Air Control Directorate, Environment Canada, Ottawa, 1973.

Table 4.12. U.S. Federal Emission Standards for automobiles:
Specifications of the Clean Air Act Amendments of 1970 and 1977.
Values shown are in grams per mile.

Amend-ment	Beginning in Model Year	Hydro-carbons	Carbon Monoxide	Nitrogen Oxides
1970	1977	1.5	15.0	2.0
	1978	0.41	3.4	0.4
	1978-1979	1.5	15.0	2.0
1977	1980	0.41	7.0	2.0
	1981	0.41	3.4*	1.0

*The administrator (of EPA) may adjust the 3.4 requirement for carbon monoxide up to 7.0 upon a finding that the technology for control is not available, as determined by cost, driveability, fuel economy, and other factors. Source: U.S. Environmental Protection Agency.

4.1.7 Control of Air Pollution

The control or prevention of air contamination is a complex and often expensive problem. Although much is said about the cost of controlling air pollution, **far too little has been said about the cost of failure to control it.** The total cost of damage from air pollution in the United States is estimated at about $10 to $12 billion per year, or about $56 per person. This includes damage to property, plants, and animals and to the cost of treating smog-caused illnesses. Of course, the cost of air pollution is not borne just by those who produce it but by all of us. Many political questions now revolve around who should bear the cost of pollution control.

CONTROL OF AUTOMOTIVE POLLUTION

Federal and provincial efforts to take active steps to control pollution have occurred in the U.S.A. and Canada. Gasoline-powered vehicles have been equipped with emission control devices, designed to filter out 30% of hydrocarbon emissions. The problem of auto pollution, unfortunately, cannot be solved completely by this method. It will take some time before most cars are equipped with anti-pollution devices. Since these devices are not completely effective, future increases in the number of cars being operated ultimately will erase any benefits achieved in the short term. In consideration of these facts, gasoline-powered vehicles eventually may be replaced by electrically-powered ones. Several low-polluting steam-powered automobiles have already been invented. Neither type of vehicle has yet been mass produced. At the same time, gasoline manufacturers have worked hard researching the possibility of pollution-free gasoline.

CONTROL OF FACTORY AND POWER PLANT POLLUTION

Through legislation and voluntary compliance in both Canada and the United States, many industries and power plants have begun installing pollution control devices. For example, oil refineries have developed a technique to capture sulfur dioxide. The steel industry has begun replacing open-hearth furnaces with oxygen furnaces to reduce emission of iron oxide. Electrostatic precipitators installed by the electric power industry are catching a major portion of the fly ash emitted. The substitution of low-sulfur fuel, higher smokestacks, and the use of chemical scrubbers and charcoal filtration techniques are aiding in the control of sulfur dioxide emission and odor.

Controversial as it is, atomic energy is currently being explored as a potential means of generating electricity without the hazards of air contaminants. As new techniques are developed, further emission control will be accomplished.

CONTROL OF REFUSE DISPOSAL

Outdoor burning of rubbish and garbage, which discharges massive pollution into the air, is now being curtailed in many areas. The private citizen plays a significant role in controlling pollution by avoiding burning leaves or trash in backyards and by keeping home furnaces in good repair.

4.2 WATER POLLUTION

By definition, **water pollution** means the presence in water of any substance that impairs any of its legimate uses—for public water supplies, recreation, agriculture, industry, the preservation of fish and wildlife, and esthetic purposes.

In many communities direct threats to human health arrive through the faucet as well as through the air. It is believed that water should be safe to drink if it is chlorinated and filtered. Unfortunately, though, the water in many cities often is unsafe to drink. Believe it or not, the drinking water that flows from the tap in some localities has already passed through seven or eight people. Although chlorination may help, there is growing evidence that high content of organic matter in water may somehow protect viruses from the effects of chlorine. Infectious hepatitis is spreading at an alarming rate in the United States, and a major suspect of the route of transmission is the **toilet to mouth pipeline** of many water systems not made safe by chlorination. Recently, the safety of purifying water with chlorine has been questioned by geneticists because certain chlorine compounds, which are sometimes formed by the chlorination process, can cause mutations that may lead to hereditary defects (in this case they are called mutagens or teratogens), or they may cause cancer and therefore be known as carcinogens. But considering the high level of dangerous germs in many of our water supplies, we probably have to continue to accept the risks involved in chlorination, at least for the time being, since it rids the water of most of these germs.

4.2.1 Principal Sources of Water Pollution

DOMESTIC WASTES

Domestic wastes include everything that goes down the drains of a city into its sewer system: used water from toilets, bathtubs, and sinks and washings from restaurants, laundries, hospitals, hotels, and other businesses. On the average, each of us uses 40 gallons of water per day for personal washing and toilet flushing. Each minute in the shower uses 5 gallons of water; each load of laundry requires about 30 gallons.

Pollutants in domestic wastes are mostly organic compounds, including protein, fat, and carbohydrates, in suspended colloidal and dissolved forms. Detergents and soap also are potential pollutants.

INDUSTRIAL WASTES

Perhaps 60% of water pollution in North America may be attributed to industry. A Sunday newspaper is made with 150 gallons of water while brewing a barrel of beer requires 1,000 gallons of water. An amount as high as 29 million gallons is needed to manufacture the aluminum in one large jet aircraft. Industry uses water to clean manufacturing processes and to cool machines. Hot water introduced into a cool stream (thermal pollution) can kill aquatic life adapted to cool water. Warm water contains less dissolved oxygen, and at high temperatures it destroys oxygen demanding bacteria, thus damaging the ecological balance of the stream. Many chemicals discharged by factories into local streams are toxic, such as acids, pesticides, plastics, radioactive materials, oils, grease, and some animal and vegetable matter.

AGRICULTURAL WASTES

Several routine farming practices also pollute water. Irrigation water acquires salts and minerals as it seeps into the ground. In the same way, the water may accumulate chemical pollutants from pesticides and herbicides, which are considered a potential hazard to various forms of living organisms. Runoff from poorly sloped farmland leaches the soil of valuable nutrients and erodes the banks of rivers and streams, resulting in an increasing sedimentation rate in reservoirs. Animal wastes, discharged into streams, destroy stream life. Fish die from the increased levels of nutrients (mainly phosphates and nitrates) which are present in animal manure.

NAVIGATION CRAFTS

Many recreational crafts and commercial ships release raw sewage and galley waste into the water. Exhaust materials, such as oil, discharged from motor boats also contaminate water surfaces. Larger ships pollute the environment with bilge and ballast water, garbage, sanitary wastes, and littering. The pollutants released into the water are hazardous to shellfish and to recreational areas. Oil spills from breaks in pipelines, ship-wrecked oil tankers, or off-shore oil wells are particularly hazardous to wildlife. Oilsoaked beaches are extremely difficult and expensive to clean, and much of the damage cannot be reversed.

Table 4.13. Effects of water pollution on human health.

Pollutant	Effect
Human	Contains pathogens of many diseases, such as typhoid, wastes, cholera, shigellosis, salmonellosis, hepatitis, amebic dysentery, parasitic worms.
Mercury	Methyl mercury poisoning through concentration through food chains.*
Lead	Lead Poisoning.
Cadmium	Cadmium poisoning when concentrated through food chains.
Arsenic	Arsenic poisoning.
Fluorides	Mottling of teeth when present in excess.
Nitrates	Converted to nitrites in digestive tract. Nitrites combine with hemoglobin to form methemoglobin, which is incapable of carrying oxygen. Causes severe anemia in infants, elderly people, and people with heart or respiratory disorders.
Other chemicals	Oils and phenols, for example, may make water toxic or unpleasant to drink.

* A food chain is the transfer of mass and energy from one organism to another by eating and being eaten.

4.2.2 Harmful Effects of Water Pollution

HUMAN HEALTH CONCERNS

Many diseases such as typhoid fever, dysentery, and intestinal disturbances are transmitted through contact with polluted water. Other ailments may be caused by the cumulative toxic effects of chemical and metal particles entering the body through drinking water or eating poisoned fish or shellfish. Sodium ions are suspected of being related to heart disease, and chlorides may aggrevate high blood pressure. The presence of cancer-producing agents in polluted water is also considered a possibility. Table 4.13 summarizes some of the effects of water pollution on human health.

Water pollution also may contribute to poor health in less direct ways. Bad taste and odor, for instance, are likely to reduce the water intake of people who already consume too little liquid. And contamination of recreation areas makes it impossible for people to swim and engage in other healthy water sports.

LAKE EUTROPHICATION

Eutrophication means the process by which oxygen is removed from water by the excessive growth of algae. When large quantities of organic waste, rich in nitrogen and phosphorus nutrients, are dumped into a lake, the algae population grows rapidly. Algae may collect on the surface and become thick enough to impede boating and swimming. Also, it will result in bad-tasting drinking water. When algae die they are decomposed by aerobic bacteria that need oxygen to live. Eventually they may seriously deplete the dissolved oxygen in the water. Fish and aquatic life will die as a result. When the oxygen level drops to the point where aerobic bacteria cannot decompose the waste, anaerobic bacteria, which do not require oxygen, replace them and produce unpleasant odors (stagnant water).

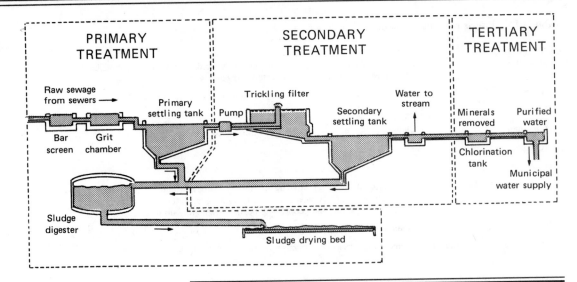

Figure 4.9. A three-stage sewage treatment process.

OTHER EFFECTS ON AQUATIC LIFE

Mine acid, a chemical by-product of coal mining, is one of the greatest dangers to fish and aquatic life. In sufficient amounts, it may corrode bridges, boats, and structures built on the water. Particles and sediments may kill plant and animal life when settled, and cloudy water prevents sunlight from reaching aquatic plants.

As mentioned earlier, oil spills primarily affect birds, which become covered with oil and subsequently starve to death because they are unable to fly. Oil also coats the respiratory surfaces of fish and other organisms, killing them.

4.2.3 Water Quality Standards

Historically, there have been three types of standards established for the maintenance of environmental water quality: drinking-water standards, surface-water standards, and effluent-quality regulations. Some of the chemical limits for drinking water in Canada, U.S., and other countries are summarized in Table 4.14.

In the last decade despite efforts to clean up U.S. surface waters the total amount of pollutants entering surface and ground water stores seems the same. Congress has continually failed to give the EPA authority to control ground water contamination (World Almanac, 1986).

The Canada Water Act, first proclaimed in September, 1970, provides the framework for joint federal-provincial management of Canada's water resources. Water quality objectives are a basic feature of water management in Canada. They are statements by governments of the quality levels suited to the uses intended for a specific body of water. When coupled with targets for their achievement, they become the basis for determining the kind and degree of waste treatment and waste control measures needed on ship or shore.

4.2.4 Control of Water Pollution

Municipal sewage should be treated until its water content is pure enough to drink. A three-stage sewage treatment process including primary, secondary, and tertiary treatment, as described in Figure 4.9, is

Table 4.14. Drinking water standards—chemical limits in $mg \cdot l^{-1}$ (parts per million, weight basis).

Chemical	United States 1962(a)	1969(b)	1975(c)	Canada 1968(d)	International 1963(e)	Europe 1970(f)
Arsenic (As)	0.05	0.01	0.05	0.01	0.05	0.05
Barium (Ba)	1.0	1.0	1.0	1.0	1.0	
Cadmium (Cd)	0.01	0.01	0.01	0.01	0.01	0.01
Chromium (Cr^{+6})	0.05	0.05	0.05	0.05	0.05	0.05
Cyanide (CN)	0.2	0.01		0.01	0.2	0.05
Lead (Pb)	0.05	0.05	0.05	0.05	0.05	0.1
Mercury (Hg)			0.002			
Selenium (Se)	0.01	0.01	0.01	0.01	0.01	0.01
Silver (Ag)	0.05	0.05	0.05			
Phenolic substances (as C_6H_5OH)	0.001	0.001		0.002	0.002	0.001
Nitrate (as N)	10.	10.	10.	10.	10.	
Boron (B)		1.0		5.0		

Sources:
(a) **Drinking Water Standards**, U.S. Public Health Service, 1962.
(b) **Manual for Evaluating Public Drinking Water Supplies**, U.S. Public Health Service, 1969.
(c) **Interim Drinking Water Standards**—Federal Register, Dec. 1975.
(d) **Canadian Drinking Water Standards & Objectives**—1968, Dept. of National Health and Welfare, Ottawa, October, 1969.
(e) **International Standards for Drinking Water**, 2nd ed., World Health Organization, Geneva, 1963.
(f) **European Standards for Drinking Water**, 2nd ed., Regional Office for Europe, World Health Organization, Copenhagen, 1970.

typically used for this purpose. In primary sewage treatment, raw sewage is screened to remove large objects and clumps of waste. Next, particulate matter is allowed to settle. Bacteria are then mixed with the sludge to **digest** it. The processed sludge is then released into the environment and the sediment is burned, buried, or sold as fertilizer. This process removes about 40% of the organic matter. In secondary sewage treatment, the partially decomposed sludge is filtered through several feet of gravel and sand, and chlorine is added to disinfect the now-liquid waste. Most of the organic matter has been removed by this time, and though many minerals remain and the water is unfit for drinking, it may be used for irrigation. In tertiary sewage treatment, the excess minerals are removed and the water is purified to levels acceptable for human use. Unfortunately, few cities provide all three treatments (see Table 4.15). Less than 30% of all Canadian municipalities provide even primary treatment, while the remainder dump raw sewage directly into the fresh-water rivers and streams! The obstacle to providing better treatment that usually is claimed is the high cost of constructing the treatment facilities.

Pollution problems may also be reduced by more specific control on the offending industries. Hot water pollution, for instance, may be reduced by insisting on the use of cooling towers or ponds, by selecting appropriate sites for plant construction, and by improving plant efficiency.

Strong legislation with strict law enforcement and heavy fines could reduce contamination from industrial waste, agricultural waste, and oil spillage. Improvement also would result from an increased emphasis on the reuse of water, the use of upstream land, restoration of land, land treatment, forest replenishment, topsoil conservation, and the conversion of sea water to drinking water. Sewage from watercraft can be eliminated by trapping it in holding tanks and disposing of it ashore. In Canada's inland waterways, such as the St. Lawrence Seaway, laws concerning the disposal of this sewage already exist.

Table 4.15. Treatment of municipal sewage in Canada.

a. within regions

Region	% of population served by sewers	None	% of population served by a given treatment Primary or Septic Tank	Lagoon	Secondary
Canada	39.6	41.2	20.7	7.9	30.2
Maritimes	30.8	89.9	3.5	3.4	3.3
Quebec	12.0	91.5	6.2	0.4	1.9
Ontario	40.2	6.3	30.6	4.1	59.0
Prairies	69.6	8.9	23.8	29.2	38.0
West Coast	71.0	46.3	29.8	12.8	11.0

b. within major urban areas

Urban Area	Population (1,000's)	% served by Treatment Facilities	% waste Water Treated	Type of Treatment
Toronto	1,800	100%	100%	Secondary
Montreal	2,436	8.4%	8.4%	Primary 2.6% Secondary 5.8%
Vancouver	940	37.0%	41.0%	Primary
Ottawa (not including Hull)	300	100%	100%	Primary
Edmonton	430	98.0%	100%	Primary 46.5% Secondary 53.5%
Hamilton	300	100%	100%	Primary
Quebec	300	NIL	NIL	None
Calgary	370	98.5%	100%	Primary
Winnipeg	520	96.0%	100%	Primary

Source: **Environmental Management**, J.W. MacNeill, Information Canada, 1981.

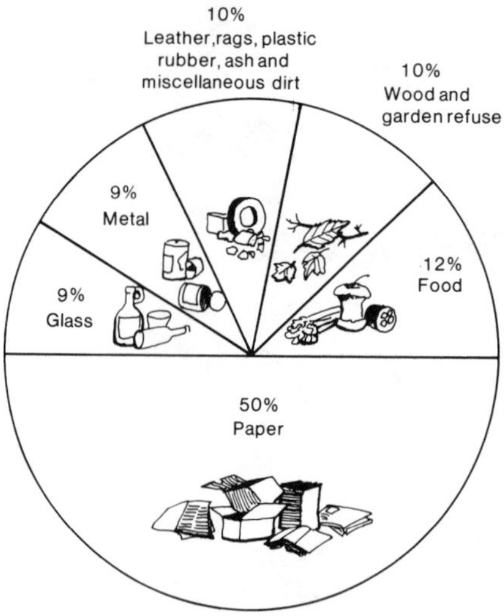

Figure 4.10. Composition of municipal waste. Much of the material we throw away can be recycled or reclaimed—if the price is right. "Consume less, recycle the rest" is a formula that could solve many of our waste disposal problems.

(Pie chart labels:)
10% Leather, rags, plastic rubber, ash and miscellaneous dirt
10% Wood and garden refuse
9% Metal
12% Food
9% Glass
50% Paper

4.3 LAND POLLUTION

Solid wastes produced by the household and industry amount to approximately four to five pounds per person each day. As cities grow it becomes more and more difficult to find out-of-the-way places to dump solid wastes. The amount of waste has increased in recent years and new products are presenting different disposal problems.

4.3.1 Sources of Land Pollution

There are three basic sources of land pollution: agricultural waste; industrial waste; and residential, commercial, and institutional waste.

Agricultural waste, the largest amount of solid waste, consists of manure, dead animals, and non-edible portions of plant crops.

Industrial waste includes all the waste products of manufacturing, particularly chemicals, mine tailings, and demolition debris.

Residential, commercial, and institutional waste consists of containers, paper, large appliances, and sewage (see Figure 4.10).

No matter what the source, waste is either **organic and biodegradable** (i.e., food, paper products, manure, sewage), **inorganic** (non-biodegradable), **organic and combustible** (such as rubber and plastic containers), or inorganic and non-combustible (i.e., cans, metal, appliances, bricks, and cement).

4.3.2 Health Effects from Solid Wastes

As raw, untreated garbage accumulates and rots, rodents, flies, and mosquitoes are attracted to the area and begin to multiply. These populations are potential carriers of communicable diseases. Open dumps may ignite spontaneously, and the resulting fires produce noxious odors and smoke. In addition, waste may leach through the ground and contaminate the water supply. Unsafe chemical waste disposal (i.e., radioactive material, PCB's, and heavy metals) are potential health hazards to humans. The incineration of such wastes also causes air pollution.

4.3.3 Control of Land Pollution

Resolving the land pollution problem requires a cooperative effort on the part of government and private citizens. A variety of approaches is needed to reverse the trend and protect the nation's land from further contamination. The first step is the salvaging and recycling of solid waste. Unfortunately, salvage work and recycling plants often are not profitable. Incentives are needed to encourage proper disposal of solid wastes that can be burned, buried, flushed, re-used, or just thrown away. Air, land, and water pollution are increased by burning, burying, and flushing, but economic pressures have almost eliminated the re-use of solid wastes. Thus, the worst method, merely throwing solid wastes away remains the most common.

Better designed incinerators can reduce air pollution from solid wastes. Also, manufacturers also should produce items (such as cans) capable of being re-used or recycled, or biodegradable containers.

4.4 PESTICIDES AND RELATED COMPOUNDS

Pesticide: A pesticide is defined as any substance capabable of killing or limiting the growth of insects, rodents, and other pests (Edlin and Golanty, 1988).

Insects and other pests can do a great deal of harm to humans, animals, and plants. Most of this harm is from damage to food supplies and agricultural products; the remainder is from transmitting communicable diseases. The development of pesticides has done much to ease this situation. They have greatly increased the quantity of our food and reduced the extent of malaria world-wide.

Over 900 basic chemical compounds are now used in commercial pesticides. The public usually identifies pesticide chemicals by their trade names such as Aldrin, Dieldrin, Endrin, Malathion, and Parathion. Most of these are chlorinated hydrocarbons. The best known is DDT (dichlorodiphenyltrichloroethylene). Billions of pounds of DDT have been used in the last 20 years to kill insects. Although its use has been

*No tolerance limits for PCB's have been
set in human food supplies, and their
cancer-causing properties remain undetermined.*

beneficial to agriculture, it also has created serious environmental and health problems. Consequently, DDT was banned from use in Canada and the United States a few years ago.

Recently, another class of chlorinated hydrocarbons, polychlorinated biphenyls (PCB's), also have been found to be serious pollutants. These chemicals show up in the milk of nursing mothers. They are highly toxic to humans when inhaled as vapors. No tolerance limits for PCB's have been set in human food supplies, and their cancer-causing properties remain undetermined.

4.4.1 Harmful Effects of Pesticides

For several years, only the positive effects of these chemicals were recognized until health problems began to develop in areas of heavy use. Recently, greater understanding and concern has developed regarding pesticides. Their harmful effects on human and other living organisms are summarized below:

- Destruction of beneficial insects (parasites, which feed on harmful bacteria, honeybees)
- Outright killing of birds, fish, and other wild animals
- Interference with the reproductive processes of birds, fish, and other wild life (i.e., preventing eggshells from hardening)
- Inhibition of photosynthesis in plants
- Concentration in fish to unsafe levels for human consumption
- Induction of new pesticide-resistant pests
- Increasing solubility in fats and oils, for example. That is, they easily mix and accumulate in fatty tissues in the body
- Presence in cow's milk, human milk, drinking water, fruits, and vegetables in very low concentrations. Greater amounts are present in meat, fish, and eggs—sometimes at levels above the legal tolerance for human consumption
- Contribution to birth defects in animals and people

- Production of sterility in humans
- Impairment of health in people who work with pesticides
- Cause of illness and death of laborers in recently treated crop areas
- DDT is a suspected carcinogen (cancer-inducing substance) in humans (incidence of increasing liver cancer in mice has been shown). Exposure to chlorinated hydrocarbons (e.g., DDT or PCB's) may cause changes in the central nervous system, inhibition of some enzymatic activities, and developing sterility in humans. Remaining unanswered is the long-term effect of human exposure to low concentrations of pesticides and the extent of the latter's biological accumulation in the human system.

4.4.2 Alternative Methods for Pest Management

A variety of new techniques for pest control are under study. Some of these are listed below.

- The use of certain lights, sounds, or odours to lure insects into traps or to confuse the mating process;
- Insect sterilization with radiation or chemicals;
- The use of predatory insects or parasites to control some insects;
- The spread of certain bacteria on crops to kill insects without leaving residues toxic to other forms of life;
- Development of pest-resistant crop varieties,; and
- Cultural practices (rotating crops, timing, planting, and harvests to escape insect attack).

   While these alternatives appear promising at present, they can only augment, not replace, chemical insecticides.

4.5 HEAVY METAL POLLUTION

Lead, mercury, cadmium, nickel, manganese, arsenic, and beryllium constitute a group of elements, known as heavy metals, commonly contained in the waste effluents of industrial processes. They are increasingly polluting the air, land, rivers, and seas of the environment. These

The developing embryo and the young child are particularly susceptible to injury from heavy metal pollution because they are in a rapid phase of developing their tissues and organ systems.

wastes are taken up by plants and animals lower in the food chain and many finally may be ingested by humans. Mercury-containing waste, for example, has frequently been dumped in the sea. There, it is taken up by microorganisms concentrating, even converting, it into compounds more toxic. Microorganisms in turn are eaten by higher organisms until the toxic compound invades and concentrates in human tissue, where it has pronounced detrimental effects. Mercury poisoning causes symptoms of muscle weakness and lack of co-ordination; advanced stages cause intermittent paralysis, increasing deafness and blindness, and pronounced mental retardation.

Lead, in addition, is an important airborne contaminant. It is given out in the exhaust fumes of cars burning lead-added gas. If it deposits on ground used for agriculture, it may enter the body through the food chain or else it may be directly ingested from the air. The body is not able to excrete lead and it accumulates there. High levels cause widespread damage by disrupting the structural protein materials of tissues and enzymes systems. The blood of an average adult living in a big city contains 100 times the normal (.25 micrograms (mcg)) background amount of lead.

The developing embryo and the young child are particularly susceptible to injury from heavy metal pollution because they are in a rapid phase of developing their tissues and organ systems.

4.6 RADIATION

Radiation is defined as the emission of energy caused by the splitting of an atom.

Radiation is an insidious pollutant; it cannot be identified by human senses. In other words, you cannot see, feel, taste, or smell it. However, the effects of radiation may be seen and are very serious even though they are not well understood by the general public. These effects may become apparent years later in the form of cancer or birth defects.

4.6.1 Sources of Radiation Exposure

NATURAL BACKGROUND RADIATION

We all live in what has been called a **sea of natural radiation**. This radiation comes from cosmic rays, radioactive substances in the earth's crust, and other radioactive agents in the atmosphere, resulting from sun-flares, which give off **solar particle beams**. Natural radiation amounts to an average of 0.08 to 0.15 rad per person per year (**the rad** is the measure for doses of ionizing radiation).

MAN MADE RADIATION

Exposure to radiation that is considered **man-made** can be classified according to its three main sources which are described below.

1. **Medical and Dental Uses.** Over 90% of the artificial radiation to which we are exposed is attributed to the medical and dental uses of x-rays for diagnosis and therapy. Medical radiation exposures today may be causing between 3,000 and 30,000 unnecessary deaths annual-ly in the U.S. alone!

2. **Fallout from Nuclear Weapons.** Up to 3% of all the man-made radiation exposure today is fallout from the testing of nuclear weapons in the atmosphere. As you probably are aware, the potential for this source of exposure to very suddenly change, from this small percentage to catastrophic levels, is uncomfortably real. This chapter has not the scope to address fully the problems associated with this but rather will discuss briefly the ways in which radiation, at its present levels in our environment, does affect human health.

3. **Nuclear Reactors.** A potentially important source of radiation ex-posure is the use of nuclear reactors to provide electric power. Nuclear power can result in the release of radioactivity into the environment in a number of ways. These include the mining and processing of the fuel, the operation itself, the transportation and reprocessing of spent

fuel elements, and the storage of long-lived radioactive wastes. In addition, there always is the possibility that an accident at a nuclear plant will release large quantities of radioactivity. On March 28, 1979, at Three Mile Island, Pennsylvannia, a nuclear accident occurred that has greatly affected the attitude of the public toward development and use of nuclear power. People have begun to realize that the potential for large scale destruction is very real if similar accidents occur again. Now the Chernobyl Power Station in the Soviet Union lies buried beneath tons of sand, lead, clay, and boron to contain the radiation set free when its number 4 reactor blew up on April 26th, 1986. Between the 26th of April and the 6th of May, 1986 it is estimated that some 50 million curies of radioactivity were released into the environment. Doses greater than 100 rads were suffered by several plant personnel and firefighters. In all, some 135,000 people within a 20 mile radius of the reactor may have been affected. Follow-up studies on radiation effects over many years, in 45,000 of the most heavily exposed, may be cause for an international research collaboration on a topic that is of vital concern to the whole world. Despite these catastrophies, nuclear power development is unlikely to cease. Mr. V. Legasov, leader of the Soviet delegation to the International Atomic Energy Agency (IAEA), spoke in Vienna in August, 1986. Discussing Chernobyl, he indicated to the meeting that the economic case for proceeding with further development was **absolutely compelling**. Dr. Hans Blix, the IAEA's Director General agreed, indicating that the production of power from atomic energy has passed the point of no return.

4.6.2 Effects of Radiation

Ionizing radiation causes **mutations**. Mutations are random changes in the structure of DNA, the long molecule that contains the coded genetic information necessary for the development and functioning of all organisms, including humans. A mutation in a gene can cause birth defects.

When a mutation occurs in the reproductive cells,
it may be passed on to future generations.

When a mutation occurs in the reproductive cells, it may be passed on to future generations. When a significant amount of radiation comes into contact with general body tissues, the individual may be severely damaged and may even die. Such consequences include cancer and the shortening of lifespan, irrespective of cause of death.

It is clear that individuals differ in their susceptibility to radiation. The kind of radiation, dose, and length of exposure also make a difference. If the doses are small and infrequent, the body can replace radiation-damaged cells. The chances of serious damage increase as the doses become more concentrated, but also, radiation damage is not always immediate. Between 1955 and 1969, children who survived the bombings of Hiroshima and Nagasaki were found to have seven times the normal incidence of cancer (this was discovered 10-15 years after exposure). Similar results have been found with American GI's who were exposed to high doses of radiation during nuclear bomb tests in the 1950's.

4.6.3 The Risks of Ionizing Radiation
The dangers and long-term effects of radiation are not yet fully understood. However, we do know that atomic accidents do happen. Aircraft carrying atomic weapons can, and have, crashed. Nuclear power plants can, and do, catch fire or leak radioactive material. Waste from nuclear power plants may stay radioactive for millions of years. Nuclear wastes are stored either in underground steel tanks or in sealed vaults and dumped at sea. Recent research shows that up to 25% of these containers have leaked! Many alternative disposal methods have been proposed for radioactive wastes, but so far there is no safe and economical technology for their effective disposal.

4.7 NOISE POLLUTION
In the context of environmental stressors, **noise is a meaningless, unwanted and irregular sound.** It is a by-product of human activ-

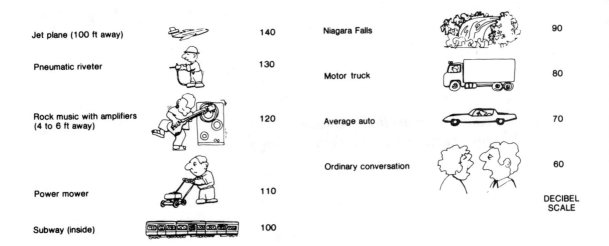

Jet plane (100 ft away)		140
Pneumatic riveter		130
Rock music with amplifiers (4 to 6 ft away)		120
Power mower		110
Subway (inside)		100
Niagara Falls		90
Motor truck		80
Average auto		70
Ordinary conversation		60

DECIBEL SCALE

Figure 4.11. Common sounds and their decibel ratings.

ity. At some point sounds become a nuisance or a distraction, and we are faced with them as a problem of **noise**. Modern living has intensified noise pollution. In the street, in our homes, and on the job, the noise of daily living can be frustrating and harmful to our well-being. In fact, the average volume of sound in our environment is doubling every 10 years. At this rate, we are fast approaching the point at which more noise will be intolerable to the human auditory system.

The intensity of sound is measured in decibels. **One decibel (dB) is the smallest difference in sound intensity detectable by the human ear.** Common sounds range from a whisper (30 dB) to the roar of a jet plane (135-150 dB), with normal conversational tones at a middle range of 60 dB. Sounds below 85 dB are generally considered safe. Unfortunately, many of the sounds we hear every day are much louder (Figure 4.11).

4.7.1 Sources of Noise Pollution

1. **Transportation:** The noise of automobiles, trucks, trains, motorcycles, buses, and airplanes is a common nuisance. Heavy traffic conditions do produce dangerous noise levels, often 90 dB and more.
2. **Construction:** The sounds of engines and equipment being used in construction and demolition are another source of stress producing noise. Intense sounds produced by a pneumatic hammer (108 dB), a rivet gun (110 dB), and a drop hammer (130 dB) can be very hazardous, particularly when workers are exposed to them for prolonged periods. Construction workers themselves indeed suffer the most from this hazard.
3. **Household Appliances:** Dishwashers, blenders, vacuum cleaners, air conditioners, stereos, and television sets are among household noise makers. The kitchen is likely to be the noisiest room in the house. Even a small device such as a food blender may operate at 93 dB, which is above safe levels. A power lawn mower operates at 96 dB and may expose neighbours to intolerable levels of noise.

4. **Industry:** The machinery of many industries is extremely noisy, and in many cases employees must work long hours in noisy environments. For this reason, particularly, deafness is considered an occupational hazard in some kinds of work.

4.7.2 Harmful Effects of Noise

We are so accustomed to noise in our environment that most of us have become insensitive to the damage our bodies may be inccurring from it. However, the effects on human health are real and, in the long term, may be very serious. Here is a list of some of the known health effects of noise:

• hearing loss and deafness over long periods of exposure;
• rise in blood cholesterol;
• rise in blood pressure;
• constriction of blood vessels;
• dilation of pupils of the eyes;
• unnatural rhythm of brain waves;
• prevention of healthful, deep sleep and relaxation;
• psychological symptoms such as irritability, fatigue, tension, and nervous exhaustion;
• accelerated heart rate.

4.7.3 Control of Noise Pollution

Much of the noise made by machinery and human activity, generally, is considered a necessary, if unfortunate, by-product of our activities. However, something can and should be done to control it. A few suggestions are offered below. *Can you think of others?*

• Changing the design and construction of engines and other machines;
• Sound-proofing to confine noise to acceptable areas;
• Wearing protective devices for the ears;
• Introducing laws to control noise, particularly in situations where workers must be exposed to high levels of noise over prolonged periods.

*Refusal to purchase from the known polluters
in industry could bring about mass
changes in manufacturing.*

4.8 GOALS FOR THE FUTURE ENVIRONMENT

Present efforts must be greatly increased if pollution is to be eliminated or even controlled. A complete appraisal of the present extent of pollution is urgently needed to give direction to future efforts. To accomplish this goal, better instruments of pollutant measurement and better research techniques must be developed and used. More information must be amassed on the nature of the pollutants themselves, their interactions, and their immediate and long-term health effects. Research is needed to develop methods of dealing both with man-made pollutants now in existence and with those that will appear with new technology. *What can you, as an individual, do to help preserve environmental quality?*

4.8.1 A Plan to Stop Pollution

In spite of the rapid growth of pollution in our environment accompanying the advance of technology, some progress is being made. Important legislation has been passed to establish and maintain national air and water quality standards. At present, more vigorous enforcement of the law is needed and efforts from individuals must gain momentum. A suggested plan for each of us to contribute positively in the fight to stop pollution may be summarized as follows:

1. **Study the problem.** Learn the local rules and regulations of air, water, and land pollution. This chapter is a good beginning!
2. **Call the problem to the attention of the proper authorities.** Contact the community newspaper, city editor, local conservation group, and city hall. Make your feelings regarding environmental quality known to your elected representatives—one letter can make a difference.
3. **Exercise your voting rights.** Vote for candidates who are known to be concerned with environmental quality.
4. **Consider taking legal action.** Identify a site of pollution and submit some supporting documents such as photos or letters from a local conservation officer, along with a statement to a consumer group or authorities who can pursue legal steps effectively.

5. **Exercise your consumer power.** Refusal to purchase from the known polluters in industry could bring about mass changes in manufacturing. Improved product design, forced on manufacturers by consumers, would eventually eliminate all non-recyclable and non-biodegradable packaging.

6. **Minimize your contribution to air pollution.** Automobiles are major sources of air pollution and consumers of energy. You might:

   a) select a small model when purchasing an automobile;

   b) keep your car tuned and in good repair;

   c) use other means of transportation for short distances, such as walking, bicycling, or public transportation systems.

7. **Minimize** your use of pesticides on lawns and gardens.

8. **Conserve** energy by every possible means.

4.9 REFERENCES

Air Pollution in Canada. Air Control Directorate, Environment Canada, Ottawa, 1973.

Brown, L.R. et al. **State of the World.** New York: Norton, 1984.

Canadian Drinking Water Standards & Objectives—1968, Department of National Health and Welfare, Ottawa, October, 1969.

Chiras, Daniel, D. **Environmental Science: A Framework for Decision Making.** Menlo Park, CA: Addison-Wesley, 1985.

Committee on Indoor Pollutants, Board of Toxicology and Environmental Health Hazards, Assembly of Life Sciences, New York: National Academy Press. p. ix-40, 1981.

Drinking Water Standards. U.S. Public Health Service, 1962.

Edlin, G. and Golanty, E. **Health and Wellness,** 3rd ed. Jones and Bartlett Publishers, 1988.

Ehrlich, P.R. **The Science of Ecology.** New York: MacMillan, 1987.

Ehrlich, P.R. and Ehrlich, A.H. **Population, Resources, and Environment: Issues in Human Ecology** (2nd ed.). W.H. Freeman Co., 1972.

European Standards for Drinking Water (2nd ed.). Regional Office for Europe, World Health Organization, Copenhagen, 1970.

Indoor Pollutants. Committee on Indoor Pollutants, Board of Toxicology and Environmental Health Hazards, Assembly of Life Sciences, National Academy Press, p. IX-40, 1981.

Interim Drinking Water Standards, Federal Register, Dec. 1975.

International Standards for Drinking Water (2nd ed.). World Health Organization, Geneva, 1963.

National Air Pollution Control Administration, Department of Health and Human Services, DHHS Publication, Washington, D.C.: U.S. Government Printing Office, 1982.

MacNeill, J.W. **Environmental Management,** Information Canada.

Manual for Evaluating Public Drinking Water Supplies. U.S. Public Health Service, 1969.

Murphy, E.M. The Environment to Come: A Global Survey. Washington, D.C. Pop. Reference Bureau, 1983.

Miller, C.D. **Health, The Science of Human Adaptation,** 2nd ed. Dubuque, Iowa: W.C. Brown, 1979.

Robinson, E. and Robbins, R. Emissions Concentrations and Fate of Gaseous Atmospheric Pollutants. In Air Pollution Control Part II, W. Strauss (ed.). New York. Wiley Inter-Science, 1972.

Ross, R.D. (ed.). **Air Pollution and Industry.** Litton Educational Publishing, Inc., 1972.

Stern, S.C. (ed.). **Air Pollution** (2nd ed.). New York: Academic Press, 1968.

U.S. Department of Health and Human Services: National Air Pollution Central Administration, 1982.

Williamson, S.J. **Air Pollution,** Reading, Mass: Addison-Wesley, 1973.

World Almanac. New York: Newspaper Enterprise Association Inc., 1986.

4.10 SUGGESTED READING LIST

Crossland, J. The Wastes Endure, **Archives of Environmental Health 19:** p. 9, 1977.

Dubos, Rene. Health and Environment, **American Lung Association Bulletin 59**: 10-12, 1973.

Ehrich, Paul R. **The Population Bomb**. New York: Ballantine Books, 1968.

Environmental Proctection Agency. **Health Effects of Environmental Pollution** (Washington, D.C.: The Environmental Protection Agency), p. 9, 1973.

Fators, EDPA Air Programs, U.S. E.P.A. Research Triangle Park, W.D., 1972.

Harrison, R.M. and D.P.H. Laxen. Natural Source of Tetraakyl-lead in Air, **Nature 275**: p. 738, 1978.

Holdgate, M.W. **A Prospective of Environmental Pollution**. Cambridge Univ. Press, 1979.

Lee, D. (ed.). **Metallic Contaminants and Human Health**. National Inst. of Env. Health Sciences.

Lesher, Delores C. and Bamberger, Audrey S. Experience at Three Mile Island, **American Journal of Nursing 79**: 1402-1408, 1979.

Linnemann, Roger, E. Medical Aspects of Power Generation, Present and Future, **Medical Research Engineering 13**: 1402-1408, 1979.

Norwood, Cristopher. **At Highest Risk**. New York: McGraw Hill Book Co., 1980.

U.S. Department of Health, Education and Welfare, DHEW Publication, Washington, D.C.: U.S. Government Printing Office, 1982.

U.S. Energy Research and Devel. Admin. **The Environmental Impact of Power Generation: Nuclear and Fossil**. 1975.

Waldbott, George L. **Health Effects of Air Pollutants**. St. Louis: C.V. Mosby Co., 1973.

Westone, Gregory S. The Need for a New Regulatory Approach, **Environment 22**: 9-14, 1980.

4.11 STUDY QUESTIONS

1. Describe the sources and health effects of the major kinds of air pollutants in large cities.
2. What are the major constituents of air pollution? What potential health effects are produced by each?
3. What causes indoor pollution? How is it different from outdoor pollution?
4. Explain how a herbicide sprayed in a forest could wind up in the breast milk of a woman living hundreds of miles away.
5. What are the health consequences of the extensive use of automobiles in North America?
6. Discuss the advantages and disadvantages of the use of nuclear power in energy generation.
7. Explain the concept of a healthful environment.
8. Give some examples of particulate matter. How do some of these pose hazards to the body?
9. Name some diseases that are associated with unclean drinking water. How many are still a threat to North Americans?
10. What would be the effect on food production if pesticides were banned? Is this a logical answer to this environmental problem?
11. What steps must be taken to preserve the environment from noise pollution?

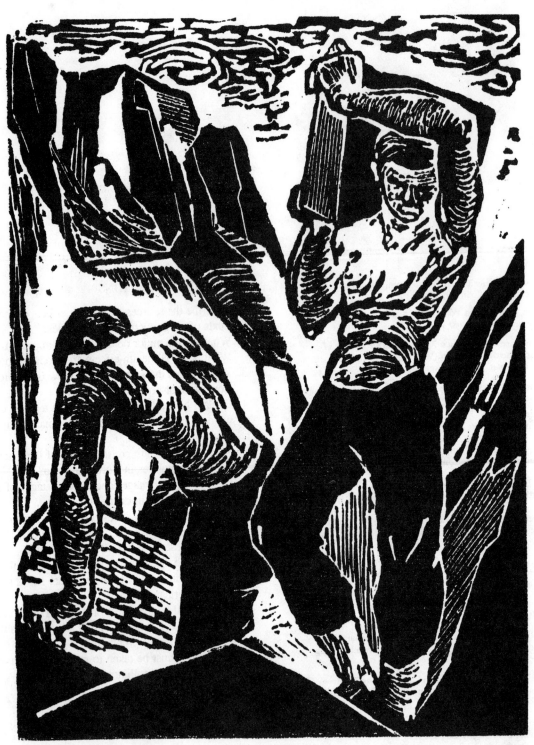

Ortizpaliente

5

Work and Health

Fit the job to the worker,
not the worker to the job.

OBJECTIVES

When you have completed this unit, you should be able to:

- **Define** and **discuss** the concepts of occupational health, industrial hygiene, human factors, and ergonomics.
- **Describe** the major sources of occupational stress and occupational diseases.
- **Discuss** occupational hazards in relation to working women.
- **Outline** the roles of workers, management, and the Workers' Compensation Board with respect to controlling hazards and providing a safe workplace.

KEY TERMS

airborne	intoxication
alveolitis	mesothelioma
biologic limit values	mutagen
chemical dusts	organic dust
chronic exposure	phenol
dermatitis	pneumoconioses
ergonomics	solvents
hyperthermia	teratogen
hypothermia	threshold value limits (TVLs)
industrial hygiene	time-weighted average concentration over 8 hours (TWA 8)

KEY CONCEPTS/DEFINITIONS

Here are some of the terms which you will need to be familiar with as you study this unit.

Occupational Health: Those work-related factors affecting workers' health, the resulting effects, and the programs for the promotion of health in the work place.

Safety: Freedom from hazards. Hazard management and accident prevention.

Table 5.1. Essential differences between occupational and community exposure to air contaminants.

Exposure Factor	Occupational Exposure	General Community Exposure
Exposure to toxic contaminants	Excessive	Not excessive
Proportion of population affected	Smaller number and selected groups only	Total population
Exposure schedule	Intermittent (8 hrs/day)	Continuous
Levels of toxic agents to which one may be exposed	High levels	Low levels
Variability over time	Low variability (confined)	High variability (temperature, wind velocity, moisture)
Controllability	Easy to control	Hard to control
Relative susceptibility of individuals	More susceptibility due to other stressors in work environment	Relatively less susceptibility
Locus of control of exposure	Voluntary exposure (employees accept risk)	Involuntary exposure

Occupational Disease: A disease peculiar to a particular industrial process, trade, or occupation and to which an employee is not ordinarily subjected or exposed outside of or away from his employment.

Industrial Hygiene: The science of recognition, evaluation, and control of occupational hazards.

Ergonomics/Human Factors: The design of a job or machine to fit human use ("human factored" design)—application of the concept, "fit the job to man, not man to the job."

5.0 INTRODUCTION

Risk is inherent in everything we do. But why are job risks especially crucial? Occupational health hazards contribute to a large number of deaths and injuries, particularly for those between 15 and 40 years of age. Each day millions of workers are fighting against the poisonous chemicals they work with and the working conditions that place serious mental and physical stress upon them. Work can be dangerous to the workers' health; nonetheless, it is still considered essential for maintaining a healthful mental, and physical state. Thus, it may be more helpful to make the work environment a healthier place than to make people work fewer hours, fewer days per year, or retire younger.

Occupational environments have been a major source of excessive exposure of people to toxic chemicals. While the populations exposed are much smaller than those exposed to contaminants in community air, drinking water, and foods, the **levels of exposure** are potentially much larger. The occupational environment is less variable in many ways than the community environment outside the factory walls, and the patterns of activity tend to be more routine. On the other hand, the proximity of air contaminants in some work environments can cause drastic changes in air contaminant concentrations to which workers are exposed. Workers also may be more susceptible to intoxication because of the stresses that result from maintaining tight work schedules and shift work that conflicts with normal circadian rhythms. Some of the essential differences between occupational exposure and general community exposure are outlined in Table 5.1.

*How do the harmful substances to which
industrial workers are exposed enter the body?*

5.1 OCCUPATIONAL EXPOSURE

One reason why it is sometimes hard to recognize an occupational disease is that the symptoms may come on so gradually that they are not noticed by the worker. This slow onset of symptoms is typical of a chronic disease resulting from long term exposure (i.e., 8 hours a day, 5 days a week for many years) to low levels of contaminants, sometimes known as **chronic exposure**. This is different from **acute exposure** which is an exposure to high levels of contaminants for a short period of time, causing an acute reaction. An acute reaction occurs immediately upon exposure, and may be severe.

5.1.1 Routes of Exposure

How do the harmful substances to which industrial workers are exposed enter the body? There are three major routes.

SKIN CONTACT

Skin contact is a common means of industrial poisoning or illness, which occurs when the body is directly exposed to toxic, that is, poisonous or harmful, substances. Some chemicals, like phenol, can penetrate the skin without being felt. Others can burn their way through the skin barrier. Sometimes a substance may react with proteins of the skin and cause an allergy. A chemical that passes through the skin can be absorbed directly into the blood stream and can be carried throughout the body, seriously damaging other organs.

INHALATION (through the respiratory tract)

This is the major route of occupational exposure. Poisons enter the body by being breathed in. Substances like chlorine and ammonia can cause local irritation of the airways and lungs. Other substances may not do their damage locally, but they may be absorbed from the lungs into the blood stream and may cause damage to other organs. Finally, insoluble substances tend to remain in the lungs for long periods of

After years of government neglect, a set of
occupational exposure limits has been
established by the American Conference of
Governmental Industrial Hygienists in the U.S.A.

time. There, they may cause serious local reactions either immediately or many years after the initial exposure. Among these substances are dusts like silica, asbestos, and Beryllium.

DIGESTION (through the mouth and digestive tract)
This is a less common route of entry for occupational toxicants than the respiratory tract or skin, but mouth contact with contaminated hands, foods, and cigarettes does occur and is very dangerous to workers who have been handling extremely toxic substances like lead, arsenic, and pesticides. Once swallowed, the substances enter the digestive tract where they are absorbed slowly and in small amounts into the blood stream. The toxic substance then goes directly to the liver, which attempts to change the substance chemically to make it harmless to the body. The liver does not always succeed, however, and in fact, it may be damaged by trying to handle too many toxic substances.

The level of exposure normally is determined by the **Time-Weighted Average Concentration** of the substance for a total of 8 hour periods (TWA 8 hours). This means its measured concentration in the body over 8 hours. This value then may be compared to the maximum permissible concentration for safe exposure, as determined by health and safety regulatory agencies.

5.1.2 Occupational Standards and Exposure Limits

After years of government neglect, a set of occupational exposure limits has been established by the American Conference of Governmental Industrial Hygienists in the United States (ACGIH). A list of recommended **Threshold Limit Values (TLVs)** was developed, which contained standards for more than 600 chemicals. Threshold Limit Values refer to airborne concentrations of substances. They represent conditions under which nearly all workers may be repeatedly exposed without adverse effect. The Threshold Limits Committee has annually updated and expanded its list of recommended TLVs. These lists were conceived as guidelines for professionals who understood their nature and limitations.

In the United States the first comprehensive federal health and safety act was established by the Occupational Safety and Health Administration (OSHA) in 1970. Under this act, the Secretary of Labor was directed to promulgate uniform federal standards. In comparison, Canada does not yet have federal occupational standards. The available exposure limits in Canada are only provincial levels; and they rely almost exclusively on the U.S. Standards for exposure limits to chemicals and physical hazards. Another set of useful criteria for determining the desired maximum extent of workers' exposure are **Biologic Limit Values (BLVs)**. These values represent the amount of substance to which a worker may be exposed without hazard to health or well-being, as determined by analysis of his or her tissues, fluids, or exhaled breath. Based on the concepts explained above, and those you will encounter in the rest of this unit, **five major Principles of Occupational Health** can be identified, as follows:

1. Work is dangerous to your health.
2. Paradoxically work is also essential to your health and happiness.
3. A good job is a human factored job.
4. Workers understand their work.
5. An optimal work environment is self-controlled.

5.2 OCCUPATIONAL HEALTH HAZARDS AND THEIR SOURCES

Take a look at the facts and figures listed on the following page relating to occupational health hazards. This will give you some idea of the levels these hazards have reached in our society.

For every death on the job there are
seven deaths due to job-related illness.

5.2.1 Records and Statistics

- More than 500,000 chemical products are known to exist; 3,000 are put into production each year; less than 500 have any occupational standards attached to them.
- For every death on the job there are seven deaths due to job-related illness.
- In the United States, at least 24,000 persons are killed each year while working. Of these, 10,000 die of diseases associated with their occupations.
- Asbestos workers have 7 times the expected rate of lung cancer and 1,000 times the expected rate of a rare lung cancer called "mesothelioma."
- Miners of soft coal have a death rate from respiratory disease that is five times that of the general population.
- Canada's occupational health and safety record is more than a little distressing (Long Range Planning Branch,1977; Chisholm, 1977):

  a) Incidence rates for fatal accidents in manufacturing and construction in Canada for the years 1972-1978, out of a total work force of some 9 million workers, were three to seven times higher than those in Great Britain.

  b) Work-related injuries and illnesses cost $4 billion annually, with 12 million workdays lost per year and compensation costs running at 1-15% of annual income.

  c) Workdays lost each year due to work-related injury and illness substantially exceed those lost due to strikes (Figure 5.6).

  d) Total incidence of cancer is 40,000 cases a year, from which 10,000 incidents are due to occupational exposure.

  In the same period out of a total work force of 88 million workers in the USA there were 8 million work-related injuries. These included 2.2 million bed-disabling injuries to workers. The resulting cost from accidents was estimated at $44 dollars **per day** and lost time due to acci-

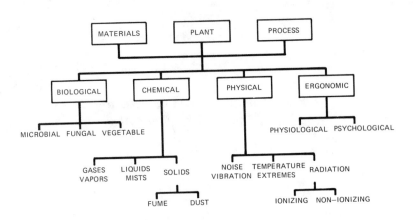

Figure 5.1. Occupational Health Hazards can be classified according to biological, chemical, physical or ergonomic sources.

dents was 2.45 million work days. Continuing rates of bed-disabling injuries in the USA are 1.8 million annually (National Safety Council, 1977).

Most of the above statistics are largely concerned with accidents and injuries, rather than occupational diseases that develop with long term exposure to noisy, dirty, hot, or cold working conditions. With these added into the picture, the hazards are major and widespread enough to demand that solutions be worked toward.

The various environmental stressors, which have been shown to cause sickness, impaired health, significant discomfort, or inefficiency in workers, may be classified as shown in Figure 5.1, according to chemical, physical, biological, or ergonomic factors.

5.2.2 Chemical Hazards

Chemical hazards arise from excessive air-borne concentrations of solvents (e.g., mists, vapours, gases), or solids that are in the form of dusts or fumes (Figure 5.2). In addition to the hazard of inhalation, many of these materials can act as skin irritants or may be toxic when absorbed through the skin.

The degree of risk in handling a given substance depends on the **magnitude** and **duration** of exposure, as well as the nature of the chemical itself. Many industrial materials, such as resins and polymers, are relatively inert and non-toxic under normal conditions of use, but when heated or machined, they may decompose to form highly toxic by-products.

Inhalation of some materials may irritate the upper respiratory tract or the terminal passages of the lungs and the air sacs, depending upon the solubility of the material. Contact of irritants with the skin may produce various kinds of dermatitis.

GASES

Excessive amounts of biologically inert (e.g., inorganic) gases, such as nitrogen and carbon dioxide, may dilute the atmospheric oxygen below

Table 5.2. Classification of lung diseases according to type of exposure.*

Type of Exposure	Disease or Disability
Inhalation of inorganic dust	Silicosis, Asbestosis Coal Miner Pneumoconiosis
Inhalation or organic dust	Farmer's Lung, Mushroom Worker's Lung Pigeon Breeder's Lung
Inhalation of dusts, fibers and toxic gases	Occupational Asthma
Inhalation of toxic gases, fumes and metals	Acute Chemical Pneumonitis Metal Fume Fever
Inhalation of dusts and gases while mining etc. (uranium, asbestos, coal tar, pitch volatiles, arsenic, nickel, chromates)	Occupational Pulmonary Neoplasms

*inherent predisposing factors include: smoking, atopy, alpha-1-antitrypsin deficiency.

the level required for normal body functioning. If the body's oxygen level falls to below the normal blood saturation value it disturbs cellular processes. Other gases and vapors (e.g., carbon monoxide and hydrogen cyanide) may prevent the blood from carrying oxygen to the tissues, thus producing chemical asphyxia. Some substances, such as certain organic solvents, may affect the central nervous system and brain.

SOLVENTS AND VAPOURS

Vapours enter the body by inhalation and skin absorption. When inhaled, they are absorbed through the lungs into the blood and are distributed mainly to tissues with a high content of fat and lipids, such as those of the central nervous system, liver, and bone marrow. Solvents include aliphatic and aromatic hydrocarbons, alcohols, aldehydes, ketones, chlorinated hydrocarbons, and carbon disulfide. Occupational exposure to solvents occurs through a variety of processes. These include the degreasing of metals in the machine industry; the extraction of fats and oils in the chemical and food industries; dry cleaning, painting, and processes in the plastic industry, including the viscose-rayon industry.

DUSTS

Dusts usually cause disease only in the lungs. Particle size in part determines its toxicity. Dusts may be classified into **chemical dusts** and inorganic minerals such as silica, quartz, coal dust, graphite, asbestos, fibrous glass and metallic dusts and fumes (beryllium and zinc); and **organic dust**, which may contain plant fibers (i.e., cotton fibers, wood dust) or fungi, bacteria, and their products. These act upon the lungs in a different manner from mineral dusts; the diseases they cause are frequently the result of allergic reactions. Table 5.2 shows typical diseases commonly associated with acute (short-term) and chronic (long term) inhalation of dusts, toxic gases and carcinogenic agents. A great deal remains to be learned about the real and potential dangers associated with exposure to such chemical contaminants as shown in Table 5.3. Many substances have been associated with cancers,

Chemical
  fumes
  dust and fibers
  mists
  vapours and gases
  liquids

Organic
  solvents
  hydrocarbons
  halogenated hydrocarbons
  cotton fibers
  pesticides
  methyl mercury

Inorganic
  metals
  acids
  alkalis
  CO
  SO_2
  NO_x
  asbestos
  glass fibers

Table 5.3 Types of chemical hazards found in the workplace.

Table 5.4. Examples of products suspected to be associated with various types of cancer.

Site of Cancer	Product or Occupation
Skin	• coal tar and derivatives (e.g., pitch, asphalt, soot, tar) • arsenic; sunlight; x-rays • petroleum oils and derivatives (e.g., tar, fuel oil, diesel oil, methylated napthalene)
Lungs and Respiratory System	• dust and fumes from asbestos, arsine gases, lubricating oils, arsenic, chromates (found in paints, wood processing, lithography), nickel, radioactive substances such as uranium, vinyl chloride, coke-ovens
Urinary Bladder	• benzidene and derivatives; beta-naphthylamine; rubber products
Liver	• production of vinyl chloride
Brain Tumors	• rubber; production of vinyl chloride
Blood-forming tissues (including leukemia)	• painters; radioactive substances (radiologists have a high incidence of leukemia), • benzol; rubber and rubber goods; paints, paint removers; rotogravure printing

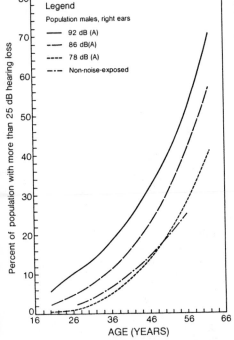

Figure 5.2. The percentage of industrial workers showing 25DB hearing loss. 6,835 workers from industries with various noise levels were examined and compared. Adapted and reproduced with permission from Stellman and Daum, **Work is dangerous to your health**, p. 117, 1973.

however, and although the data from current research must be interpreted with caution, the indications should not be ignored. Table 5.4 shows the tentative connections that have been made with respect to cancer and particular substances and occupations.

5.2.3 Physical Hazards
Problems relating to such things as noise, temperature extremes, ionizing radiation, and non-ionizing radiation are physical stresses. It is important that the employer, supervisor, and those responsible for safety and health be alert to these hazards because of the possible immediate or cumulative effects on the health of employees.

NOISE AND VIBRATION
Effects of Noise on Workers
When a sound wave hits the ear, it is transformed and translated to a nervous impulse. All parts of the ear are delicate. It may be injured easily through the noises of common everyday living. The modern industrial environment, however, often gives our ears more abuse than they can cope with. Besides the effects of noise on ears and hearing, other bodily functions are also affected by noise (see Chapter 4).

Because of the lack of control conditions in research, long-range studies of the sickness rate of workers in noisy industries do not indicate how much illness can be attributed to the effects of noise alone. There are always other factors: anxiety over danger from accidents, inadequate ventilation, vibration, hot working conditions, poor lighting, and so on. However, in one study that compared 1,005 German workers in a less noisy factory with a similar number in a more intensively noisy factory differences appeared as shown in Figure 5.2.

The graph indicates that workers in the noisier factory showed a higher percentage of hearing loss. Other data, collected in the Soviet Union (Andrukovich, 1966), show that workers in noisy heavy industry environments suffer from a higher than normal incidence of digestive and circulatory problems. These data also indicated higher proportions of psy-

Table 5.5. Examples of the negative effects of varying frequencies of vibration on particular areas of the body.

Frequency in cycles per sec	Part of Body Vibrated	Types of Effects
3	whole body	motion sickness
4-12	hips, shoulders, abdominal parts	damage to skeletal muscular systems, stomach problems
4-5	joints of the spine	damage to joints of back-bone
20-30	skull, whole body	loss of visual ability, permanent physical injury

Adapted and reproduced with permission from Stellman and Daum, **Work is dangerous to your health**, p.105, 1973.

chiatric difficulties and disturbances of the nervous system and metabolism. An Italian study showed deterioration of the digestive tract after one to two years of exposure to noise and vibration combined (Tarantola, 1960). In addition, noise interferes with communication between workers. This can create safety hazards such as the inability of workers to warn each other of imminent danger. It also limits their ability to discuss mutual work problems.

In North America many production plants do not even approach the legal standard for noise limits. **It is a sad commentary on any government that it should set a deleterious health standard that is so high that it almost guarantees eventual disability for its workers.** Insult is added to injury, though, when the same government is unable to supervise effectively enough to enforce even this inadequate set of standards!

How Vibration Affects the Body

Vibrations travel in the form of waves similar to those of sound and are transmitted to the body vertically through the feet or the hips when a person is standing or sitting on a vibrating surface. The frequency and duration of vibration are the most important factors which determine its effect on the body. Table 5.5 outlines possible effects of different frequency levels of vibration.

Workers who handle vibrating tools have been found to have four special problems:

- **Injury to the bone:** due to loss of calcium in the small bones of the wrists.
- **Injury to the soft tissue:** muscles, nerves, and connective tissue of the hands may be injured. This results in weakness in the hand.
- **Injury to the joints:** joints of the hands, wrists, and elbows may develop osteo-arthritis.
- **Injury to the circulation:** the mechanism controlling circulation in the fingers is damaged. This results in an occupational disease known as "White Fingers": The finger is white, and it is numb, except

Table 5.6. Estimated ideal temperatures for various types of work. (Relative Humidity=30-60% air velocity = 21 ft·min^{-1}.) Monotonous or repetitive work in each category is best done at temperatures a few degrees cooler than those listed.

Type of Work	Temperature
Clerical	65-72° F
Light but active industrial work	66-67° F
Heavier industrial work	55-65° F

Reproduced with permission from Stellman and Daum, **Work is Dangerous to Your Health,** p. 122, 1973.

for a tingling feeling. Movement of the finger is clumsy and painful. If circulation is severely impaired, the finger may turn blue from lack of oxygen, sometimes even resulting in gangrene. This injury occurs more frequently in workers who grip vibrating tools tightly. Many pneumatic tools have caused this type of injury, for example air hammers, compressed air chisels, compressed air drills, jack hammers, riveting guns, and stone cutting tools. People exposed regularly to vibrations become uneasy, fatigued, and irritable.

TEMPERATURE EXTREMES

The body is continuously producing heat through its metabolic processes. Since the body processes are designed to operate only within a very narrow range of temperature (around 73°F at 45% humidity), the body must dissipate this heat as rapidly as it is produced if it is to function efficiently. Relative humidity, or the amount of moisture in the air, affects the rate at which the body loses heat. A sensitive and rapidly acting set of temperature sensing devices in the body must also control the rate of its temperature-regulating processes. Table 5.6 gives some estimated comfortable temperature ranges for different levels of work activities.

Exposure of workers to high temperatures, as in mining, steel and glass manufacture, agriculture, and roadbuilding, can make workers uncomfortable, distressed, less efficient, and more careless than usual. This, in turn, means lower work quality as well as higher absence and lateness rates. The end result, of course, is decreased productivity.

Body Reactions to Temperature Extremes

Heat Stress (Hyperthermia)

Heat reactions depend on the extent and duration of exposure, the degree of activity, and the individual's own body response. Heat stroke, heat exhaustion, heat shock, fatigue, and stress are the most common heat disorders (see Figure 5.3). The body attempts to counteract the effects of high temperature by increasing the heart rate. The capillaries in the skin also dilate to bring more blood to the surface so that the rate of cooling is increased.

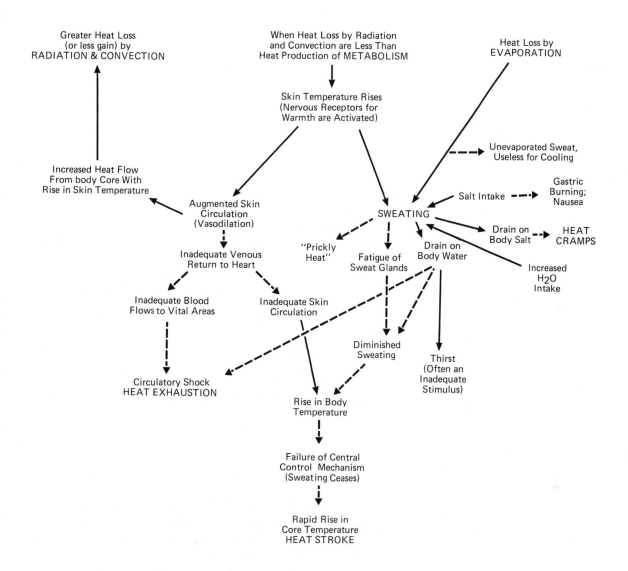

Figure 5.3. Human response to heat build-up. In Olishifski and McElroy, **Fundamentals of Industrial Hygiene,** 1979. Reproduced with permission from Department of H.E.W. Public Health Service Publication, 614.

*The healthiest light
is natural light.*

Cold Stress (Hypothermia)

Exposure to extreme cold results in local tissue damage (frostbite) and lowered body and brain temperatures, which leads to strange behaviour, unconsciousness, and coma. At a body temperature level of 64°F, the heart stops. Some research has shown that exposure to temperatures below freezing leads to chronic lung disease and sinus irritation. There is reason to believe that extreme cold may be one cause of arthritis but as yet there is no scientific proof of this fact.

General hypothermia is an acute problem resulting from prolonged cold exposure and heat loss. Use of appropriate clothing provides proper insulation to minimize heat loss, and a satisfactory microclimate may be maintained. Air movement is an important factor in a cold environment because of the combined effects of wind and temperature resulting in a condition called "windchill."

LIGHTING

Lighting the industrial environment provides the visibility of objects and the awareness of space that are needed to perform well. Advantages derived from good lighting include fewer mistakes, increased production, fewer accidents, improved morale, and better housekeeping. Visual tasks in industry vary in degree of difficulty depending on the size, the contrast (between detail and surround), the luminance of various objects, and the time available for completing each task (Off, 1973).

Considerations relating to the effects of improper lighting on the health of workers include the following:

- The healthiest light is natural light—full spectrum via windows.
- Fluorescent lighting should be placed on the sides, not in front of desks.
- Poor lighting causes eye strain, sore or swollen eyes, blurring of vision, headaches, fatigue, and stress.
- Lighting that is too bright causes glare.

*Exposure to non-ionizing radiation may
cause fatigue, headaches, palpitations,
faintness and sometimes memory loss.*

Proper lighting may be ensured by taking such measures as using spot, adjustable lights where good, natural light is not available and using matte (non-reflective surface) materials to minimize glare. At least 30-50 foot-candles of light are needed for proper office work conditions.

NON-IONIZING RADIATION

Interest in the public health aspects of the non-ionizing radiation has increased greatly in recent years due to the expanded production of electronic products, which use or emit this type of radiation. Examples of these are lasers, microwave ovens, **video display terminals (VDTs)**, infrared inspection equipment, and high-intensity light sources.

Non-ionizing radiation is that type of electromagnetic radiation that does not cause ionization in biological systems (photo energies less than 10-12 ev). This type of radiation will include ultraviolet (UV), visible, infrared (IR), microwaves (MW), radio frequencies (RF), and lasers.

It is believed that VDTs and microwave ovens may be a source of microwave radiation. Microwave radiation is absorbed by biological systems and ultimately dissipated in tissues as heat. The current American National Standards Institute sets an exposure limit of 10 milliwatts per square centimeter for exposure periods of 6 minutes or more.

Here are some of the hazards to health that are associated with non-ionizing radiation:

- Exposure to non-ionizing radiation may cause fatigue, headaches, palpitations, faintness, and sometimes memory loss.
- Microwave radiation may exert a cumulative effect on the lens of the eye, causing cataract damage.
- A possible relationship between mongolism in offspring and previous exposure of the male parent to radar has been suggested.
- Soviet investigators claim that microwave radiation produces a variety of effects on the central nervous system (CNS), with and without a rise in temperature in the organism.

The ergonomics approach goes beyond
productivity, health, and safety.
It includes consideration of the total
physiological and psychological demands
of the job upon the worker.

5.2.4 Ergonomic Hazards

The term "ergonomics" literally means the customs, habits, and laws of work. It is the application of human biological science in conjunction with the engineering sciences to achieve the optimum mutual adjustment of people to their work; the benefits being measured in terms of human comfort, efficiency, and well-being.

The ergonomics approach goes beyond productivity, health, and safety. It includes consideration of the total physiological and psychological demands of the job upon the worker.

Benefits that may be expected from designing work systems to minimize physical stress on workers include the following:
• more efficient operation
• fewer accidents
• lower cost of operation
• reduced training time
• more effective use of personnel

In our modern industrial environment, efficiency is a by-product of comfort. The enterprise that produces no sore backs, shoulders, wrists, and hips has a competitive advantage over one inducing discomfort in suffering workers. To ensure a high level of performance on a continuing basis work systems must be tailored to human capacities and limitations. How can this be achieved? First of all, the task should not require excessive muscular effort, considering the age, sex, and state of health of the worker. Secondly, the job should not be so easy that boredom and inattention lead to unnecessary errors, wasted material, and accidents.

Ergonomic stresses can impair the health and efficiency of the worker just as significantly as the other more commonly recognized environmental stresses.

MAN-MACHINE SYSTEMS

In modern society man is considered the monitoring link of a man-machine environment system. In any man-machine system, there are tasks that are better performed by man than by machine, and conversely, there are some tasks that are better handled by machines, as shown in Table 5.7. A man-machine system is an arrangement of a wide range of components that are interrelated and interact to perform some task or function. These components include machines, tools, materials, environmental factors, people, operating instructions, training manuals, or computer programs, and so on. A malfunction of any component will affect the other components, and thus degrade performance.

The question is how to achieve maximum efficiency of performance with minimum health hazards to workers? To achieve this, the system must be designed as a whole, with machines being complementary to human abilities, and vice-versa. The general physical and mental demands of the task should be designed within the expected capacity of the operator, and so reduce the load. Below are eleven Ergonomic Commandments which, if followed, will ensure a properly working man-machine environment system.

Ergonomic Commandments
1. Aim at movement (static is killing)
2. Optimize movement speeds
3. Avoid extreme movement or positions (unusual positions or movements)
4. Avoid overloading muscles
5. Avoid twisted or contorted postures
6. Vary the posture
7. Alternate sitting, standing, and walking
8. Use adjustable chairs
9. Let the small person reach, let the large person fit (General Motors designs automobiles for 90% of the population, excludes 10%)
10. Provide operational training
11. Provide optimal workload

Table 5.7. People versus machines: in an effective and efficient system the strengths of each compliment the other. Adapted and reproduced with permission from Olishifski, J., p. 425, 1971.

People Excel In	Machines Excel In
Detecting certain stimuli of low-energy levels	Monitoring (both people and machines)
Sensing an extremely wide variety of stimuli	Performing routine, repetitive, or very precise operations
Perceiving patterns and making generalizations about them	Responding very quickly to control signals
Detecting signals in high-noise levels with precision	Exerting great force, smoothly and evenly
Storing large amounts of information for long periods—and recalling relevant facts at appropriate moments	Storing and recalling large amounts of information in short time periods
Exercising judgment when events cannot be completely defined	Performing complex and rapid computation with high accuracy
Selecting own inputs	Sensitivity to stimuli beyond the range of human sensitivity (such as infrared, radio waves)
Improvising and adopting flexible procedures	Doing many different things simultaneously
Reacting to unexpected low-probability events	Reasoning deductively—from the general to the specific
Applying originality in solving problems, that is, coming up with alternative solutions	Being insensitive to extraneous factors
Profiting from experience and altering courses of action	Operating very rapidly, continuously, and precisely the same way over a long period
Performing fine manipulation, especially where misalignment appears unexpectedly	Operating in environments which are hostile to people or beyond human tolerance
Continuing to perform even when overloaded	
Reasoning inductively—specifics to generalities	

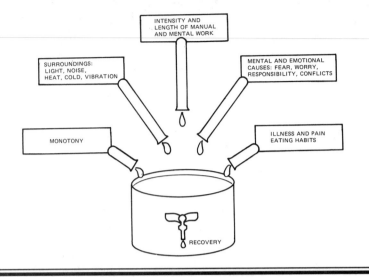

INTENSITY AND
LENGTH OF MANUAL
AND MENTAL WORK

SURROUNDINGS:
LIGHT, NOISE,
HEAT, COLD, VIBRATION

MENTAL AND EMOTIONAL
CAUSES: FEAR, WORRY,
RESPONSIBILITY, CONFLICTS

MONOTONY

ILLNESS AND PAIN
EATING HABITS

RECOVERY

Figure 5.4. Causes of fatigue. Adapted and reproduced with permission from Stellman, J.M. et al., **Work is Dangerous to Your Health,** 1973.

5.2.5 Occupational Stress: Psychological Hazards

Job stress is the biological response of the body to any demand upon it in the work environment. **Strain** is the abnormal reaction to stress. It can occur when the body has undergone prolonged periods of stress, or when one's resistance is down due to multiple stressors in the environment. Strain manifests itself in a variety of ways. The most serious are those cases where physiological damage has occurred, such as ulcers, arthritis, diabetes, or cardiovascular abnormalities. Fatigue is closely related to stress (stress is discussed in detail in Chapter 6).

Fatigue may be experienced in two general forms. Muscle fatigue is strictly physical and reflects an exhaustion of the chemical energy supply to the muscles. It is associated with a buildup of bodily waste products in the muscle tissue. General fatigue, on the other hand, is more a psychological experience, which leads to less willingness to work. This type of fatigue is due to the accumulation of individual stresses a worker faces during the day. Figure 5.5 shows the types of stresses that lead to fatigue.

Some of the factors contributing to job stress that are commonly identified are shown below.

- Physical working conditions: chemical exposure, noise, lighting, heat, including fluctuations.
- Organization: supervisory style.
- Workload: variations in workload, pace, production standards.
- Work hours: shiftwork, overtime.
- Work role: dealing with public, responsibility, job insecurity, office politics.
- The work itself: exposure to risk, quality expectations, complicated work, monotonous work.
- Career development: dead-end jobs, promotional opportunities.
- Extra-organizational: conflict between job and home responsibilities, problems of aging.

People react differently to stress at least externally, and it may be useful to use health evaluations to determine whether chronic stress reactions exist in their workforce. Health/medical examinations may reveal stress problems in people who otherwise appear healthy. Here are some other factors to think about:

- The *"be more tolerant"* reaction to problems of fellow workers may lead to fewer problems and less stress at work.
- The difficulty of problem-definition: for example, worker condition or working condition?
- Management's response when people report suffering from stress symptoms (Smith, 1979).

Once the cause of job stress has been identified, however, the final step in the process is to propose solutions. Some ways to eliminate stress include:

- re-design jobs
- rotate jobs
- improve training
- job transfer or trade
- change in shiftwork pattern
- physical conditioning program (fitness, see Chapter 9)
- professional services to help workers deal with stress and stress-related illnesses
- adjusted workloads
- promotional programs to increase motivation and morale
- early retirement options
- supervisory training, especially in interpersonal skills
- meditation/relaxation training for workers
- time management training

5.2.6 Accidents

Occupational accidents and related injuries are a major concern in overall work and health issues. Broken bones, lacerations, burns, sprains, and back and spinal problems can be caused by a poor system of work, defec-

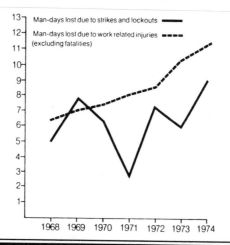

MAN-DAYS LOST: STRIKES VS INJURIES
Canadian figures in millions of man-days (18)

Man-days lost due to strikes and lockouts ━━━
Man-days lost due to work related injuries ▪▪▪▪
(excluding fatalities)

Figure 5.5. The continuing disparity between man-days lost to work related injuries relative to days lost from strikes and lockouts. Reproduced with permission from Long Range Health Planning Branch, Occupational Health in Canada—Current Status, Health and Welfare Canada, Ottawa, p. 123, 1977.

tive equipment, carelessness, and/or inattention of the employee or a fellow worker. Usually only one incident is needed to produce an injury. Thus, the source usually is identifiable and can be shown to be attributed to the work situation in many cases.

Millions of work hours are lost annually in Canada through physical injury at work due to accidents, which may range from the temporarily to the permanently disabling and often involving mutilation and death These figures may be applied proportionally to the work force of any industrialized country.

Obviously some workers are more susceptible to accidents than others, and many of the traditional female occupations are less risky than, for instance, construction or machine work. Hospitals are one kind of place where sprains, back strains, objects striking against people, falls, and scratches are plentiful, as are many factories where the work force is mostly women.

Most accidents are preventable when care is taken by the worker or the employer. Legislative bodies, management, unions, design engineers, workmen's compensation boards, medical personnel, and employees all make efforts to reduce accident rates. The whole subject of safety is well-documented, and statistics are available delineating factors according to occupation and time of day or week. In Canada, compensation for industrial accidents is available to victims or their families.

5.2.7 Biological Hazards

Harmful biological agents may be a part of the total environment or may be associated with certain occupations. Those agents found in the work environment include viruses, rickettsiae, bacteria, and parasites of various types. Many of them carry or cause disease. These diseases commonly are transmitted from animal to man. Infectious and parasitic diseases also may result from exposure to contaminated water or to insects. The following are two examples of occupational diseases caused by biological agents.

Legionnaire's Disease

This is a stressful allergic disease often contracted by office workers. It is caused by fungal or bacterial growth in humidifier systems or paper-based insulation.

Farmer's Lung

Farmer's Lung is a lung disease which is caused by dust from moldy hay. It is a hazard for agricultural workers and grain handlers.

5.3 OCCUPATIONAL DISEASES

A disease is considered occupational if:

- Medical findings are compatible with the effects of the agents to which the worker has been exposed.
- Existence of this agent in the occupational environment (past and present) is in sufficient amounts to cause disease.
- The weight of evidence supports the contention that the disease is occupational rather than of a non-occupational origin.

Occupational diseases affect all types of people in many walks of life—laborers, crafts workers, business people, and professionals. But the diseases are more common in blue-collar workers than in white-collar workers, and they are more common in small and medium sized businesses than in large concerns. Economists estimate the cost of occupational illnesses and injuries to be at least 1% of the gross national product (American Lung Association, 1979).

New evidence seems to reinforce the view that the prevalence of occupational diseases is underestimated. The National Institute for Occupational Safety and Health (NIOSH) found in a survey of a group of manufacturing industries that 28% of the 908 people examined had some occupational disease. Yet fewer than 10% of these cases had been recorded in official documents, as required by law. Put another way, more than 90% of diseases were unrecognized officially.

Table 5.8. Percentage of total industrial diseases reported by type (U.S.A.)

Percentage of Total Diseases Documented	Type of Industrial Disease
18%	skin irritation (dermatoses) (including skin cancer)
54%	respiratory conditions (lung and heart diseases, ergonomic problems)
28%	hearing loss

Most **occupational diseases** are chronic and untreatable. Their relationship to a particular occupation is often difficult to determine because the disease may not become apparent until as long as 20 years later. It is virtually impossible to keep track of former employees for such long periods, so records usually are unavailable. Moreover, not every worker is exposed to the same amount of the disease-causing agent, and the disease may be caused by the interactions of two or more agents. Thus, accurate records and sophisticated statistical analysis are required to determine many of these relationships. Because of these difficulties, countless occupational diseases may lie hidden for years until they surface.

5.3.1 Major Types of Industrial Diseases

LUNG DISEASES
Lung diseases account for more than half of all occupational deaths. Exposure to dusts, fumes, and gases can cause both acute and chronic diseases of the respiratory tract and lungs. Examples of these hazards are outlined below (refer also to Table 5.2, earlier in this Unit).
• Exposure to fumes in welding and smelting may cause **metal fume fever**. Irritant gases can cause acute bronchial irritation or even pneumonia. Miners, sandblasters, and asbestos workers exposed to coal dust, silica dust, and asbestos dust (asbestosis) commonly suffer from a chronic disease known as pneumoconioses.
• Dusts from moldy plant materials such as grain or wood may produce a disease of the lungs called alveolitis.
• Many adults suffer from a group of chronic lung disorders that have no single cause but that result in persistent air-flow obstruction. The term chronic obstructive pulmonary disease (COPD) is usually applied to chronic bronchitis, emphysema, and asthma, and their combination.
  It is important to note that asthma, chronic bronchitis and emphysema are not always caused by hazards in the workplace. In fact, chronic

The nervous system is delicately balanced,
and many of the conditions and
substances to which workers are exposed
can upset this balance.

bronchitis and emphysema most often result from cigarette smoking. This is why it is necessary to base judgements concerning occupational diseases on the evidence of each situation, rather than simply on the outcome e.g., the disease or symptoms).

SKIN DISEASES: "DERMATITIS"
There are almost an infinite number of substances that can cause skin irritation. Oils, solvents, and detergents are frequently responsible. Some substances cause **primary irritation** of the skin on contact, while others produce allergic reactions. Hands and forearms are most often affected from industrial exposure.

CANCER
There are a number of agents known to cause cancer, some of which are occupational. In most cases, where cancer is attributed to occupational hazards, an even more prolonged interval between the first exposure and development of the cancer (usually 20 years or more) is found. Cancer can be caused by physical agents, such as X-rays and ultra-violet light, as well as by chemical agents. Known cancer-provoking agents—**carcinogens**—include arsenic, asbestos, some chromate compounds, and tobacco smoke. Cancer is considered to be the prime industrial disease. A report by the World Health Organization stated that 90% of all cancers are environmentally related. About 20-40% of all cancer is considered to be work-related.

NEUROTOXIC DISORDERS
The nervous system is delicately balanced, and many of the conditions and substances to which workers are exposed can upset this balance. Noise, stress, and some chemicals (i.e., heavy metals and solvents) have direct effects on the nervous system (see Figure 5.1).

HEART DISEASE

There have been very few studies of the probable risk of contracting heart disease in different occupational groups. However, one study recently showed that rayon viscose workers who were exposed to carbon disulfide had a greater incidence of coronary heart disease than those who were not exposed (see Stellman et al., 1973, "Toxicology"). Some studies also suggest that occurrence of heart and blood vessel diseases is increased among workers exposed to high levels of noise.

Many lung disease victims also finally die from heart failure. When lung disease causes the blood to be low in oxygen, the heart tries to compensate by pumping harder at higher pressure. This causes the heart to become enlarged and eventually diseased (see Occupational Lung Diseases, American Lung Assoc., 1979).

5.4 WORK AND WOMEN'S HEALTH

All occupational health hazards are dangerous and can affect workers of both sexes. However, women now are being directly exposed to a greater number of occupational hazards than ever before. This is true for two reasons:

1. their numbers are increasing: women now comprise 38% of the work force; 9 out of 10 women now work outside the home at some time in their lives in the U.S.A.; and
2. they are aspiring toward a wider variety of occupations. Many of these occupations are, by their nature, deterimental or dangerous to health.

During this decade, increasing interest has been shown in issues concerning occupational health. However, problems of working women generally have been ignored in the research. Most of the research concentrates on male workers, and yet two-fifths of the work force is female.

There are a number of types of health hazards faced by modern working women. While many of these are shared equally by men, some differences also may be seen. For example, women in jobs which traditionally have been classified as male occupations, such as police officers or top executives, often must contend with resistance from co-workers and/or the public, in addition to the normal stresses of these jobs. This may lead to a greater risk of stress-related illness and/or danger for these women.

A second distinction between health hazards for women as opposed to men is apparent in occupations typically held only by women. These jobs, such as nursing, secretarial, or domestic work, carry their own hazards to health, which differ from those in other types of work. Finally, women workers in many occupations face hazards from agents or chemicals (i.e., radiation) which may affect fertility or reproductive functions.

In general, the physiological reactions of males and females to similar stressors or hazards are about the same. Most of the differences that are experienced may be classified in terms of differing sources of hazards or stress, rather than differences in people's reactions to the same hazard. There are two exceptions to this. One is that women, as mentioned above, can be affected in different and more serious ways than men, by radiation or other agents that affect reproductive functions (this is discussed separately below). The other exception relates to hazards, which exist or are exaggerated, because of physical forces exerted (such as in construction work, mining, etc.). In other words, some jobs simply are more dangerous or hazardous for those workers who have less physical strength than others. While some women in fact are physically stronger than some men, generally speaking this is not the case. Women tend to have less muscle mass and physical strength than men, and as a result they will face greater health hazards while doing certain kinds of work.

Occupational stress is one area where women are seen as more susceptible to illness than are men. Again, however, this is due to the

*Secretaries rate second highest in
the workforce as victims of
stress-related illnesses.*

fact that different types, amounts, and combinations of stressors are faced by female workers. One major determinant here is the fact that a great many working women maintain most or all of the responsibility for family and domestic concerns in addition to their jobs. A partial explanation for this is that about 60% of all women workers are single, divorced, separated, or widowed; and of course a large number of these women have children.

Secretaries rate second highest in the workforce as victims of stress-related illnesses. In one study, clerical workers who had children and were married to blue collar workers were found to have the highest risk of developing chronic heart disease.

5.4.1 Hazards to Pregnant Women and Fetuses

Many hazardous agents may reach an embryo or fetus after the mother's exposure to them through inhalation, digestion, or the skin. Most substances are in the mother's bloodstream may be transmitted to the embyro and fetus. Much remains to be discovered about the rate of transmission and the effects of such hazards at different stages of the pregnancy, but a particularly dangerous stage appears to be the first trimester of pregnancy.

It does not appear that the fetus and the newborn have developed the mechanisms to detoxify and excrete all poisonous materials. As a result, the mother may not show symptoms of being exposed to noxious substances but the fetus may be affected (Spyker, 1974).

It is nearly impossible to be conclusive with respect to such hazards. The fetus is exposed to numerous substances during its nine months of incubation, any number of which **may** be dangerous. The existence of some defects (such as mental retardation) may not be noticeable for a number of years after birth. This fact, coupled with serious inadequacies in reporting outcomes, which are exaggerated when the mothers do not return to work following childbirth, make accurate accounting extremely difficult to establish. Research has, however, established the causes

Table 5.9. Environmental agents known to cause damage to the fetus.

Causal Agent	Effect on Fetus
Anesthetic gases	Spontaneous abortion
Beryllium	Stillbirth
Carbon monoxide gases	Prematurity
Radiation, vinyl chloride	Carcinogenesis*
Estrogens and hormones	Mutagenesis**
Lead pentachlorophenol	Teratogenesis***

* **A carcinogen** is a cancer-causing agent. The fetus may be harmed when the agent crosses the placenta, but the effects may not be known for many years.
** **A mutagen** is an agent which can cause changes in the genetic material of living cells or in germ cells (sperm or egg). The result may be spontaneous miscarriage or the development of the fetus with genetic defects.
*** **A teratogen** is a substance which causes harm to the women. The result may be miscarriage or congenital defects.

of a number of dangers to the developing fetus and pregnant mothers. These are summarized in Table 5.9. Table 5.10 shows a number of potential risks to women from work in specific occupations.

5.5 SOCIOECONOMIC IMPLICATIONS

The social cost of occupational hazards is high, but the currently estimated monetary cost of eliminating every hazard is even higher. Some industries knowingly allow their employees to work in an environment that may produce chronic occupational diseases, simply because it is so expensive to improve working conditions. If prices have to be raised to pay for improvements, an industry may become less competitive; this is not a trivial concern for most companies!

Once a disease has been traced to occupational factors, the company is liable for the cost of treating the employees suffering with it. As a result, many owners of coal mines, for instance, refuse to recognize the relationship between black lung disease and coal mining; and owners of uranium mines refuse to recognize the significant correlation between high rates of lung cancer and the radioactivity in the mines. As a general rule, though, large companies are better able to afford safe working conditions than are smaller companies.

With respect to working women, the economic, legal, educational, political, and social forces concerning occupational health hazards faced by women are in a sort of equilibrium. To change one component means that the others must alter. If women are permitted to make their own choices about the hazards to which they subject themselves and their unborn children, then these choices must at least be educated ones. If persistent demands are made upon the legal system and compensation boards to recompense people retroactively, for damage done negligently to them before birth, then employers will be reluctant to hire women for fear of later legal suits, costing money and reputation. Furthermore, pressure upon employers to provide completely safe working conditions may result in fewer jobs being made available to women and men alike.

Table 5.10. Examples of female workers in various occupations who may be at risk.

Occupation	Risk/Hazard	Agents to which Workers may be Exposed
Nurses/first aides	Miscarriage Birth defects in children Infections	anesthetic gases, ozone, alcohols, viruses, soap, bacteria disinfectants, radiation
Office/clerical workers	Lung diseases Allergies Chronic headaches	ozone, dust, solvent ammonia, alcohol, radiation
Laundrers/dry cleaners	Skin diseases Carcinogenic/ Teratogenic effects	solvents, soaps, bleaches
Laboratory work toxic chemicals	Bone marrow damage Reproductive problems Liver damage Blood cell damage	radiation
Electrical/ electronic workers	Heart disease Fetus abnormalities, Lung disease	arsenic, mercury, asbestos, beryllium, solvents
Sawmill/plywood mill workers	Asthma Premature babies Allergies Teratogenesis Liver damage Cancer	wood dust, carbon monoxide, formaldehyde, pentacholorophenol, solvents, vinyl chloride
Farmers	Reproductive problems Cancer	pesticides
Teachers	Infections	bacteria and viruses
Hairdressers	Skin diseases Respiratory disease Cancer	hair tonics, detergents, nail polishes, dyes, hair spray

All of these factors combined paint a complicated picture. The problems from every perspective are real and serious ones. Solutions must be thought out carefully, in light of sound evidence concerning the hazards and societal and health priorities. Above all, both employers and employees must see themselves and hold themselves responsible for these issues.

5.6 RECOMMENDATIONS FOR CONTROL OF THE WORK ENVIRONMENT

In general, employers and employees alike should insist upon:
- Process control: familiarity with the contaminants, their sources, and their effects on health, and development of techniques to avoid contact with them.
- Use of protective equipment for eyes, nose, skin, and so forth where appropriate.
- Proper general ventilation, which guarantees the entry of adequate fresh air to dilute the contaminants to safety levels.
  a. Regular check up of ventilation performance
  b. Adequate exhaust ventilation
- The use of air cleaners to remove dusts, gases, and vapours.
- A cautious approach to using new chemicals in any manufacturing.

Employees must
- take initiative to become aware of health hazards,
- share their concerns,
- organize for solutions.

Employers/Manufacturers must have
- awareness of research on health hazards,
- fairness in response to health complaints,
- responsibility for minimizing health hazards in machine products,
- investment in development of machines that involve human factors, for example that reduce vibration, noise, radiation, and so forth.

5.7 REFERENCES

American Lung Association. **Occupational Lung Diseases: An Introduction**, 1979.

Anticaglia, J.R. & Cohen, A. **American Industrial Health Association Journal**, 1(3): 227, 1970.

Andrukovich, Gig. Tr. Prof. Zabol. Vol 9 (1965), p. 39. N.N. Shalalov, A.O. Sailanov, and K.V. Glotova. **Report T-411-R, N-65-155577** (Toronto, Canada: Defense Research Board, 1962) A.B. Strakhov. **Report N-67-11646** (Washington, D.C.: Joint Publications Research Service, 1966).

Chisholm, D. Occupational Health: A Priority and a Challenge. **Canadian Journal of Public Health, 68**: 189-191, 1977.

Epstein, Samuel, S. **The Politics of Cancer**. Garden City, New York: Anchor Press, 1979.

Geiser, Kenneth. Health Hazards in the Microelectronics Industry in International Journal of Health Services 16(1), 1986.

Long Range Planning Branch. **Occupational Health in Canada—Current Status Health and Welfare Canada,** Ottawa, 1977.

National Safety Council. **Accident Facts**, Chicago, Illinois, 1977.

NIOSH. **The Industrial Environment: Its Evaluation and Control**. Washington, D.C. U.S. Department of Health, Education & Welfare. National Institute for Occupational Safety and Health, 1974.

Off, John. Health and Light: Full Spectrum Lighting. Old Greenwich, Connecticut: Devon-Adair, 1973.

Safety Levels of Microwave Radiation With Respect to Personnel. Committee C95-1, U.S.A. Standards Institute. (now American National Standard Institute) New York, N.Y., 1966.

Sigler, A.T., Lilienfeld, A.M., Cohen, B.H., and Westlake, J.E. Radiation exposure in parents of children with Mongolism (Down's Syndrome). **John Hopkins Hospital Bulletin, 117(6)**: 374-399, Dec. 1965.

Smith, M. Recognizing and Coping with Job Stress Symposium for Worker Educators, October, 1979.

Spyker, J.M. Occupational hazards and the pregnant women. In: **Behavioral Toxicology Early Detection of Occupational Hazards**. Ximtaras, C. et al., (Eds.) U.S. Dept. of Health, Education and Welfare, Washington, D.C. 1974.

Stellman, J.M. and Daum, S.M. **Work is Dangerous to Your Health.** New York: Vintage Books, 1973.

Tarantola, A.; A. Grignari et al.,. **Lavoro Umano (Naples), 20(6)**: 245, 1960.

Tolgskaya, M.S. and Gordon, Z.V. **Trans. Institute of Labor Hygiene and Occupational Diseases of the Academy of Medical Science**, 99, 1960.

5.8 SUGGESTED READING LIST

Olishifski, J.B. and McElroy, F.E. (Eds.) **Fundamentals of Industrial Hygiene**, 2nd ed. Chicago: National Safety Council, 1979.

Patty, F.A. (Ed.) Industrial Hygiene and Toxicology, 2nd Edition, Vol. 2, **Toxicology**. New York: Interscience Publishers, 1973.

Rothman, H. **Murderous Providence: A Study of Pollution in Industrial Societies**. Indianapolis: Bobbs-Merrill Co., 1972.

Stellman, J.M. and Daum, S.M. **Work is Dangerous to Your Health.** New York: Vintage books, 1973.

U.S. Department of Health, Education and Welfare. **Occupational Diseases: A Guide to Their Recognition**. W.M. Gafafer, editor. Public Health Service Publication No. 1097, Washington, D.C.: Government Printing Office, 1966.

Worker's Compensation Board, 1981. **Regulatory Standards**. British Columbia, Canada.

5.9 STUDY QUESTIONS

1. What is ergonomics? Outline the contribution ergonomics can make to the quality of life.
2. Describe several chemical health hazards faced in various occupations. How might these hazards be avoided or controlled?
3. Discuss "carcinogens" in terms of the work place—what are they, what occupations are the most dangerous in this respect, and how can society, industry, and/or individuals effectively deal with them?
4. What is noise pollution? What kinds of physical problems have been shown to be related to excess noise in human environments?
5. Describe some of the potential hazards associated with non-ionizing radiation.
6. What is an "occupational disease"? Name at least three types of industrial disease which have been documented.
7. Name several substances known to be dangerous to unborn fetuses. What are the implications of this information for women in the workplace?
8. Discuss possible ways in which your own community and the industries in it can improve the health of its workers. What could you do personally to help achieve these ends?

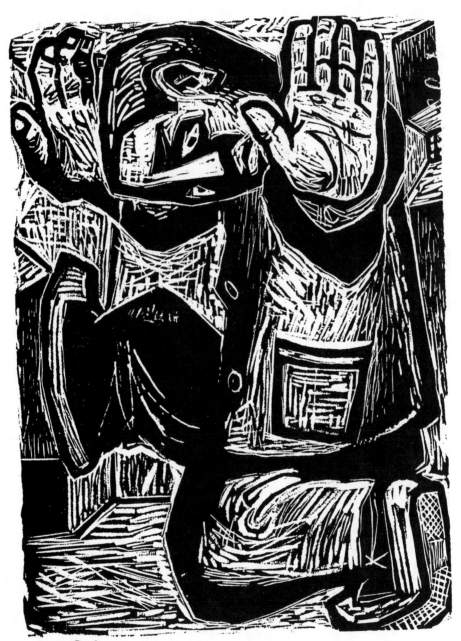

J.G.ORTEGA

6

Stress

For each of us, we must gauge our stress carefully
and know both when and how to retreat from the breaking point.

Table 6.2. Physical and chemical manifestations of the body's preparation to cope with stress.

- stored fats, and sugars mobilized for action
- breathing rate increased more than normal
- red blood cells (RBC's) mobilized
- heart rate is increased
- blood clotting mechanism is activated
- muscles tense and ready to act
- digestion ceases, all blood is needed by muscle for physical action
- perspiration is activated
- increased circulating hormones in blood, especially adrenaline for fight or flight

OBJECTIVES

When you have completed this chapter you should be able to:
- **Define** and **evaluate** stress as it occurs in everyday life
- **Understand** the physical and psychological responses associated with stress
- **Recognize** that stress can be healthy but where necessary can be changed
- **Explain** why too much stress is not good even though some stress is good
- **Discuss** stress management strategies
- **Describe** the General Adaptation Syndrome (GAS) and explain its consequences

Table 6.1.
Human correlates of stress.

Non-Stress
apathy
boredom
decline
illness
anxiety

Optimal Stress
vitality
awareness
stimulating activity

Excessive Stress
anxiety
illness
debilitation
degeneration
premature aging
aggression

KEY TERMS

adaptation	response
adrenaline	GAS
change	stress management
coping	type A behavior
fear	

6.0 INTRODUCTION

Stress is often an overused term. During the mid 40's when Hans Selye first studied this topic in relation to humans the word had greatest relevance in physics or engineering. It's application in describing human overload both physically and psychologically was just beginning.

Stress is the overall process that can lead to mental and physical dysfunction. One of the principle components of stress is the change in ourselves that is needed to adapt to new situations of either an acute or chronic nature. A little change induces only a little stress, a large change induces a great deal of stress.

Does this mean that our goal should be to eliminate all stress? If indeed we were unfortunate enough to succeed in this dubious effort of

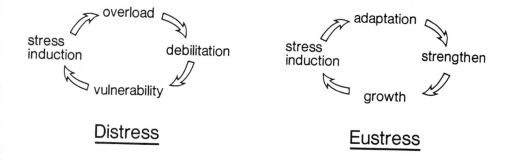

Distress   Eustress

Figure 6.1. Positive feedback effects of stress, defined by Selye, leading to distress (breakdown) or eustress (accommodation).

total stress elimination, the world would be a very dull place indeed, and might also lead to physical dysfunction as well (Table 6.1).

Stress is not often occasioned by change itself, but by the rate at which accommodation to it has to take place. There are of course individual limits in the adaptation to stress but life is full of change and therefore it is stressful in a greater or lesser degree to everyone, and we must all learn to cope with it.

Many individuals function at a very high level of stress, the variety and complexity of activity in their daily lives is very high and for them, the rewards of such stress can be very satisfying. Probably they did not reach this level of stress overnight, but rather built upon their stress levels one stage at a time. For each of us, we must gauge our stress carefully and know both when and how to retreat from the breaking point. Understanding stress, how to recognize it, measure it, cope with it and decide how much we will tolerate is a skill increasingly important for us to attain in order to reach our best potential in life.

Hans Selye (1974) showed us that certain definite physical illnesses could develop as a result of the body/mind's effort and failure to cope with stress. Table 6.2 shows some common physical and biochemical signs of stress. Stress, and the life changes that are associated with it, lead to an accelerated rate of wear and tear upon the body to which it either succumbs or accommodates (Figure 6.1).

6.1 SELF-EVALUATION

6.1.1 Stress Self-Assessment

How do we assess our stress? The hectic pace of day-to-day living may sometimes cloud our perspective on life. What are we doing? Where are we going? What is happening to us? Where is our life leading? Are we suffering from stress without realizing it? Are the ways we deal with life stressors healthy ones? These are all-encompassing questions that often have ill-defined answers, or none at all.

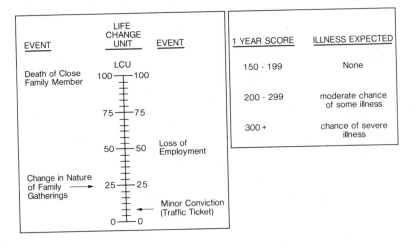

EVENT	LIFE CHANGE UNIT	EVENT

LCU

Death of Close Family Member — 100

Change in Nature of Family Gatherings → 25

Loss of Employment — 50

Minor Conviction (Traffic Ticket)

1 YEAR SCORE	ILLNESS EXPECTED
150 - 199	None
200 - 299	moderate chance of some illness
300 +	chance of severe illness

Figure 6.2. Relation between stress (Life Change Units) and expected illness. Adapted and reproduced with permission from Homes and Rahe, 1967.

6.1.2 Change Equals Stress

All change is stressful, but without a baseline of stress we would be bored or depressed. Perhaps the most consistent human endeavor across all ages, races, and cultures is the pursuit of change. The status quo is not fun. In fact, man's rise from the jungle has been built on his capacity to accommodate change. But what are our limits?

This concept of change has lead to the development of simple scales to quantify stress (Homes and Rahe, 1967). Figure 6.2 shows some common life experiences which in fact are elements of stress, in that each experience is actually an accumulation of circumstances that have led to the "event". Some changes are positive and thus less stressful in a negative sense, they are given low scores on the scale. As you go through such a list, you could add other equivalent events from your own life and give them proportional value somewhere between the death of a spouse rated as the "criterion" 100 point level negative stress, and a minor traffic violation.

As we have already indicated the response to stress is also a matter of accommodation. An event may be very stressful when first experienced, but subsequent exposures may be quite routine. For example, a pilot landing at a strange airport for the first time might feel considerable stress, but after frequent landings at the same field the stress level will become minimal (hopefully never to the point of inducing carelessness). Strangely we often seek out stress in our lives; it can be compellingly exciting and fulfilling as well as harmful. Positive success with risk-taking often induces bigger risk taking-and bigger stress. It is characteristic of the human spirit that it seeks challenges and dangers in almost every conceivable kind of endeavor (stock market, sport, exploration, industry, arts and entertainment, politics, etc.).

Susceptibility to stress, reflected in the body's organic reaction to a current stressor, results from the complex interaction of inherited weak or strong characters (psychological traits), and environmental influences

Hans Selye identified
three stages of response to stress as
alarm, resistance and exhaustion

(current trauma, illness, other responsibilities or state of debilitation). For these reasons an individual's degree of susceptibility at any one time is unpredictable since it depends upon the balance between, or the predominance of, any of the above factors. On average, the higher the stress level the more likely an individual will experience some ill effect from it. The final effect therefore varies with the current circumstance and previous experience and thus is susceptible itself to management strategies. These are discussed later in the chapter.

Some measure of an individual's susceptibility to stress-provoking activity may be assessed from a simple, subjective questionnaire about personal events, associations, habits, etc.in their life (Figure 6.3).

6.2 RESPONSES TO STRESS

When faced with difficult problems or acute change in circumstances, our responses are quite stereotyped. With few exceptions, we react in similar, well-defined ways. In 1956, Hans Selye identified three stages of response to stress as 1) alarm, 2) resistance, and 3) exhaustion. Later he named this trilogy of effects the "General Adaptation Syndrome, or GAS (Selye, 1975).

6.2.1 Physiological Responses

ALARM PHASE
The initial alarm phase is two-fold, characterized by:
• Secretion of adrenaline, which causes a "fight or flight" reaction. This is the thumping heart, cold sweat, rapid respiration, tense muscles, and a reaction that rushes us into rage or causes us to escape with utmost haste. Adrenaline release may trigger part 2 of the alarm phase, ACTH secretion.
• Secretion of adrenocorticotropic hormone (ACTH). This pituitary hormone is released after a stress situation, and in turn causes the adrenal gland to release cortisone.

1=Always
2=Often
3=50/50
4=Seldom
5=Never

Score
1 2 3 4 5

Eat 3 well balanced meals per day? |_|_|_|_|_|
Get 7-8 hours sleep per night, 5-6 times week? |_|_|_|_|_|
Have an affectionate/intimate relationship? |_|_|_|_|_|
Can rely on some other person implicitly? |_|_|_|_|_|
Exercise 3 times a week for 30 minutes? |_|_|_|_|_|
Financially secure? |_|_|_|_|_|
Happy in own convictions and/or religion? |_|_|_|_|_|
Club/social activities regularly undertaken? |_|_|_|_|_|
Possess several close friends and/or acquaintences? |_|_|_|_|_|
Possess one or more friends who will give personal council? |_|_|_|_|_|
Possess good physical health? |_|_|_|_|_|
Possess tact and strength to speak out on issues? |_|_|_|_|_|
Am able to discuss problems of living with family? |_|_|_|_|_|
Able to do "fun" things, at least once a week? |_|_|_|_|_|
Organized and productive? |_|_|_|_|_|
Organize relaxation time, at least once a day? |_|_|_|_|_|
Smoking (pack/day)?
        1=none, 2=none but around smoker, 3=<1, 4=≥1, 5=≥2 |_|_|_|_|_|
Alcohol (1 oz)? 1=none, 2=<5 oz, >3=10 oz, >4=20 oz, 5=alcoholic |_|_|_|_|_|
Coffee? (cups) 1=none, 2=<3, 3=<6, 4=<10, 5=≥10 |_|_|_|_|_|
Weight (from optimum)?
        1= ±10%, 2=±30%, 3=±60%, 4=obese, 5=anorexic |_|_|_|_|_|

TOTAL: _____

Scoring:
    <50 not vulnerable
    50-80 moderate vulnerability
    >80 high vulnerability

Figure 6.3. A simple "vulnerability to stress" rating scale.

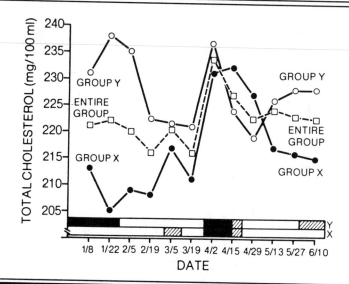

Figure 6.4. Elevated average serum cholesterol during stressful intervals in groups of accountants. Friedman and Rosenman, **Type A Behavior and Your Heart.** New York: Alfred A. Knopf, 1974.

RESISTANCE PHASE

Cortisone is a chemical which reduces the body's reaction to stress. It is an anti-inflammatory drug of great power. It tends to settle the initial alarm response over the next few hours or days after the initial arousal stage. It helps us cope with physical shock.

EXHAUSTION PHASE

If the stress continues for extended periods of time, ACTH, and thus cortisone, continue to be secreted. In time, the adrenal gland becomes larger and larger in response to ACTH stimulation, but excess cortisone production over prolonged periods has very damaging effects upon the body—sometimes including death.

Among the chemical mediators of stress deserving special interest are the endorphins, which provide a controlling influence. In people who exercise regularly, the endorphins, besides calming the mind, modify the secretion of the stress chemicals.

Specifically, endorphins inhibit excess adrenaline secretion—and ameliorate ACTH action. It is suspected that the resistance phase of GAS is less intense in well conditioned people (Allen, 1983). Nature, it seems, provides a convenient and simple chemical system to protect itself from the ravages of stress—but good physical shape is needed to activate these defenses.

A typical reaction to stress is shown in Figure 6.4. The figure shows how serum cholesterol is elevated intermittently in groups of accountants, reflecting the times that specific groups are especially busy. In periods of less activity stress-related organic response diminishes. The cholesterol concentration is elevated coincidently in both groups during the time of the general public tax return which is a common busy accounting period. The changing serum cholesterol concentration; its high levels patterning closely in both groups the stressful activity period of each, is compelling evidence for the dose/response connection between stressful activity and the concomitant organic reaction.

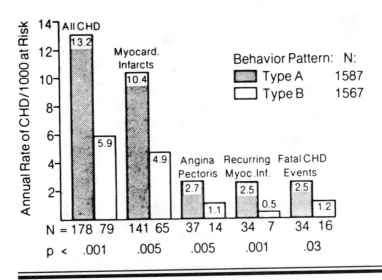

Figure 6.5. Comparison between Type A and Type B individuals in the incidence of coronary heart disease (CHD). Reproduced with permission from Friedman and Rosenman, **Type A Behavior & Your Heart**. New York: Alfred A. Knopf, 1974.

In recent years a characterization of overt behavior has developed defining busy, high achieving, industrious, driving personalities as Type A individuals, and their opposites the more placid and relaxed; Type B.

The so-called Type A pattern is shown in Figure 6.5. A high attendant risk of cardiovascular disease has been associated with the Type A profile, however, this association has been made without real regard for the effect of adaptation and with little evaluation of initial susceptibility of the individuals or groups studied to any possible negative effects of their activity. Thus, the characterization of all Type A individuals as being "at risk" by reason of their behavior is too simplistic. It omits consideration of the underlying complex interaction of inherited, learned, and environmental factors which, as noted previously, define vulnerability to organic dysfunction from stress.

Major Stress Related Disorders

Several major disease states shown in Table 6.3 have been associated with stress. This is the stress of ordinary daily living, for some, as well as the inordinately high stress levels identified with other specific activities or jobs.

It must be remembered however that the etiology of these diseases (i.e. the historical sequence of events leading to the final clinical manifestation of symptoms) is complex. Direct responsibility for an effect is often difficult to ascribe unequivocally to a single cause. The latency in development of several disease states also makes identification of the direct precipitating factors difficult. It was previously theorized that the stress played a major causative role in all of the disorders mentioned, but it is now accepted that stress is only a very minor factor in the evolution of these illnesses. The role of stress is primarily that of exacerbating an existing disorder.

Table 6.3. Organic stress related disorders.

Major organic stress related disorders	Minor organic stress related disorders

• Cardiovascular Disease
  heart attacks
  stroke
  angina pectoris
  (chest pain radiating from the heart)
• Ulcers (more frequent in men but increasing
  in frequency in women)
• Diabetes—adult onset (pancreatic exhaustion)
  25 in every 10,000 Americans 35-60 years old
  suffer from this disease
• Disorders of the immune system
  (increased susceptibility to infection)
• Asthma
• Cancer
	• Headaches
	• Urticaria (eczema)
	• Migraine headaches
	• Rhinitis (hayfever, runnynose)
	• Muscle pains (low back, shoulders)
	• Menstrual irregularity

6.2.2 Psychological Responses

The psychological indicators of stress are manifest in oneself as:
• inability to concentrate
• difficulty in making decisions
• poor priorization of activities (tasks) to be done
• loss of self-confidence
• irritability and anger (aggression)
• a specific craving e.g. for a food, a cigarette, etc.
• nervousness (anxiety)
• insomnia
• fear of rage
• emotional outbursts of tears or laughter

They may be recognized in others by:
• the efficient worker becoming careless
• the casual worker becoming compulsive
• the frugal person becoming lavish
• the generous person becoming selfish
• the friendly person becoming aloof
• the group participant becoming lonely
• the kind person becoming mean

Such signs of frustration may be reflected in absenteeism, high accident rates, sickness, strikes and occasional violence in the workplace. Productivity declines. Job frustrations may even invade the homelife, leading to domestic disputes, violence, and drug or alcohol abuse.

Possession of a positive attitude is a great help. One 40 year longitudinal study of university graduates showed that those with a high positive score on a measure of mental attitude survived better (i.e. were robust and healthy) than those with a negative mental attitude (i.e. were often ill or even died) (Vaillant, 1979). All subjects studied were of similar social, cultural, racial and religious backgrounds and all had similar activity/exercise patterns at the beginning of the study. Those who died did so from a variety of causes, but inevitably in the long term, the ill and the dead were those with a history of negative self image.

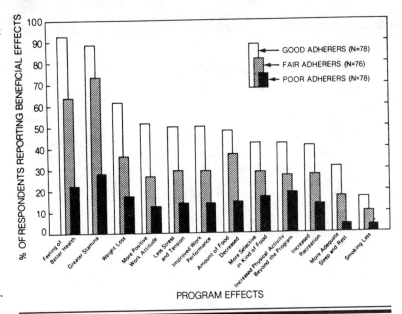

Figure 6.6. Program effects of exercise. Reproduced with permission of Durbeck et al., 1972.

6.3 PHYSICAL ACTIVITY AND THE HEALTHY MIND

"A healthy mind in a healthy body" is a well worn phrase, but recent evidence suggests that it may be true (Shephard, 1983). In an effort to enhance the quality of life rather than just its length, physical activity is being promoted in communities, and particularly in the workplace. Physical activity programs may increase life satisfaction through an immediate increased alertness as well as a long-term enhancement of self-esteem and body image.

The physical, psychological and social benefits of exercise are many. In young children, the competition associated with sports and games may sometimes cause excessive tension, but long term adverse effects are rare. Children quickly learn to cope with increased tension and anxiety generated by their sporting activity and in fact learn to cope, not only with the exercise stress, but with other stressors as well. A similar response is noted in adults, who have reduced anxiety and increased feelings of well-being resulting from regular physical activity.

Regular exercisers have a reduced frequency of minor complaints and less absenteeism from work (Durbeck et al., 1972). The positive attitudes demonstrated by the good adherers to the training regimen in this study is shown in Figure 6.6. This type of program is not only good for the individual, but has a positive effect on the overall social climate of the work place (naturally, there are secondary economic benefits expected to accrue to the company too).

Physical activity programs also help to correct the reactive depression that accompanies conditions such as heart attacks. Interest in physical activity should be stimulated from the earliest years of primary school. The allocation of curricular time to physical education does not hamper academic achievement, but rather produces the opposite effect; physically active individuals tend to attain greater scholastic achievements. In the final analysis, it seems that one cannot separate the mind's activities from those of the body; they are interdependent parts of the same person (Collis, 1977; Shephard, 1983).

Those who exercise regularly tend to order their lives better. They tend not to clutter their minds with unneccessary trivia, thus leaving themselves time and effort to concentrate on productive goals. Exercise may help the stress syndrome by giving the mind a break. During exercise, we are physically and often mentally removed from other concerns. Good study/work habits suggest limiting an individual session to only 45 minutes followed by a 10 minute break. The brief break is as "good as a rest", and provides "freshening" time before starting the next session. This sequential approach improves knowledge retention and productivity. It also reduces the dreariness of doggedly sticking to a project. Taking an exercise break is a stimulating and proven manner of retaining vigor and freshness of approach to a job. Many large corporations evidently subscribe to this notion as shown by the fact that they now invest considerably in providing employee fitness facilities based on a feeling that work habits improve and less absenteeism results. However, few studies are able to document this situation unequivocally.

It may be this "time away" allows the mind to think freely and solve problems. It is now well established that vigorous exercise elevates circulating endorphin levels in the body (Allen 1983, 1987). This neuroactive chemical produces an overall calming effect. Exercise is now considered an excellent therapy for stress and other psychological disorders.

6.4 MANAGEMENT OF STRESS

In recent years there have been as many methods for stress management proposed as there are stressors. The more credible stress management approaches require:

• Adoption of a positive, realistic attitude to problems.
• Recognizing the futility of self-deception and the similar or equal susceptibility of oneself to the same stresses others experience;
• A readiness to modify behavioral patterns to defuse or avoid possible stressful events (Watzlawick 1974);

The ideas presented in the "Stress Prevention Strategies" are based on the information and techniques developed for the Institute for Human Performance at Simon Fraser University, for the management of stress in widely different groups of competitors (e.g. swimmers and pistol shooters) by Dr. Wolfgang Luthe. Dr. Luthe was associated with the Institute from 1981 until 1983. The methods are unique in the sense that elements of stressful events (inducing anxiety or aggression) and recuperative acts (sleep or relaxation) are quantified (scored) and evaluated, objectively, rather than qualitatively. Thus, specific strategies taken to modify the impact of such events or problematic elements of habit (self-stress) may be evaluated through the serial (regular) measurements being undertaken.
This type of interactive, continuously responsive strategy in stress management is much more likely to produce positive results than any phasic (occasional) measurement and intervention in lifestyle. It is a pleasure to pass on these thoughts of Dr. Luthe, who died in 1985. They honor an eminent scientist/physician in the field of psychosomatic medicine and a gentle, friendly man.

- Adoption of certain basic elements of lifestyle, such as:
  a. adequate sleep
  b. adequate nutrition
  c. adequate exercise
  d. adequate sociability
  e. moderation of indulgence
- Setting and planning long and short term goals and priorities

6.4.1 Stress Prevention Strategies

When we talk about stress and stress prevention strategies, many people are inclined to think of environmental factors. They think of stress at work, of responsibilities, of job satisfaction, of job-home interaction, of interpersonal relationships and perhaps of so-called Type A behavior.

Such perspectives seem to indicate that stress prevention strategies must emphasize changes in the environment. Of course, stress prevention strategies that focus on environmental changes are useful and desirable. However, there is another area which is easily underestimated or forgotten when stress prevention is discussed. From a medical perspective, it is important to look at the impact of stressors from inside the organism. Any consideration of stress reactions inside the organism leads to the conclusion that the ability of the natural forces of inner self-regulation are actually the factor which decides whether we are going to suffer from stress disorders or not.

In other words, when the capacity of natural forces of inner self-regulation are overburdened, they cannot maintain a normal range of function. The consequence is the onset of functional disturbances. Such functional disturbances may be of a general nature, such as feeling sick, or they may involve specific mental or bodily activities.

This actually means that stress prevention strategies must include an approach that assists and facilitates the beneficial work of those self-regulatory systems nature has designed to keep our mental and bodily functions in order.

From this perspective, stress prevention generally consists of two interacting tasks:

• Conducting our daily life in such a manner that we avoid undue exposure to demands that overtax the capacity of our self-regulatory systems, and

• Doing whatever we can to facilitate the function of our inner forces of natural self-regulation.

Directly stated, this means modifying behavior, defined from the analyses described below, which overtaxes the self-regulatory system.

6.4.2 Recuperation and Stressor Effects

Throughout the world of living organisms we can observe a natural pattern of alternation between activity and rest. A lack of adequate recuperation is known to be followed by disturbances of various mental and bodily functions. Adaptation functions deteriorate, and the health-disturbing effects of various types of stressors increase. The system's resistance is progressively reduced and susceptibility to fatigue increases. A vicious cycle begins implying an increased probability of mental and bodily stress reactions. If the vicious cycle of events is are allowed to continue, functional breakdowns increase at various levels of activity and more mental and bodily disturbances become prominent.

All this means that the natural forces of self-regulation within ourselves have gradually lost their habitual power to maintain a normal state of functional harmony. Adequate recuperation is essentiall in order to reduce the adverse effects of stress.

WHAT IS ADEQUATE RECUPERATION?

Adequate recuperation varies essentially with:

• The peculiarities of the systems involved (e.g., eyes, coordination, muscular work, attentional functions, decision-making),

• The workrate to which each of the systems is exposed,

• The existing degree of training and habituation,

You should make it a point to
listen to the messages from inside yourself.

• Other co-existing functional situations (e.g., virus infection, anxiety, family conflicts) that consume a part of the vital energy which maintains the work of our natural forces of inner self-regulation.

Thus, **adequate recuperation** varies greatly from one person to another. A typical example is sleep. There is no explicit rule specifying that an adult person needs 6, 7, 8 or 9 hours of sleep (people also need different amounts of sleep in order to function properly and feel comfortable).

While sleep is nature's most obvious device of recuperation, there are many other situations during daily activities where natural forces of inner self-regulation demand or impose periods of rest in order to meet a need for recuperation (daydreaming is an example). In fact, studies have shown that about every 90 minutes our mind drifts into a lull—a daydream. This period may last for 5 to 10 minutes before things move back into focus. We all experience the moment when we've read a page, but upon reaching the bottom realize we absorbed nothing—a blank. Our mind was elsewhere—it needed a break. This is our mind's natural "ultradian" rhythm. When you recognize this happening to you, don't fight it. Lean back, close your eyes (if possible) and relax. This period is akin to autogenic training, Transcendental Meditation (TM), progressive relaxation, or self-hypnosis. Take advantage of such intervals to recharge your body. It is unlikely that you will be very productive at that time anyway (Lavie, 1982). Systematic application of stress protection strategies begins with the adequate management of these minor episodes of everyday life. In practice this means that you should make it a point to listen to the messages from inside yourself. This we call **receptivity**.

As you maintain a sharp sense of receptivity and respect for the fact that your eyes feel tired for instance, and you decide to give them a chance to rest and recuperate, they will work better for you. However, if you have turned off your receptivity and you keep overruling the mes-

If you chronically generate stressful situations for yourself, then stop complaining about all the stressful situations around you.

sages from inside, you are in fact generating a stressful situation for your own system. Moreover, if you have drifted into the habit of over-ruling all kinds of other messages from inside, **you very well may be the most important source of stress for your own system.**

So think for a minute.... in case you may be one of those "willpower people" who, like a stubborn dictator, does not care to respect internal signals, if you chronically generate stressful situations for yourself, then stop complaining about all the stressful situations around you. Stop imposing these stressful decisions on your own system and develop receptivity. Respect and be nice to your system, and your system will be nice to you.

Normally high performance periods will alternate with rest periods. It is not intelligent to over-rule the recuperative needs and the well-being of one's own system.

In the area of stress-prevention a variety of mental methods can effectively support our natural forces of self-recuperation. Some of these strategies can be practiced intermittently whenever you have a minute for yourself. Other methods require a bit more time, and may for example, be used to enhance and facilitate the onset of sleep.

We will discuss and practice both types of approaches. Since sleep is the most important natural form of recuperation sleep promotion strategies are discussed first before other stress prevention strategies.

ADJUSTMENT OF SLEEP PATTERNS: THE SLEEP CHART
In order to support nature's self-regulatory sleep functions it is necessary to make systematic recordings of your sleep pattern. Once you have a clear picture of your sleep profile in front of you it is easier to decide where adjustments are indicated. Try the following procedures for tracking your own sleep patterns.

		DAY OF WEEK						
Name:		S	M	T	W	Th	Fr	S

CODES

sleep: _____

rest: ....

sleep interruption: xxxxxx

other activities: oooooooo

TOTAL REST: time (mins.) spent in bed

S	=	Sleeping Pill
D	=	Other drugs
A	=	Alcohol
C	=	Coffee
BSE	=	Body Space Exercises
BR	=	Bathroom
T	=	Tea
Rd	=	Reading
TV	=	Television

RECUPERATION

Very rested, full of energy	= 5
Reasonably well rested	= 4
Relatively rested	= 3
A bit tired	= 2
Very tired	= 1

DREAMS

Very agreeable	= 5
Agreeable	= 4
Neutral	= 3
Disagreable	= 2
Very disagreable	= 1

DREAM RECALL

No recall	= 0
Vague memory	= A
Some parts	= B
Detailed recall	= C
Very detailed recall entire dream	= D

Week Begining: _____

I.D. NUMBER

8PM 9PM 10PM 11PM 12PM 1AM 2AM 3AM 4AM 5AM 6AM 7AM 8AM 9AM

	S	M	T	W	Th	Fr	S
TOTAL REST (min.)							
SLEEP (min.)							
Score RECUPERATION:							
Score NATURE OF DREAMS:							
Score RECALL OF DREAMS:							

Figure 6.7. The Sleep Chart.

Procedural Details:

1. Study the sleep chart (Figure 6.7) which shows how to proceed.
2. Indicate the periods during which you are in bed (lights off) without sleeping by a vertical dotted line (the space between each dot is equivalent to 5 minutes).
3. Indicate periods of actual sleep with a vertical solid line in each column for each day.
4. Indicate sleep interruptions by changing the vertical line to crosses equivalent to the time of the interruptions.
5. Add text abbreviations at the appropriate times for the events shown or define your own.
6. Use appropriate abbreviations for noting pre-sleep activities and the consumption of sleep inhibiting beverages.
7. After getting up in the morning, evaluate your feeling of recuperation by using the 5-point "Recuperation" scoring system printed on the left side of the form.
8. Indicate the appropriate scores for dream activities. Use "0" in cases where no dreams are remembered.
9. Calculate the total of all recuperation scores for a 7-day period.

   Scoring these aspects of sleep allows evaluation of the adequacy of a major recuperative phase for the body defining:

- the sleep onset latency period defined as the time from when the head is on the pillow to when you remember falling asleep,
- duration of actual sleep per night and per 7-day periods,
- duration of total rest period (i.e., resting in bed without sleeping plus actual sleep period),
- number and nature of sleep interruptions,
- quality of recuperation experienced when getting up in the morning,
- probability of increased susceptibility to stress-related reactions and onset of functional disturbances (e.g. recuperation score below 20 for a 7-day period, see sleep chart),
- occurrence and general nature of dreams.

*The practice of the Body-space Exercise is
designed to reduce and largely
eliminate participation of the left-hemispheric
information systems.*

Regular weekly measurement of the same details allows on-going evaluation of the effectiveness of any strategies implemented such as:
• changes in dream-related, awakening episodes after beginning relevant mental approaches (i.e. training to awake on disagreeable dreams and using Body-Space Exercises (BSE) to fall asleep again),
• sleep onset improvement after practicing sleep-promoting mental strategies (BSEs),
• changes in the relationship between pre-sleep activities, sleep pattern and the quality of recuperation (reducing drug reliance, reducing activating stimuli e.g., TV).

THE BODY-SPACE EXERCISE (BSE)
This **mental** exercise is based on research in the area of hemispheric specialization (e.g., **left hemisphere systems:** work with words, numbers, analytical logic, classification, logic linear information processing; **right Hemisphere systems:** work with non-linear information processing, intuition, holistic, "Gestalt"-type, spatial elements, symbolism, colors, music, melodies).

The practice of the Body-Space or Mental Exercise is designed to reduce and largely eliminate the participation of left hemispheric information systems. It induces a recuperative situation for left hemispheric information systems and promotes mental and bodily relaxation. Furthermore, BSEs are helpful in facilitating sleep onset functions (e.g., at bedtime, after waking up during the night) and it enhances recuperation. You may wish to practice BSEs yourself using the following procedures.

BSE Procedure:
Adopt a comfortable recumbent or sitting posture, eyes closed (disconnect the telephone). Begin with thinking about the space between your **right shoulder and left knee** .. (5-10 seconds) then imagine the space between your **left knee and right heel.**. (5-10 seconds) then

the space between your **right heel and left earlobe..** (5-10 seconds) then the space between your **left earlobe and right wrist.**.(5-10 seconds). Continue for 5 to 20 minutes.

Essential Technical Points:
1. Try to alternate between points on the right and left side of the body (i.e. involvement of interhemispheric conditions).
2. Use each point of reference as a point of departure for the next step (e.g., right shoulder-left knee,... left knee-right heel,...right heel-left elbow).
3. The task is to proceed with your own pattern in an almost effortless manner. As you add one step to the next, do not "force" anything, but rather adopt the attitude that you are serving sets of stimuli to certain parts in your brain.
4. Do not force yourself to visualize, because the facility to "see in mental pictures" varies greatly among persons and may constitute a special effort for you (i.e. stress).
5. The mental task is focused on "the space between" and not on "the distance between").
6. Do not use the eyes or parts of the brain or upper part of the head (except earlobes) for points of reference.
7. Do not use the "inside of the body" (e.g. heart, stomach, liver) for points of reference.
8. Stop when anything uncomfortable occurs.
9. When awake or disturbed, terminate in three steps by:
   (a) bending both arms vigorously,
   (b) taking a deep breath,
   (c) opening both eyes (also when practicing in darkness).
10. In case you should fall asleep or when intending to sleep, you do not need to worry about the termination procedure, because the sleep mechanism will terminate the exercise automatically.
11. If you start yawning or begin to feel sleepy during or after an exercise, you have a sleep deficiency and you need more sleep.

*Two types of stressors that
are of particular medical concern
are aggression and anxiety.*

12. Indicate in your Sleep chart when and how long (appoximately) you practiced BSEs (use the designation "m" for BSEs).
13. You can also use this exercise for very brief periods (e.g., 1 or 2 minutes) in your office, in the washroom, while riding on a bus.
14. Do not practice BSEs at a red light, or while responsible for machinery, because you may fall asleep.
15. Do not practice this exercise when intoxicated or under the influence of drugs.

6.4.3 Reduction of Exposure to Stress-Promoting Stimuli

Sleep and BSEs are mainly concerned with supporting and facilitating the self-regulatory activities that attempt to cope with stress-producing situations already existing within our system.

Now let us focus attention on the stressful situations and stimuli not yet recorded in the brain which we must attempt to avoid. Two types of stressors that are of particular medical concern are aggression and anxiety. In order to understand the significance of the following discussion better it is helpful to note a few facts.

1. Our brain records automatically whatever is going on, including many things of which we may not be aware.
2. These recordings remain in the brain throughout one's life. They are not dead, they remain active to variable degrees. In other words we have to live with them.
3. Our brain mechanisms are able to engage in "Play-back" activities if given an opportunity to do so. Such self-regulatory "play-backs" tend to contain an astonishing amount of detail.
4. From studying such self-regulatory play-back functions we have learned many things. For example, we know that our brain has certain classification systems. Events with stimuli of similar natures are functionally interrelated. Furthermore, we learned that new incoming stimuli do at least two things: they add more of the same to material already present in the brain and they activate material of similar nature, previously accumulated.

5. In case the exposure to new stimuli coincides with the nature of brain-disturbing material that previously caused functional disturbances, then, these disturbances will be reactivated and increased.

Such stress-promoting effects that occur within our mental system are sometimes obvious. However, in most instances nothing in particular is noticed, unless sensitive research instruments are in place to record the response.

The situation is rather like the accumulation of particles of dust. Each particle is of negligible significance. However, as accumulation continues, the sensitive parts of the machinery begin to show functional disturbances. In a way, we are talking about "brain pollution" by stress-promoting stimuli. In psychosomatic medicine both the acquisition of unexpressed aggressive reactions and the anxiety dynamics generated by brain-disturbing events are known as severely health-disturbing types of "brain pollution". Therefore, if we want to fight stress, we must take care of situations and stimuli that add and activate aggressive dynamics and anxiety material.

Consider the dynamics of aggression. The accumulation of aggressive material is particularly health-damaging because of the increasingly possible potentiating effect of otherwise well controlled unexpressed reactions of hostility and direct aggression. Such stress promoting accumulation of aggressive reactions is a characteristic feature of people who manage to maintain a certain degree of politeness under the most aggravating circumstances. This is no coincidence. Many people would not permit themselves to vocalize for example, four-letter words. However, from self-regulatory discharge dynamics we know that certain systems of the brain are highly loaded with impulse materials designed to express such terms when accompanied by related reactions. And, of course, as the accumulation of such brain-disturbing material continues, the functional situation is prone to become more delicately balanced and easily upset. There are avariety of technical approaches that may be learned and used to neutralize and unburden such overloaded brain systems.

In all such instances the desired adjustments always involve two types of procedures. One procedure is designed to help reduce the disturbing potency of accumulated aggressive material already in the brain. The other type is aimed at reducing new additional loading of systems that are already a source of functional disturbances or dysfunction.

One of these approaches which you can use immediatley to reduce activation and accumulation of aggression promoting stimuli is the Aggression Control Inventory.

6.4.4 The Aggression Control Inventory

Figure 6.8 shows this inventory and the procedural details for its use are outlined below:

Step 1: Begin by looking over the scoring system printed in the lower left corner of the form. The "Intensity of Activation" of aggressive dynamics which reach your awareness range from being a bit annoyed (1 point) to being infuriated (5 points).

Step 2: Make a list of all those situations that activate your aggressive reaction systems. In the model form you see a list of such situations. Usually a complete inventory comprises about 40 to 70 items listed on 3 or 4 forms.

Step 3: Next, determine the "Intensity of Activation" for each of the items on your list. For example, look at item 1 of the model sheet: "Messiness in the kitchen". The "Intensity of Activation" varies between "clearly irritated" (2 points) and feeling "somewhat angered" (3 points). These "Intensity of Activation" scores are listed in the first column (i.e., Intensity 1-5).

Step 4: Estimate how many times each episode occurs per week or month. In this example, annoying "Messiness in the kitchen" occurred about twice a day. That makes 14 times per week, So you would write "14" in the column for "Frequency per week". You should determine at the start whether you will calculate frequencies by the week or month and then be consistent (as far as possible) across all types of episodes.

Item No.	INVENTORY (situations, stimuli)	Intensity 1 → 5	Frequency Day ☐ Wk ☒ Mth ☐	Activation Score Day ☐ Wk ☒ Mth ☐	Control evaluation after 1 week	2 wks.	3 wks.	4 wks.

STRESS MANAGEMENT: AGGRESSION CONTROL INVENTORY

Subject ID #

Name: _____

	Date #1	Date #2	Date #3	Date #4	Date #5
1	11	1x11			

Item No.	INVENTORY (situations, stimuli)	Intensity 1 → 5	Frequency	Activation Score	1 week	2 wks.	3 wks.	4 wks.
1.	Messiness in kitchen	(2 – 3)	x 14	= 35				
2.	Loud record players		x	=				
3.	Lateness in others		x	=				
4.	Messiness in bathroom		x	=				
5.	Lying in others		x	=				
6.	Rudeness in others		x	=				
7.	Insincerity in others		x	=				
8.	Smoking (local pollution)		x	=				
9.	Unauthorized "borrowing"		x	=				
10.	Prejudice in others		x	=				
11.	Poor restaurant service		x	=				
12.	Lack of initiative in others		x	=				
13.	Injustice (real or perceived)		x	=				
14.	Playing games (physical)		x	=				
15.	Petty revenges		x	=				
16.	Annoying sequences in films, plays		x	=				
17.	Petty officialdom hastles		x	=				
	TOTAL			357	260	190	120	107

*Intensity of Activation

1 = bit annoyed
2 = clearly irritated
3 = somewhat angry
4 = very angry
5 = Infuriated

Figure 6.8. Stress Management: Aggression Control Inventory

Step 5: Now you can determine "Activation Score", multiplying the "Intensity of Activation" score by the "Frequency per week". In this example the intensity score is about 2.5 on the average, and the frequency per week is l4. So, the "Activation Score" is 35 (l4 x 2.5 = 35).

Step 6: Repeat the initial 5-step procedure for each item in your list.

Step 7: Once the sheet is full, calculate the total of all "Activation Scores". In our example the total is 357 for l7 items.

Step 8: Continue with a new sheet, and make an exhaustive inventory of all those apparently trivial and not so trivial things that are stress-promoting and harmony-disturbing to you.

Step 9: After listing most of the aggression-promoting situations of your daily life, look at the items on your list. Some are more important than others. Some are relatively easy to approach, while others appear to be very difficult or impossible to adjust. Begin to think about what you can do to reduce or eliminate such health-disturbing sources of mental pollution. Thus by carefully observing and recording the stressors in your life now you can begin to **develop your own strategies to reduce exposure to stress-promoting situations around you.** Keep at it, do it gradually and systematically. Progress may be slow but patience and persistence will usually bring success.

Step l0: It is normal to discover new items as the days go by. Some of these aggravating situations occur perhaps only once a week, or only once per month. These **low frequency episodes must also be included in your inventory**. They all add up and contribute to stress-promoting brain pollution.

Step 11: A week after you started your first listing, sit down again and do a "Control evaluation". The "Control evaluation" permits you to see in which areas you managed to obtain improvements, and which items require more effective strategies. **In order to do your "Control evaluation"** you simply repeat the initial 5-step procedure for each item and note the **Activation Score** in the first column of

*If your Aggression Control Inventory
lists less than 20 items, you are either very
lucky or your are kidding yourself.*

the "Control evaluation" section. then, as before, calculate the total of all "Activation Scores". The progress you made within a week is reflected in a lower total for the second week's calculation.

Step 12: Again, one week later, do your second "Control evaluation" and see where you stand. You should continue with this program until you have maintained a comfortably low total for at least three weeks.

Other Technical Information:
• Most people are able to reduce the initial total of the "Activation Scores" 70 to 80% within 4 weeks.
• If you achieved a 50% reduction within four weeks, you've made good progress, but should try to achieve further reductions.
• If your improvement during four weeks is less than 30% you are either in a very difficult and rather stressful situation, or, you may want to see your doctor or clinical psychologist to discuss your difficulties.
• Do not expect to reduce the total of the "Activation Scores" to zero.
• If your Aggression Control Inventory lists less than 20 items, you are either very lucky or you are kidding yourself.

While control of aggression-promoting stimuli is important the other area of stress-promoting "brain pollution" concerns the accumulation of anxiety material and the ensuing activation of anxiety dynamics.

In order to help reduce your exposure to anxiety- activating situations and stimuli, an Anxiety Control Inventory may be used.

6.4.5 The Anxiety Control Inventory
Figure 6.9, represents the Anxiety Control Inventory. The procedures for using this approach are similar to those for the Aggression Control Inventory we have just discussed. The scoring system for indicating the "Intensity of Activation" of anxiety dynamics reaching your awareness is printed in the lower left corner of the form. The 5-point scoring system ranges from "slight feelings of uneasiness" (1 point) to feeling

					STRESS MANAGEMENT : ANXIETY CONTROL INVENTORY					Subject ID #

STRESS MANAGEMENT : ANXIETY CONTROL INVENTORY

Subject ID #

Item No.	INVENTORY (situations, stimuli)	Intensity 1 → 5	Frequency Day ☐ Wk ☐ Mth ☐		Activation Score Day ☐ Wk ☐ Mth ☐	Control evaluation after			
						1 week	2 wks.	3 wks.	4 wks.
1.	Reading about burglaries, holdups, muggings	(1 - 2)	x	25	= 38	10	4	4	4
2.	In a car, fast driver	(1 - 3)	x	5	= 10	0	0	0	0
3.	Sudden noise during the night	(1 - 4)	x	10	= 30	30	30	20	16
4.	Telephone ringing (night)	(1 - 3)	x	5	= 10	10	10	0	0
5.	Thunderstorms, lightning	(3 - 4)	x	2	= 7	7	7	7	7
6.	Worry about losing my boyfriend	2	x	20	= 40	40	40	8	0
7.	Worry about losing my job	2	x	10	= 20	20	20	10	10
8.	Being late (missing bus)	2	x	15	= 30	8	8	8	8
9.	Gaining more weight	(1 - 2)	x	20	= 30	30	20	12	8
10.	Spiders	(2 - 3)	x	8	= 20	20	10	0	0
11.	People quarrelling, fighting	(1 - 3)	x	10	= 20	8	8	8	8
12.	Certain T. V. programs (murder, violence)	(1 - 3)	x	12	= 24	12	8	8	4
13.	Stock market news	2	x	16	= 32	32	32	0	0
14.	Height, looking down	(3 - 4)	x	8	= 28	12	12	12	12
15.	Bad news from family	2	x	3	= 6	6	6	6	6
16.	Not recalling whether I turned the stove off	2	x	10	= 20	0	0	0	0
17.	Losing my purse	(1 - 2)	x	60	= 90	45	45	20	20
			TOTAL		455	290	260	123	103

Name: _____ Date Jan. 5, 1981 Date Jan. 12 Date Jan. 19 Date Jan. 26 Date Feb. 2

1   1 1   1x1 1

*Intensity of Activation

1 = slight (uneasy, apprehensive)
2 = somewhat (clearly worried, anxious)
3 = moderate (feeling of moderate anxiety)
4 = strong (quite frightened, scared)
5 = very strong (panic, very badly frightened)

Figure 6.9. Stress Management: Anxiety Control Inventory.

"very badly frightened" (5 points). The procedural instructions are the same as those listed for the Aggression Control Inventory.

You are now in possession of two instruments that can help you fight stress-promoting "brain pollution" in a systematic manner. However, it should be emphasized that your fight against stress-promoting brain pollution should not be limited to the particular items listed in the control inventories.

There are all kinds of everyday situations that involve elements of aggression and anxiety which, like particles of dust are automatically recorded and accumulated by your brain. For example, much anxiety can come from radio news, television scenes, violence in movies, colorful pictures of massacres, war reports and stories about murders and burglaries. All are sources of stimuli contributing to the accumulation and reinforcement of stress-producing "brain-pollution".

Furthermore, research has shown that amusement machines, risky driving, and competitive or dangerous sports (e.g., judo, football, skydiving or downhill skiing) are in many instances quite disturbing to our brain function. Similarly, disturbing effects may also result from viewing accident scenes, burning homes, injured or dying animals, or, just listening to vividly described tragedies.

In all these areas of daily life you can develop your own strategies to reduce the progressive accumulation of brain-disturbing stimuli in a significant manner.

6.5 SUPPLEMENTARY STRESS MANAGEMENT TECHNIQUES

While basic changes in lifestyle habits effect the greatest reduction in organic stress, some learned strategies can also be effective. Considerable clinical research has been reported in the last decade which describes various stress reduction techniques applicable to specific situations.

6.5.1 Biofeedback

During the late 1960's, biofeedback devices were found to be useful in the management of some stress related disorders (Brown, 1974). The term biofeedback was well chosen, for the system monitors biological signals (skin temperature, EEG, brain waves, respiration, etc.) from the body or mind and uses a different biological system (hearing, sight) to inform the mind of the events that are occurring. For example, an electromyograph (EMG can monitor the activity in the frontalis muscle (forehead) and the EMG signal can be converted to a buzzing sound. When the frontalis muscle is tense, the biofeedback monitor will buzz at a very fast rate. If the muscle is only slightly active, a slow frequency buzz is heard, and if the muscle is totally relaxed, then the monitor is silent. Sound is usually the preferred feedback signal. It can be used to provide audible information on different functions such as muscle tension, brain waves, blood pressure, or perspiration.

During the course of therapy, the subject concentrates solely on reducing the audible signal, effectively reducing the physiological signal at the same time. This type of demonstration, training the mind to control undesirable physiological responses, promised to be a valuable aid to many in controlling their vulnerability to stress, but unfortunately all the hoped-for benefits did not accrue (Hume, 1981). This is because although biofeedback training may significantly influence bodily function the control doesn't seem to last outside the laboratory. The sessions tend to be long, expensive and require highly trained people; yet the benefits are uncertain. The place for biofeedback training seems best relegated to certain muscle contraction headaches (which are not as common as doctors initially thought) and to only a few low back pain disorders. Hypertension or migraines are poor responders to biofeedback. Some long term low back pain sufferers can benefit from biofeedback training in order to relax more and to learn to live with their disorders.

*Each one of us possesses a very potent healing
capacity, however, we are not always
aware of it or able to activate it.*

6.5.2 Hypnosis

There are a number of induced or self-induced states of individual awareness which have been used in order to reshape a particular lifestyle.
Such altered states are not strictly sleep or wakefulness, nor anything in
between. They have many names: hypnosis, progressive relaxation,
alpha thought, Zen state, Transcendental Meditation (TM), charismatic
prayers, autogenic training, and day-dreams. It would appear that all
normal minds pass through altered states about every 90 minutes during the day and night. The cycle starts with the first REM (rapid eye
motion) sleep of the night and occurs in conjunction with these REM
or dream sleep phases every 90 minutes. During the day as we have
noted, we call them daydreams. They reach a peak of intensity in early
afternoon. It is assumed that these periods are very important natural
events, but science has not yet determined their exact cause or function.
During such states, a person is physically more relaxed, muscles
become less tense (in fact during REM sleep the muscles are paralyzed)
and he/she is hypersuggestible. This state of mind can be very useful to
a person for formulating an overall personal policy, getting a "feel" for
their situation, producing self-instructed changes, motivation or
formalizing specific goal directed behavior. Some of our most creative
ideas are brought into our consciousnes during these dream-like phases.

These states, by whatever name, are very powerful tools for stress therapy. This latter strategy illustrates the very potent healing capacity that
each one of us possesses but which we are not always aware of nor able
to activate. The previous discussion on Body Space Exercise is an example of activating an altered mental state to achieve relaxation or sleep.

6.6 SUMMARY

Stress comes in many forms. We feel it as an everyday event which
shapes our lives. Many seek out stressful activity as a necessary ingredient of their lives, while others retreat from challenges and are unwill-
ing to accept much stress. We can assess our levels of stress (aggres-

sion, anxiety) as well as the level of recuperation from it (sleep) and thus formulate strategies to control and optimize its level.

However, many of the so-called stress related illnesses are not caused by stress. More likely stress from the illness itself creates behavioral signs of stress. In other words, illness often occurs first, and stress and personality changes occur secondarily. Additional stress from other sources however, will often exacerbate the symptoms of many illnesses, but we should not be deluded into concluding that the "additional" stress is the actual cause of the illness.

Stress creates very definite physiological enhancement in body functions which may in fact lead to a beneficial, adaptive and ultimately protective response against the negative aspects of stress. But unremittingly repeated stress, allowing no recuperative periods, is ultimately debilitating and leads to the breakdown of some organ systems and poor health results. Loading the system with enough—but not too much—stress is a delicate balancing act. Those who surpass individual limits suffer the consequences. Each person's limit is different and each must explore their own.

Physical activity seems to produce a number of beneficial physiological effects related both to improving the functional capability of many bodily tissues (e.g. muscle, blood vessels, etc.) and enhancing levels of circulating chemicals (e.g. endorphins) which exert calming effects within the brain.

The management of stress initially requires a means of assessing the level of stress—is it high enough to be a negative factor in the long term health of the individual? How high is too high? Thus the physical response to stress must be accurately defined. In some cases, adopting simple basic strategies may be all that is required to reduce stress. Sometimes biofeedback may help in specific situations. Hypnosis may be effective in bringing about inner policy changes. Professional counselling or psychiatric help may be required in more serious cases where self-help has not proved effective.

6.7 REFERENCES

Allen, M.E. Activity Generated Endorphins, Their Role in Sports Science. **Can. J. Appl.Sports Science, 8(3):** 115- 133, 1983.

Allen, M.E. and Cohen, D. Blockade of Running Induced Mood Changes by Naloxone: Endorphins Implicated. **Annals of Sports Medicine** 3(3): 67-93, 1987.

Brown, B. **New Mind, New Body: Biofeedback, New Directions for the Mind.** Harper and Row, New York, 1974.

Brown, B. **Between Health and Illness.** New York: Bantam, 1984.

Collis, M.L. **Employee Fitness.** Minister of Supply and Services Canada, Ottawa, 1977.

Durbeck, D.C., Heinzelmann, F., Schacter, J., Haskell, W.C., Payne, G.W., Moxley, R.T., Nemiroff, M., Limoncelli, D.D., Arnold, L.B. and Fox, S.M. The National Aeronautics and Space Administration—U.S. Public Health Service and Enhancement Program. **American Journal of Cardiology,** 30: 784-790, 1972.

Edlin, G. and Golanty, E. **Health and Wellness: a Holistic Approach,** (3rd ed). Jones and Bartlett Publishers, Boston, 1988.

Fortune Magazine. Keeping fit in the company gym. pp.8, October, 1975.

Friedman, M. and Rosenman, R.H. **Type A Behavior and your Heart.** New York: Alfred A. Knopf, 1974.

Holmes, T.H., & Rahe, R.H. The social readjustment rating scale. **Journal of Psychosomatic Research,** 11: 213- 218, 1967.

Hume, W.I. **Biofeedback,** Vol.III. Human Sciences Press, New York, 1981.

Lavie, P. Ultradian rhythms in human sleep and wakefulness. In **Biological Rhythms, Sleep, and Performance.** Webb, W.B. (ed.), Wiley & Sons Ltd. 238-72, 1982.

Patterson, G.R. Families. Champaign, Ill.: Research Press, 1971. Seyle, Hans. **Stress Without Distress.** New York: Lippincott, 1974.

Seyle, Hans. **Stress Without Distress.** New York: Lippincott, 1974.

Shephard, R.J. Physical activity and the healthy mind: A Current review. **Canadian Medical Association Journal,** 128: 525-530, 1983.

Skinner, B.F. **Beyond Freedom and Dignity.** New York, Bantam/Vintage, 1972.

Smoking or Health. The third report from the Royal College of Physicians of London. Pitman Medical, 1977.

Vaillant, G.E. Natural history of male psychological health. **New England J. Medicine,** 301: 1249-1254, 1979.

Watzlawick, P., Weakland, J., & Fisch, R. **Change: Principles of Problem Formation and Problem Resolution.** New York: W.W. Norton, 1974.

Weeks, G.R. & L'Abate, L. **Paredonical psychotherapy: Theory and practices with individuals, couples, and families.** New York: Bruner/Mazel, 1982.

Weinstein, M.S., Conry, R.F. & Neidhardt, J. Introduction to Stress and Stress Management. Western Centre Health Group: Vancouver, 1982. Woods, D. Does your office put you off? **The Financial Post,** Nov: 76-82, 1979.

Woods, D. Does your office put you off? **The Financial Post,** Nov: 76-82, 1979.

Woods, D. The big squeeze. **The Financial Post,** March: 43-48, 1980.

6.8 STUDY QUESTIONS

1. Who popularized the expression "stress" as we use it today? What does it mean?
2. Comment objectively on the results of your self-assessment with regard to stress.
3. Compute your life change risk of stress (LCU self-evaluation).
4. Describe someone you know who demonstrates so-called Type A behavior. What behavior patterns do they show which define them as such?
5. Discuss job fulfillment and its implications for your life and the life of our nation.
6. Describe an event in your life which, as a child, set you up for problems (it's OK, we all have them!) relating to stress.
7. List five psychological conditions which could be improved with physical fitness.
8. Discuss the three stages of the GAS by Selye.
9. What are the common psychological responses to stress?
10. List the five basics of good mental and physical health.
11. Discuss some strategies to avoid or alleviate the negative affects of stressful events in our lives.
12. Fill out a sleep chart on yourself.
13. Calculate your aggression control inventory.
14. Calculate your anxiety control inventory.

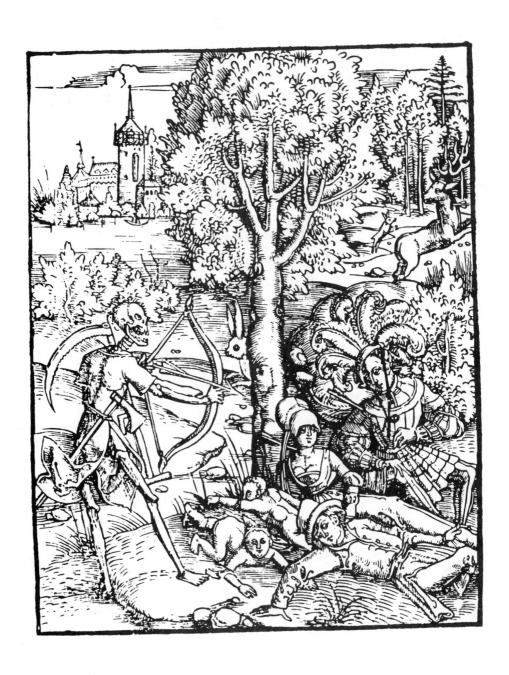

7

Disease

A disease state is no longer a simple one cause and effect event but an interactive physical, biological, socio-cultural and life-style complex of factors.

OBJECTIVES
When you have completed this chapter you should:
- **Understand** the types of disease that afflict people at different stages of their life.
- Be able to **distinguish** the typical disease states that are prevalent in developed and developing countries.
- **Understand** the contribution an individual's constitutionality (genetic inheritance) makes to the contraction of disease.
- Be able to **explain** the term congenital disease.
- Be able to **discuss** the immune response to the body's infection by micro-organisms.
- Be able to **distinguish** six types of micro-organisms which can invade the body and describe their effect.
- Be able to **write** an account of the comparative importance of infectious and non-infective disease in the modern world.

7.0 INTRODUCTION
The science of the study of disease, its nature, causes, processes, development and consequences derives from the Greek pathalogia, the study of passions. The branch of medicine specifically associated with this activity is called pathology.

In a delightful introduction to the text **Mechanisms of Disease** (1985) its author Ruy Perez-Tamayo traces the development of the subject from the Egyptians, Greeks and Chinese to the present day. The early Mediterraneans attributed different diseases to the confluence of the "humors" air, fire, water and earth. However, it was not until the early renaissance period of Leonardo de Vinci (1548) that quantitative relationships between disease and morbid changes evoked within the body's anatomy, began to be understood. It was realized that disease or death did not just happen, but were due to prior events which could be measured. The Italian Anatonio Benivieni (1440-1502) is generally accorded the founding role in anatomical (organ structure) pathology. He classified the facts on organs in health and disease and established relationships between the site, cause, and outcome of pathologic processes. Succeeding anatomists (Fernel, 1497-1558; Bonettus, 1620-1689) continued this work based upon innumerable autopsies performed by each of them. Later with the work of Giovanni Morgagni (1682-1771) the dominant era of the organ as the sole seat of disease passed, although the clear concept remained that symptoms of disease were always accompanied by definite anatomical alterations. The next advance was in 1800, when Bichat, a French physician (1771-1802), established that organs were formed from tissue. From organ to tissue to cell, finally it was Virchow (1821-1902) who composed the scattered theory of cellular components and their interaction into a coherent account of cellular pathology and in 1858 proposed (Cameron, 1952):

• Cells are the unit of life,
• The tissues and organs of living organisms are composed of cells,
• The organism is thus a cell state,
• Cells are nourished by blood vessels,
• Cells are the units of disease,
• Cells possess irritability as long as they live. Response to irritation may be of 3 different types: functional, nutritive, and formative,
• **Functional** disturbances result in fatigue and exhaustion; **nutritional** upset is shown by hypertrophy, cloudy swelling and inflammation, or passive changes such as necrobiosis (gradual degeneration). **Formative** disturbances yield hyperplasia (cellular profusion), pus formation, tuberculosis and neoplasms (cancers).

During several recent decades our understanding of the living cell has extended to subcellular, molecular and even to atomic levels. Perez-Tamayo (1985) argues however that these atomic divisions are not the seat of disease processes. They lack both the necessary complexity of organization and prescribed existence in time, possessed by the living organism, which is needed to demonstrate the typical time course of evolution and resolution of the disease process. Molecules or atoms have no temporal restriction and do not develop illness, but their accretion into the network which becomes complex living tissue affords them that privilege.

7.1 THE CONCEPT OF DISEASE

A precise definition of disease is hard to make since almost every temporary departure of bodily function from a prescribed homeostatic condition may be deemed abnormal, diseased, or potentially life threatening. This is especially so if any of the regulatory mechanisms of the body fail, e.g. those constraining core temperature changes between 32°C to 42°C, or the acidity of the blood between pH 6.9 to 7.9.

While acknowledging its inadequacy, we will define disease as an infection or ailment causing a departure from generally accepted normal bodily structure and function. In addition the symptoms shown may not be immediately contained by naturally acting regulatory mechanisms or reversed by external supplementary actions such as medical intervention or removal of the inducing stressor.

The disease process may be effected by endogenous (from within, either constitutional or genetic) or exogenous (from without, environmental) forces or their combination. As an example of the former, defective inheritable traits may be recognized as an abnormality of function early in life (deformations at birth) when they are termed congenital, or later as a predisposition to illness which is often influenced by the environment, such as degenerative atherosclerotic plaques in blood vessels.

Some forces from without (exogenous) are in the form of viruses, bacteria, protozoa etc., which are the ever present agents of infection. Paradoxically some of the very mechanisms marshalled to fight infection (the immune response) may boomerang pathalogically. Immunological hypersensitivity to some antigens (which are invasive agents recognized as non-self and thus marked for destruction by the body) may sometimes cause severe reaction and even death in sensitized people. This is a consequence of antibody (one of the body's defensive agents) action on certain

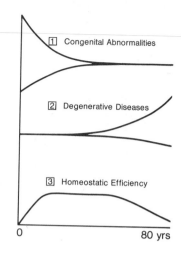

1. Congenital Abnormalities

2. Degenerative Diseases

3. Homeostatic Efficiency

0   80 yrs

Figure 7.1. Three important factors which determine the frequency and effect of disease. Reproduced from **The Physiology of Disease** by I.C. Roddie and W.F.M. Wallace ©1975. Reprinted with permission of Year Book Medical Publishers Inc.

cells of the body in addition to their action against the invading antigen. For example, vasoactive secretions from immunologically hypersensitized mast cells can cause sudden peripheral blood vessel vasodilation, a fall in blood pressure, loss of fluid from the vascular system, and poor perfusion of tissue (shock). Bronchial constriction (airway obstruction) also occurs. The condition is termed anaphylactic shock (Greek: ana - against, phylaxis - protection).

Another complication occurs whenever a pathogenic (disease producing) bacteria is engulfed but not killed by a phagocytic white blood cell (a polymorphonuclear leukocyte or a macrophage described later) the phagocyte, in effect, becomes an armour and carrier for the bacteria, protecting it from other potentially effective defenses or chemoagents, and transporting it wherever the phagocyte travels. This can allow wide dispersion of the disease and is thought to occur in some types of chronic infections such as tuberculosis. A variation of this type of disfunction is associated with AIDS.

7.2 STUDY OF DISEASE

7.2.1 Distribution by Age

The frequency, pattern and effect of disease upon the host varies distinctively throughout life. Roddie and Wallace (1975) categorized three important factors (Figure 7.1) which determine the frequency and effect of disease: congenital abnormalities, degenerative diseases and homeostatic efficiency.

7.2.2 Congenital Abnormalities

These encompass both biochemical and structural abnormalities which, while compatible with life, are too severe for the latter's extended survival outside the womb, Figure 7.1(1). Infant mortality is high in these cases and especially high in underdeveloped countries. Five hundred children in

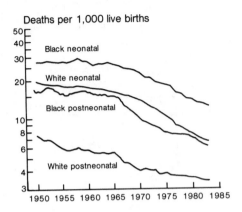

Deaths per 1,000 live births

Black neonatal

White neonatal

Black postneonatal

White postneonatal

Figure 7.2. Showing infant mortality differences between racial groups in the United States between 1950 and 1985. Reproduced with permission from U.S. Dept. of Health and Human Services, Public Health Service, Health United States, Maryland, 1985.

every 1,000 never reach the age of 5 years in some Third World Countries. Even within developed countries among certain ethnic groups infant mortality is high (Figure 7.2). Undoubtedly these high death rates will decrease as more, and better procedures are developed for early diagnosis and surgical treatment of the worst abnormalities. Encouragingly, the survival of the least impaired of those suffering from congenital abnormalities at birth, differs little from those normally born (see the stem end of Figure 7.1(1)). Crucial future ethical decisions, not yet addressed however, may determine the extent of future medical effort directed at extending the survival of the most severely mentally and structurally handicapped. In much of the world, however, a much more urgent task than the one of delicate ethics just discussed is one of providing adequate nutrition, primary health care and immunization against infectious diseases for all infants and children. The World Health Organization (WHO) currently has a long range plan, begun in 1974 and extending to 1990, to immunize all the children of the world, while also strengthening primary health care support in many Third World Countries. Figure 7.3 shows the mortal infectious diseases of childhood which the above program is attempting to eradicate (Henderson, 1987).

7.2.3 Degenerative Disease

At the opposite end of the age spectrum, degenerative tissue diseases are brought about by aging, environmental or self-inflicted abuse. Both the onset and progress of such disease is usually insidious. The manifestation of clinical symptoms are latent and not obvious.

The above diseases are the most frequent causes of death in middle to old age (Figure 7.1(2)).

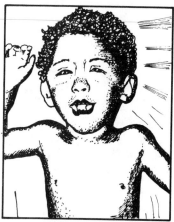

Measles

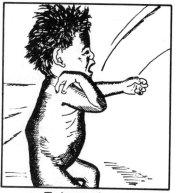

Tuberculosis

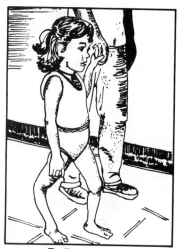

Poliomyelitis

Every 15 seconds a child dies from **measles:** two million children die each year. Virtually every unprotected child will contract the disease, which may be fatal for those already weakened by malnutrition or chronic diarrhoea. Complications occur in about 30 per cent of cases, and include ear infections, diarrhoea, blindness, and encephalitis.

Diphtheria kills between 10 and 15 per cent of its victims. It causes membranes to develop in the throat, and death may follow from asphyxiation. Diphtheria bacilli in the throat also produce a toxin which, in the bloodstream, may attack the heart or nervous system with fatal results.

Some 51 million children contract **pertussis** (whooping cough) every year; over 600,000 of them die from it. The disease got its common name from the "whoop" children make while desperately trying to inhale after coughing spasms. Complications include: malnutrition (due to excessive vomiting after coughing), permanent brain damage and pneumonia.

Neonatal **tetanus** is estimated to cause 800,000 deaths a year. Nearly 100 per cent of newborn babies who get it will die. It is caused by unsterile methods of cutting the umbilical cord or by applying germ-laden substances to the stump. Immunization of the mother will give protection to the baby.

Annually, about 275,000 children are affected by **poliomyelitis**. It is the major cause of lameness in the Third World, where nearly all children get polio before they are three. Although only one out of every 200 infected children develops typical symptoms, among those with recognised polio, one in ten will die

Tuberculosis attacks as many as ten million victims a year, and is particularly lethal for infants. In the lungs, TB can trigger a rapidly fatal pneumonia or a slow wasting disease. In the bone, it can lead to severe deformities. When TB occurs in the brain, the results are usually fatal.

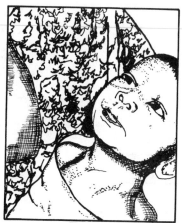

Tetanus

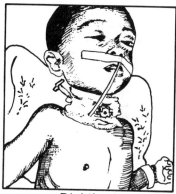

Diphtheria

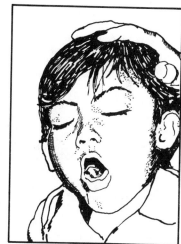

Pertussis

Figure 7.3. Shows six killers of children. Reproduced with permission from Henderson, R.H., **World Health**, 4-7, 1987.

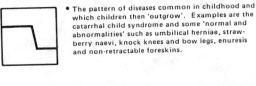
• The pattern of diseases common in childhood and which children then 'outgrow'. Examples are the catarrhal child syndrome and some 'normal and abnormalities' such as umbilical herniae, strawberry naevi, knock knees and bow legs, enuresis and non-retractable foreskins.

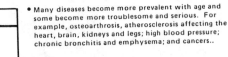
• Many diseases become more prevalent with age and some become more troublesome and serious. For example, osteoarthrosis, atherosclerosis affecting the heart, brain, kidneys and legs; high blood pressure; chronic bronchitis and emphysema; and cancers..

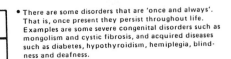
• There are some disorders that are 'once and always'. That is, once present they persist throughout life. Examples are some severe congenital disorders such as mongolism and cystic fibrosis, and acquired diseases such as diabetes, hypothyroidism, hemiplegia, blindness and deafness.

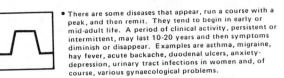
• There are some diseases that appear, run a course with a peak, and then remit. They tend to begin in early or mid-adult life. A period of clinical activity, persistent or intermittent, may last 10-20 years and then symptoms diminish or disappear. Examples are asthma, migraine, hay fever, acute backache, duodenal ulcers, anxiety-depression, urinary tract infections in women and, of course, various gynaecological problems.

• For completeness' sake, this pattern includes collections of symptoms most prevalent in the young and the old. This pattern includes: acute wheezy chests, hydrocoeles, herniae and constipation.

Figure 7.4. A classification of the natural history of disease in humans shows the changing pattern of disease between child- and adulthood. From **Common Diseases**, 4th ed., by H.J. Fry ©1985. Reprinted with permission of MTP Press.

7.2.4 Homeostatic Efficiency

The regulation of bodily functions within a narrow range determines our healthy existence. Continued growth and development of organs and systems into the third decade of life confers considerable plasticity, reserve and control of responses by the body to both internal and external stressors up to this time. Depending upon heredity and life style, effectiveness of function can remain relatively constant for years before finally declining in old age.

The outcome to the stress of a disease process will often be determined by the efficiency of the body's homeostatic mechanisms. The known greater susceptibility of both the very young and the very old to the adverse effects of infections reflects the immaturity or decline of their respective homeostatic systems typically represented by the solid line of Figure 7.1(3). A similar, slightly more extensive classification of the natural history of disease in humans due to Fry (1985), is shown in Figure 7.4.

7.2.5 Epidemiology

Epidemiological science has grown gradually from its original narrow base of inquiry into the etiology (history of development) and progress of infections, epidemics, diseases such as cholera, plague, typhus, polio and typhoid, to the broad based study of all human afflictions (Glass, 1986). Included now, are chronic disease states such as bronchitis and emphysema, either environmentally caused or self-induced. Others which might also be viewed as self- or nutritionally-induced are degenerative cardiovascular disease and cancer. Diseases attributed to the social problems of the time such as drug abuse, violence (including both deaths and injuries from illegal and legal (police) interventions), accidents, suicides and unintended pregnancies have also increased in modern society. Table 7.1 reflects a changing evaluation of society's loss from disease, from one counting only the number of years in life, to one numbering the Years of Potential Life Lost (YPLL) by the premature death of individuals before

Table 7.1. Causes of deaths in the U.S.A. in 1984 ranked by estimated years of potential life lost before age 65 and by deaths per 100,000 population.

Cause of death	Years of potential life lost (rank)	Deaths per 100,000 (rank)
All causes (total)	11,761,000	866.7
Unintentional inj.	2,308,000 (1)	40.1 (4)
Malignant neoplasms	1,803,000 (2)	191.6 (2)
Heart diseases	1,563,000 (3)	324.4 (1)
Suicide, homicide	1,247,000 (4)	20.6 (7)
Congenital abnorm.	684,000 (5)	5.6 (10)
Prematurity	470,000 (6)	3.5 (11)
Sudden infant death	314,000 (7)	2.4 (12)
Cerebrovascular dis.	266,000 (8)	65.6 (3)
Chronic liver diseases and cirrhosis	233,000 (9)	11.3 (9)
Pneumonia, influenza	163,000 (10)	25.0 (6)
Chronic obstructive pulmonary diseases	123,000 (11)	29.8 (5)
Diabetes mellitus	119,000 (12)	15.6 (8)

Reprinted with permission from **Centers for Disease Control**, 35: 1986.

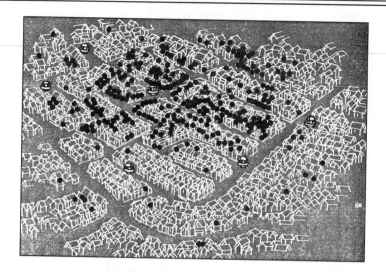

Figure 7.5. More than 100 years ago John Snow determined how cholera spread in London from contaminated public drinking water at the Broad Street Pump. Reproduced with permission from Life and Health, CRM Books, 1972.

the conclusion of a normally productive life. This is defined as one lasting for 65 years. Ranked in this way, quite a different view of a disease's importance may be recognized (Centers for Disease Control, 1986).

Epidemiological investigations of any sort still follow a similar deductive course as the one first introduced by John Snow more than 100 years ago. He determined how cholera spread in London from contaminated public drinking water at the Broad Street Pump (Figure 7.5).

Now, modern methods of analytical epidemiology assist in the prevention of diseases of yet undetermined cause, e.g. Reye's syndrome (a childhood disease characterized by brain and visceral degeneration). This disease was linked epidemiologically to aspirin therapy taken during flu or **chickenpox** illness in children. Although the mechanism of its action still remains unknown, elimination of the use of aspirin has reduced the prevalence of the already rare syndrome (Barrett et.al., 1986; Remington et al., 1986).

An alliance between epidemiological investigation and modern laboratory methods is becoming especially fruitful in the identification and characterization of new diseases such as: toxic shock syndrome (TSS) identified with the toxin from a bacterium (Shands, 1980), **Staphylococcus Aures**, found in women using a certain brand of tampon; diseases from a family of viruses producing Legionnaire's Disease (**Legionella pneumophila**) and outbreaks of nonbacterial gastroenteritis (**Norvalk virus**); a Human Immunodeficiency Virus (HIV) from the association of **Pneumocystis Carinii Pneumonia** (a marker for immunodeficient hosts) to high risk diverse groups of homosexuals, intravenous drug users, hemophiliacs (from transfusions), all of whom subsequently showed the AIDS virus. Similarly significant advances in biostatistical treatment of data have proved vital in the completion of large complex epidemiological studies, such as the Framingham study (1967-87) of risk variables for coronary heart disease (Truett et. al., 1967), and the study of the effects of smoking in 34,440 British doctors (1951-1971) carried over several years (Doll and Peto, 1976).

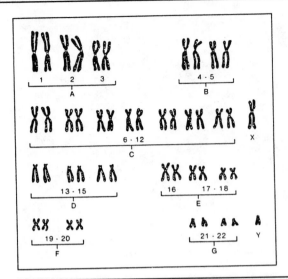

Figure 7.6. Showing a karyotype prepared from lymphocytes of a human male obtained during the metaphase stage of cell division. Reproduced with permission from **Gray's Anatomy**, 36th ed., 1980.

7.3 CAUSES OF DISEASE

Deterioration of normal cell function into disordered or abnormal states constitutes a condition we have defined as ill or diseased. This state may derive separately from intrinsic or extrinsic factors or from a synergistic interaction of both these effects.

7.3.1 Intrinsic Factors

Intrinsic factors arise in two ways, first from aberrations in transcription and expression of genetic information which controls tissue growth or species reproduction, and secondly from abnormal hypo-or hyper-sensitive reactions to invading antigens.

GENETICS: THE PROCESS OF INHERITANCE

Fundamental to good health is a requirement that the structural integrity and metabolic activity of the organism is precisely ordered and controlled from the cell level.

The instructions ordering normal cellular function reside in the DNA (deoxyribonucleic acid) of the cell nucleus. The original fertilized cell, a zygote, acquires all its DNA from the fusion of the male sperm with the female ovum each termed a gamete. Human gametes have their total DNA complement shaped into 23 bodies called chromosomes one of which is a distinctive sex chromosome (an X chromosome for female; a Y for male). In the human species the 23 chromosomes in each gamete pair with each other on fusion so that each zygote contains 23 pairs of chromosomes, 22 pairs of which are called autosomes because they appear as equals. Two remaining chromosomes may both be X chromosomes, one each from the female gamete (ovum), and the male gamete (sperm) respectively, or one X from the female and one Y from the male. Thus, the new cells from this union will either be female (22 pairs of autosomes and an X and X) or male (22 pairs of autosomes and an X and Y). The 23 pairs of chromosomes in the new living cell gain stability not only from the genetic integrity of the

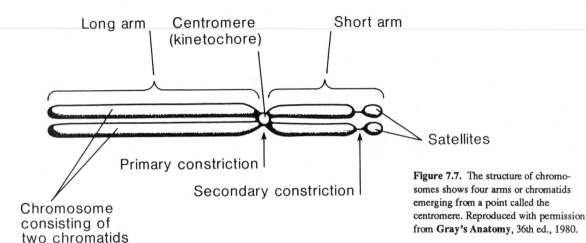

Figure 7.7. The structure of chromosomes shows four arms or chromatids emerging from a point called the centromere. Reproduced with permission from **Gray's Anatomy**, 36th ed., 1980.

immediate parent's (since they had themselves, survived long enough to procreate), but also from the general genetic diversity contained in the total gene pool of the human species developed over centuries. This has allowed for a continuous healthy evolution of the species and its adaptation to the surrounding environment. In the repeated cycle of growth, death and reproduction, new germ cells which differentiate from the zygote will again each contain only half the chromosomes needed in the cells of a new organism. Thus, 23 pairs of chromosomes result each time from a union of sperm and ova as a new life is formed. All cells of the human species always contain 23 pairs of chromosomes except sperm and ovum which contain 23 unpaired chromosomes. During growth, the single original cell of the zygote divides repeatedly, growing and differentiating into daughter cells. These eventually differentiate (develop) into every sort of cell, tissue and organ found in the human, e.g. heart, liver, muscles, nerves, etc., according to instructions bound in the original 23 pairs of chromosomes inherited from the male and female parents. Every cell thus formed in the organism contains in its nucleus the karyotype (fingerprint) of the original zygote. Figure 7.6 shows a karyotype prepared from lymphocytes of a human male (one X and one Y sex chromosome with 22 autosomal pairs).

GENETICS AND HEREDITABLE TRAITS

An appreciation of genetic influence on disease states requires some understanding of cellular growth and reproduction. The process of cell division and growth is called mitosis and the formation of germinal cells for reproduction and the transfer of hereditable traits is meiosis. The structure of chromosomes, best seen during cell division typically shows four arms or chromatids emerging from a point called the centromere (Figure 7.7).

The chromatids are each composed of regularly repeating units of purine-pyrimidine base molecules with sugar and phosphate residues, called deoxyribonucleic acid (DNA). Each unit is a triplet combination of 3 out of 4 possible bases used, guanine (G) cystine (C) adenine (A) and thymine (T) (Figure 7.8).

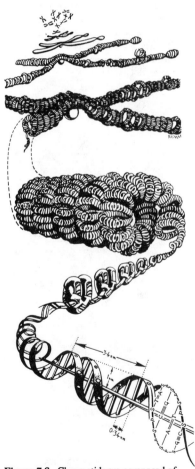

Figure 7.8. Chromatids are composed of regularly repeating molecules called DNA. Reproduced with permission from **Gray's Anatomy**, 36th ed., 1980.

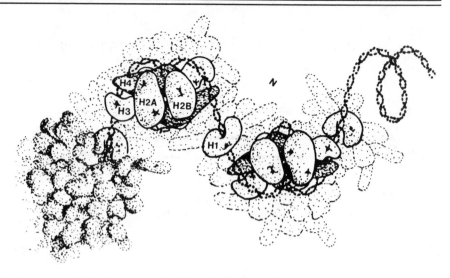

Figure 7.10. Histones and non-histones form part of the chromatin of the nucleus. From **The Genetic Basis for Human Disease**, by K.H. Muench ©1979. Reprinted with permission of Elsiveir, North-Holland Inc.

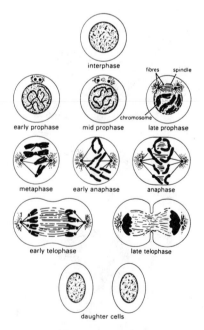

Figure 7.9. Mitosis, the duplication of cells. From **The Genetic Basis for Human Disease**, by K.H. Muench ©1979. Reprinted with permission of Elsiveir, North-Holland Inc.

Different combinations of bases e.g. C.A.T. or G.A.C. etc., code for the assembly of any 1 of 20 essential amino acids, from molecules available in the cytoplasm of the cell. Sixty-four triplet combinations of base linkages are possible but since only 20 are needed to code for the 20 essential amino acids it is likely that particular amino acids are coded by 2 or more triplets. Sets of triplet sequences or codons, often numbering in the hundreds, are able to assemble proteins which are composed of many amino acids linked together. The aggregations of triplet or codon units coding for an individual protein or protein enzyme is called a gene. Thus, a protein like hemoglobin, containing 300 amino acids, requires a length of DNA (a gene) 900 bases long (300 x 3) to command its formation. The total number of single genes coding for structural and enzymatic proteins in humans number some 50,000, all of which are contained in the 46 chromosomes (23 pairs) of the cell.

Before cells duplicate in mitosis (Figure 7.9) the DNA content of the cell doubles so that each daughter cell carries the exact information in its DNA to instruct formation of the next cell generation (growth) in the exact image of the parent cell (zygote). Various cells and organs of the body develop differently in order to perform a specific function e.g. digestion or respiration. As discussed previously this process is called differentiation and both the sequence and exact timing of different forms of the original cell appearing in the organism e.g. skin, nerve cells, is ordered by information specified in the original 46 chromosomes (the genome) of the parent cell (zygote) and carried on from one generation of cell to another.

Some DNA of the nucleus has no function in coding for a specific protein. It occupies space (spacer DNA), between genes and may have a function in timing the on and off signals controlling key differentiations of the cell into new tissues and organs. Other proteins called histones and non-histones also form part of the chromatin of the nucleus, only 15% of which is actually nucleic acid DNA (Figure 7.10).

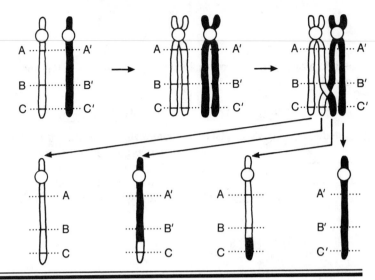

Figure 7.11. Meiosis, cells reproduce but daughter cells contain only 1/2 the DNA content of the parent cell. Adapted from **Principles of Human Genetics** by Curt Stern. Copyright 1949 ©1960, 1973. Reprinted with permission of W.H. Freeman and Company

Within the germ cells, during the meiosis phase of reproduction, (Figure 7.11) autosomal chromosomal pairs, come together to form bivalent chromosomes. Four chromatids appear in the bivalent chromosomes and genetic information is exchanged between them by successive intertwining, breaking and rejoining of chromatids from each autosome (Figure 7.11). The bivalent chromosome is then segregated into two distinct cells each with only 1/2 (haploid content) the DNA of the parent (diploid content) cell. Subsequent division of these haploid cells, each still with the haploid 1/2 DNA content of the parent cell finally produces 4 germ cells with the haploid DNA content ready to fuse with a haploid DNA content of another germ cell. This union (at fertilization) restores the full diploid DNA content of the zygote from which all the tissues of a new organism differentiate. The only non-homologous chromosomes not available for pairing in the initial stage of meiosis are the X and Y chromosomes, the sex chromosomes, and these attach only at limited points producing segmental pairing along their length.

This seemingly complicated method of producing progeny in all animal species ensures a large variation in the total gene pool of that species. Each parent offers 2^{23} (8 million) possible chromosome combinations to their gamete thus each set of parents offers 2^{23} x 2^{23} possible chromosome combinations to an offspring. Genes at the same locus, on homologous chromosomes, ordering the same protein or enzyme formation are called alleles and a further variation in offspring chromosomal gene content is due to the crossing over phenomena taking place in meiosis, shuffling and segregating alleles at linked loci. This provides a truly unlimited number of possible autosomal combinations.

GENE DOMINANCE AND RECESSION
Since one of a homologous pair of autosomes comes from each parent, genes at specific loci on each chromosome may be different versions (alleles) of a gene coding for an enzyme, influencing eye colour for

Table 7.2. Possible progeny from autosomal heterozygous dominant (G) and recessive (g) genes.

Parents	Sperm and Ova	Combinations/Offspring
Heterozygous male	G———GG	homozygous dominant trait shown
	g———Gg	heterozygous dominant trait shown
Heterozygous female	G———Gg	heterozygous dominant trait shown
	g———gg	homozygous recessive trait shown

example. When alleles are different the cell is heterozygous for that gene. If alleles are identical this determines the homozygous condition for that gene. If only one of the two different alleles determines the outcome of gene expression. i.e. the protein, enzyme or visible trait produced, this gene is the dominant one of the two (and is referred to by the upper case of a single letter allocated to the particular genetic trait); the other is recessive (referred to by a lower case letter). If autosomal heterozygous alleles exist in both parents for a specific trait, one of which (G), is dominant and the other a minor variant of the trait, (g), which is recessive, their off-spring have various possibilities of showing either trait (Table 7.2).

AUTOSOMAL SINGLE GENE-DEFECT DISEASE

It is clear that the processes of mitosis and meiosis are sufficiently complicated and variable in their final product that there is abundant room for error in the transcription of DNA during both cell replication and germ cell formation. If an error in only a single base of an active gene causes impairment or non-production of a vital structural protein or enzyme, a serious structural or metabolic disease may result.

Chemical action, radiation, even the processes of intertwining, breakage and readjustment of allele DNA and its rejoining during crossover in meiosis, produce substitution or modification (mutation) of an allele and determine a number of alternative genetic expressions which may quite possibly be detrimental in character.

Mutation is more serious when it occurs in a germinal cell since any defect is then passed on to progeny. A single abnormal gene may result in disease depending on whether:

- the abnormal gene is dominant or recessive,
- the protein or enzyme, now unable to be coded by the aberrant gene is vital to function.

Fetuses with single-gene aberrations formerly coding for an important protein will often abort or be still-born. Defects, in coding for a less

Table 7.3. Both parent's heterozygous for the recessive aberrant gene (f) and the normal gene (F).

Parents	Sperm and Ova	Combinations/Offspring
Heterozygous Male	F ⎯ FF	homozygous dominant normal
	f ⎯ Ff	heterozygous dominant normal
Heterozygous Female	F ⎯ Ff	heterozygous dominant normal
	f ⎯ ff	homozygous recessive abnormal

important protein probably has little effect. However, the survival (by whatever means) and later parenting (reproduction) of persons with genetic disorders often causes serious medical problems, which are often life-threatening to both the mother and fetus. Some single-gene aberrations produce well-recognized diseases. They are caused either by the presence of one dominant or two recessive defective genes on homologous chromosomes.

DOMINANT-GENE DISEASE

Serious disease caused by a dominant gene defect is rarely passed on to the next generation since a person with such an affliction is always suffering from it, is ill and generally debilitated and tends not to reach the age for procreating. In addition, either by design or due to illness, the person often has not reproduced. Some less serious, dominant gene defect-diseases may allow the sufferer to live long enough to reproduce. Some are also caused by mutations in DNA arising spontaneously later in life from environmental influences. Examples of some dominant gene diseases are:
• **Osteogenesis Imperfecta** which is imperfect bone formation due to a defect in formation of the protein collagen,
• **Huntington's Chorea** (Saint Vitas Dance) causes a gradual loss of intellect (dementia) and deterioration of the nervous system.
Dominant-gene defects are easy to trace since they occur in every generation (The Open University, 1985).

RECESSIVE-GENE DISEASE

In order for this type of disease to be manifest, each parent must provide at least one abnormal-recessive gene to an autosomal pair in the zygote. Thus, each parent may be heterozygous for the gene and a recessive aberrant allele silently carries the disease while the other dominant allele of the pair expresses the normal condition. 25% of their offspring will be affected (Table 7.3). In the case that one affected parent is homozygous for the aberrant-recessive gene and one parent heterozygous for the gene, 50% of their offspring will be affected (Table 7.4).

Table 7.4. One parent Homozygous and One parent heterozygous for the recessive aberrant gene (f).

Parents	Sperm and Ova		Combinations/OffSpring
Homozygous Female	f	fF	heterozygous dominant normal
	f	ff	homozygous recessive abnormal
Heterozygous Male	F	fF	heterozygous dominant normal
	f	ff	homozygous recessive abnormal

Disorders caused by enzyme defects are generally inherited in the recessive mode. Examples of recessive-gene diseases are:

- **Cystic fibrosis,** a defect of surfactant causing excessively thick and viscous mucus formation in the lungs and pancreas. It occurs in 1 of 2,000 live births.
- **Tay-Sachs disease,** an enzymatic disease causing fat accumulation in the brain resulting in blindness, convulsions and death at an early age. Occurs in 1 of 2,000 live births.
- **Sickle-Cell anemia,** a structural defect in the hemoglobin causing problems due both to blood flow and to anemia. This is not completely a recessive-gene disorder. Strangely enough, it protects a person against malaria!
- **Phenylketonuria,** caused by a defective gene normally coding for a liver enzyme, which breaks down phenylalanine, a substance otherwise accumulating in the brain, to produce brain damage and mental retardation. The disease is managed by controlling the environmental conditions. In this case maintaining a phenylalanine free diet.

SEX-LINKED, SINGLE GENE-DEFECT DISEASE

X and Y chromosomes are different in length and carry different genes. A defective gene may occur on either sex chromosome. A dominant gene on one X chromosome of a pair in the female will obscure the effect of an aberrant, recessive, defective-gene present on the paired X chromosome. In males with only one X and one Y chromosome such a blockage of a recessive gene defect is not possible. Thus diseases, due to both aberrant genes, may be observed in the male.

Recessive aberrant genes do not show the disease in females but they still function as carriers passing an aberrant recessive gene to male offspring. Thus, hemophilia is caused by a recessive aberrant gene carried on the X chromosome and occurs only in males.

Table 7.5. Sex-linked gene disease carried on the X chromosome where x is the aberrant recessive chromosome.

Parents	Sperm and Ova	Progency
Male	X ——— XX Y ——— Yx	homozygous dominant normal heterozygous recessive abnormal
Female	X ——— XY x ——— Xx	heterozygous normal heterozygous dominant normal

The sex-linked, aberrant recessive gene produced disease shown above in Table 7.5, is carried in the Xx condition in female progeny and manifest in male progeny.

CHROMOSOME-LINKED DISEASE

During cell division two possibilities for dysfunctional chromosomes arise. The first may be due to physical loss of part of a chromosome arising from breaks in the chromosomal material which then fails to be repaired. Diseases due to this cause are rather rare. Significantly more important are the diseases caused by the non-uniform segregation of chromosomes (autosomes or sex chromosomes) into two cells during replication.

Chromosome Non-disjunction

Separation of each chromosome of a pair into two chromatids and the subsequent migration of equal numbers of chromatids (one from each chromosome division) to poles in different halves of the dividing cell is called disjunction of the chromosome (Figure 7.12). Disjunction occurs during cell replication. Non-disjunction therefore describes failure of some chromosomes to divide and segregate into the daughter cells. Spontaneous non-disjunction of chromosome number 21 during mitosis or during reduction division in meiosis causes the presence of 3 number 21 chromosomes in one daughter cell with only 1 in the other and produces the mongoloid appearance and mental retardation observed in Down's Syndrome children. The Down's Syndrome karyotype (Figure 7.13) may be compared with the normal karyotype (Figure 7.6) The 3 chromosomes in the 21 position (trisomy 21) may be clearly seen. Sex-linked nondisjunction of X and Y chromosomes cause Turner's Syndrome (XO) seen in 1 in 500 births and Klinefelter's Syndrome (XXY or XYY), seen in 1 in 500 births. XXY patients develop as men with testes and penis, XO patients possess no female genitalia and abnormal ovaries which do not secrete estrogen. XYY males, are considered to have behavioral problems, and slightly

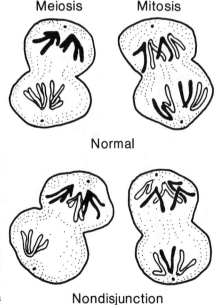

Figure 7.12. Non-disjunction is the failure of some chromosomes to divide and segregate into the daughter cells. From **The Genetic Basis of Human Disease** by H.J. Muench ©1979. Reprinted with permission of Elsevier, North-Holland Inc.

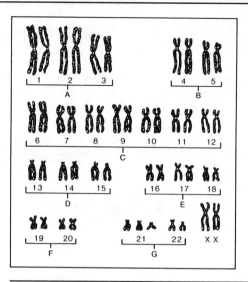

Figure 7.13. The 3 chromosomes in position 21 are clearly seen in the Down's Syndrome karyotype. Reproduced with permission from The Open University, **The Biology of Health and Disease** ©1985. The Open University Press.

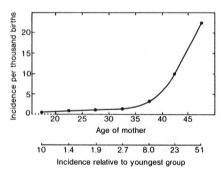

Figure 7.14. The effect of maternal age on the incidence of Down's Syndrome. Reproduced with permission from The Open University, **The Biology of Health and Disease** ©1985. The Open University Press.

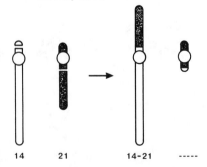

Figure 7.15. The translocation of the long arm of chromosome 21 to the short arm of chromosome 14 forming chromosome 14-21. From **Principles of Human Genetics**, 3/E. by Curt Stern. Copyright 1949 ©1960, 1973. Reprinted with permission of W.H. Freeman and Company.

lower intelligence but show no aggressive or criminal behavior. The frequency of autosomal non-disjunction in maturing ova increases with age. The effect of maternal age on the incidence of Down's Syndrome is shown in Figure 7.14. Each year an estimated 300,000 American women over 35 are pregnant and at risk of carrying a genetically defective fetus. There seems to be a particularly dominant maternal effect producing autosomal trisomy. It has been suggested that of the 750,000 oocytes present at birth, the most "fit" self-select for possible fertilization during the early fertile years after menarche, but as the years pass by only the "unfit" are left over. The dormant nature of this process contrasts with the short time course of spermatogenesis (64 days). This may render the oocyte more susceptible to non-disjunction during reduction division in gametogenesis. A preventive procedure now taken to diagnose a Down's Syndrome fetus called amniocentesis determines the karyotype of the developing fetus from sloughed off cells in the amniotic fluid and affords the parents the option of aborting a defective fetus. It is recommended that most pregnant women past 38 have this test performed.

Chromosome Translocation

Although Down's Syndrome usually arises sporadically due to nondisjunction, some cases also result from a genetic defect produced by a process termed translocation. Here a major segment of one chromosome is joined to another, to form a composite chromosome carrying enough genetic information to be recognized as the third contributor to a trisomy aggregation in a zygote. Thus, the translocation of the long arm of chromosome 21 to the short arm of chromosome 14 forms chromosome 14-21 (Figure 7.15). This is now able to form the third component of trisomy during normal mitosis. The translocation chromosome may be carried by either parent or may occur during an otherwise normal cell division in the developing fetus.

Many disease states may now be recognized as developing from inherited or mutated single gene aberrations of the genome which determines an essential enzyme or structural protein, the gene product. As described, these diseases are inherited either in autosomal dominant (1,200 known diseases) or recessive modes (1,000 known diseases); caused by errors in rejoining or repairing broken chromosomes (translocations); or are due to extra chromosomes carried in a cell nucleus (e.g., trisomy).

In addition many disorders arise from polygenic inheritance. In these cases several gene loci affect the appearance of a disorder (phenotypical expressions). Clearly the incidence of such disorders is not predictable as is single gene disorders from Mendelian principles. Recurrence rates among siblings and offspring of persons suffering this type of polymorphic defect such as cleft palate and lip, congenital dislocation of the hip, club foot and atrial septal defect range up to 7%. Generally, in polygenic disorders, the more severe the original defect, the higher the risk is of its contraction among relatives. Since the full expression of a disorder requires the presence of several genes, the mere presence of one defective one may cause only a partial expression of the disorder, this is called "incomplete penetrance" of a gene.

GENETIC/ENVIRONMENTAL INTERACTIONS
Even those diseases generally recognized as predominantly genetic in origin reveal clear environmental interactions and vice versa. Thus, people in whom there are varying levels of the enzyme aryl hydrocarbon hydroxylase (inherited according to Mendelian rules), which converts arl hydrocarbons in cigarette smoke to more potent carcingogens, may show a varying susceptibility to cancer induced by tobacco. Chemicals, radiation and viruses may all be regarded as environmental agents which act upon genetic material to produce aberrant mutations, detrimental to normal phenotypical expression. In congenital dislocation of the hip, genetic factors include familial joint laxity and acetabular dysgenesis; environmental factors include breech positioning of the fetus and positioning of the lower extremities after birth either maintained in extension and adducted (contraindicated) or abducted and flexed (therapeutic).

CANCER AND GENETICS

Many cancers develop from somatic (non-germinal) cell mutations either in autosomal dominant mode; such as **retinoblastoma, neurofibromatosis** or in autosomal recessive mode; **xeroderma pigmentosum**. Others develop from major translocations such as deletion from the long arm of one of chromosome 22 (in leukemia), usually to number 9. Lack of one chromosome from the number 22 pair is frequently associated with meningiomas; or deletion of a long arm from one of chromosome 13 pair (retinoblastoma).

Some inherited traits carried in autosomal recessive genes affect a cell's ability to repair DNA after its damage by environmental agents such as sunlight. Similarly, some cells lack a protein enzyme which is responsible for excision and repair of broken chromatids, and this leads to the development of skin cancers (Xeroderma pigmentosa).

Many viruses are thought to contribute to chromosomal abnormality and a great amount of research effort is focused on the identification of viral agents responsible for this. However, at the present time (1987), no virus isolated from tumors in humans has been found capable of causing human cells in cultures to grow uncontrollably.

The Epstein-Barr (EB) virus in humans, which is though to interact with genes at a particular locus on chromosome 14, can trigger the formation of Burkitt's Lymphoma. It also causes infectious mononucleosis, a common disease of adults in all countries. A significant difference between individuals who are sero-positive for the EB virus and those developing Burkitt's Lymphoma is that non-malignant cells do not contain the abnormal chromosome 14 noted above.

In a new type of x-linked recessive mode gene deficiency, males demonstrate an inability to resist EB viral infection. Males with this deficiency succumb to mononucleosis or from agammaglobulinemia or from a B-cell lymphoma (see later immune system pathology). The locus on the X-chromosome mediating this response is currently unknown.

The current threat to society from auto immune deficiency syndrome (AIDS) due to Human Immunodeficiency Virus (HIV) results from a RNA virus, which, through the action of a reverse transcriptase enzyme allows the virus to synthesise an exact DNA copy of the viral RNA and be incorporated directly into the transcription machinery of the nucleus of infected cells. Thus, the virus is able to code protein for its own reproduction and it replicates itself with every reproduction of the cell, eventually overwhelming and killing the cell, which is an integral part of the immune system—the T-cell (see AIDS in Chapter 12). Eventually all such T-cells are invaded and killed leaving the organism immunologically defenseless and susceptible to any opportunistic infection contracted. In this way the host quickly succumbs to otherwise non-fatal diseases such as pneumonia.

CORRECTION OF GENETIC DISEASE STATES

Treatment of gene related diseases range from:

- surgery for the phenotypical defect such as retinoblastoma, cleft lip, club foot, etc. This does not cure the cause, but does correct the result;
- removal of accumulated dangerous substrate (such as phenylalanine accumulation which leads to phenylketonuria and brain damage in the developing organism);
- provision of essential missing products, caused by the defect. Thus, giving growth hormone to a deficient subject reactivates normal growth;
- restoration of enzyme action. Defective enzyme activity may sometimes be restored by provision of massive co-enzyme therapy e.g. thiamine therapy for a genetically produced defect in transketolase, lack of which produces a neuropsychiatric disorder.
- induction of enzymes, as an example, steroid hormones seem to control gene expression, and hence induction of enzyme formation, in those cases where genetic deficiency causes the absence or inadequacy of the required protein enzyme. Thus phenobarbital is able to combat a specific type of neonatal jaundice by inducing glucoronyl transferase formation

in the liver, previously lacking in this autosomal dominant disorder called Dubin Johnson disease. More difficult techniques of intracellular enzyme replacement and enzyme modification are also being investigated.

Perhaps the most exciting technique, discussed later in Chapter 11, is popularly known as genetic engineering. Using this technique, specific genes in a DNA strand may be isolated by bacterial enzymes known as restriction endonucleases. Isolated genes formed in this manner may be annealed (spliced) to each other or inserted into a plasmid or molecule of DNA enabling it to exist in bacterial cells. The plasmid may then infect a bacterium, introducing the foreign DNA into it so that the new DNA will be reproduced in cell division and continuously cause the formation of a prescribed protein coded in its DNA structure. In this way a chemically synthesised gene coding for the human hormone somatostatin introduced by the above process into the bacterium Escherichia Coli (E. coli) was able to cause production of 5 gm of somatostatin in a colony of 100 gm bacteria raised on an 8 litre culture medium. Previously, it needed the brains of 1/2 million sheep to produce the same amount of the vital hormone. The potential for good in these techniques is countered by their potential for abuse. Recent controversy (1987) was raised in the U.S.A. when the government allowed patenting of new animal life-forms produced using bioengineering techniques (see Chapter 16).

7.3.2 The Immune Response

The term, immunology, derives from the original Latin word "immunos" which means "exempt from" and came to be used to describe those who were spared infection during the spread of highly contagious diseases. In 1906 Von Pirquet and Schick, building on the pioneering work of Arthus (1903), Richet (1902) and Koch (1890), defined allergy as an altered capacity to react to an environmental poison, brought about by previous contact with that poison.

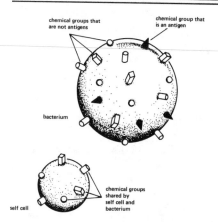

Figure 7.16. Shows normal functioning of the immune system. Reproduced with permission from Roddie & Wallace, **The Physiology of Disease,** 1975.

Figure 7.17. Shows schematically, surface antigens covering self and non-self cells. Modified and reproduced with permission from The Open University, **The Biology of Health and Disease,** ©1985, The Open University Press.

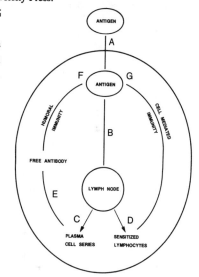

The expanding field of immunology, besides describing the protective effects and mechanisms invoked by the body against invading organisms and toxins, also examines the frequent excesses and deficiences of a system, normally considered beneficial, but which can also produce disease. This branch of the science deals with **immunopathology.**

Normally, the body's immune system protects it against foreign invading substances called **antigens.** The antigens may be either intrinsically harmful to everyone like **germs,** or else be regarded as benign by some but as an irritant or harmful by others, like **pollen** or **dust.** Antigens have a molecular weight greater than 1,000. They contain protein or carbohydrate or both and are recognized by the body as "foreign". Smaller foreign molecules called haptens which would not otherwise stimulate the immune system may combine with some of the body's own protein and become antigenic. The body's own proteins do not elicit an immune response of course, usually being recognized as "friendly".

Figure 7.16 (Roddie and Wallace, 1975) summarizes normal functioning of the immune system. An invading **Antigen (A)** is sensed by cells in the **Lymphatic System (B),** which is a second circulating system collecting and returning fluid from the extravascular spaces to the central circulation. Two defenses then develop, one is **humorally mediated** (along the line FEC) by soluble circulating proteins called **Antibodies (Immunoglobulins, Igs)** which are manufactured from **Plasma Cells** derived from **B-lymphocyte** cells of the lymphatic system. These antibodies circulate freely in the blood with the other plasma proteins. Figure 7.17 shows, schematically, surface antigens covering self and non-self cells. A specific antigen protein characterizes the invading cells and these are recognized by a circulating B cell which then directs the manufacture of specific antibodies to attach to and target the invader (Figure 7.18) for digestion by phagocytic cells; the polymorphonuclear lymphocytes and by macrophages and a variety of other methods.

A second immune response is **cell mediated,** by **T-cells** (along the line

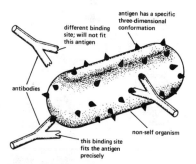

Figure 7.18. Shows that only specific antibodies attach to and target the invader for digestion by phagocytic cells. Modified and reproduced with permission from The Open University, **The Biology of Health and Disease,** ©1985, The Open University Press.

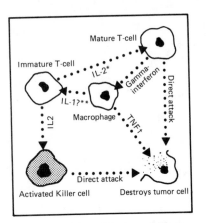

Figure 7.21. Cytotoxic T-cells are part of the induced immune response and are capable of acting against the invading organism. Reproduced with permission from **The Economist**, June, 1987.

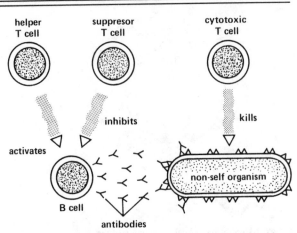

Figure 7.22 Shows T-cell mediated immunity. Reproduced with permission from Health and Disease, The Open University, **The Biology of Health and Disease**, ©1985. The Open University Press.

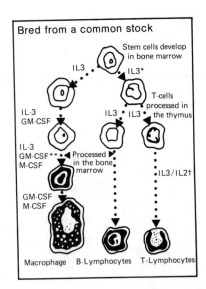

Figure 7.19 Cell mediated immune response shows how T-cells, B-lymphocytes and macrophages originate from the same precursor stem cells in the bone marrow. Reproduced with permission from **The Economist**, June, 1987.

GD, Figure 7.16) which are formed from the same precursor stem cells in the bone marrow as B-lymphocyte cells but are then developed further in the Thymus gland before being released into the blood stream (Figure 7.19). Both B and T-cells are sequestered in peripheral lymphoid tissue (in lymph nodes, spleen, tonsillar tissue, respiratory tract, urinary tract, gut, and bone marrow). Figure 7.20 (**Gray's Anatomy**, 1984) illustrates the general organization of these defensive mechanisms in responding to an antigenic stimulus. Both B-lymphocytes and T-lymphocytes are aroused directly by an antigenic stimulus which may be enhanced by the secondary effects of substances formed from defensive cells called macrophages. These substances (1L-1, 1L-2, 1L-3, etc.), activate various T-cell formations e.g. Helper T-cells which facilitate differentiation of B-lymphocytes to the plasma cells (plasmocyte), producing antibodies (the gammaglobulins), and suppressor T-cells which limit the above action thus providing a balancing effect. Cytotoxic T-cells are also part of the induced immune response and are capable of acting independently and directly against the invading organism or in conjunction with antibodies from B lymphocytes (Figure 7.21). Cytotoxic T-cells are particularly effective against viruses which shelter inside the cell itself but which leave markers at cell surface level identifying that they are there (Figure 7.22). Unfortunately, the action of cytotoxic T-cells is also to kill the invaded cell as well as the virus. Neutralization of microorganisms and other antigens invading the body is effected in various ways: by agglutination i.e. by sticking the affected cells together (agglutin antibodies), making them vulnerable for digestion by phagocytes (large lymphocytes); by lysis or disruption of affected cells (by lysin antibodies); by specific targeting of bacterial cells with opsonins, substances attractive to phagocytes so that this latter type of cell will find and digest the bacteria; macrophages and polymorphonuclear lymphocytes destroy the invader by antitoxin action of antibodies forming a nontoxic product with the invading toxin itself or with toxins released from invading microrganisms. Several of these actions, principally those acting

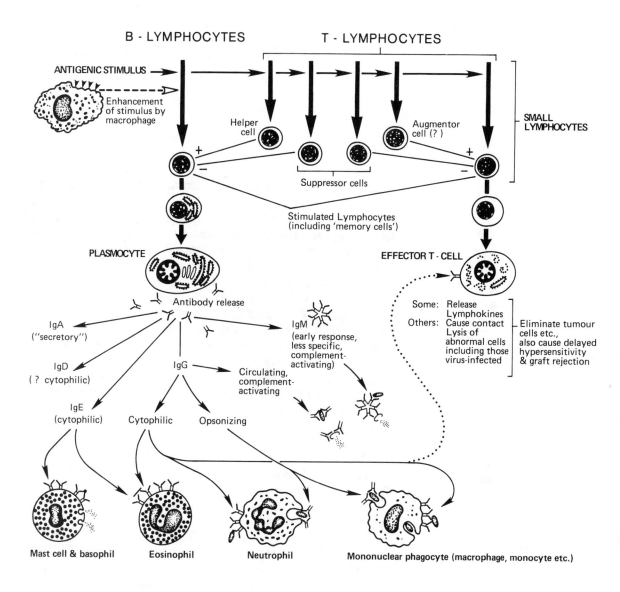

Figure 7.20. Shows the general organization of defense mechanisms in responding to an antigenic stimulus. Reproduced with permission from **Gray's Anatomy**, 36th ed., 1980.

through the antibodies IgG and IgM activate other soluble plasma proteins called **Complement** which form a membrane attack complex (MAC) capable of disrupting and digesting all cell membranes (producing a lot of cellular debri, inflammation and local temperature increase in the process).

Cell mediated immunity provided by the small lymphocytes of the T system (killer T-cells) also result from the lytic action (disruption and destruction) of factors released from lymphocytes acting on the invader. These cells are attracted to the site of antigen invasion and attach directly on the invading cell. In the case of allografts (transplants of foreign tissue or organs), the immune response has to be suppressed with drugs to allow a graft to "take". A complex, T-cell mediated immunity is thought to be a significant factor in control of cancer cells in the body since cancer cells differ antigenically from normal cells (Figure 7.22). **Interferons** are specific immunological proteins also manufactured in this latter response

IMMUNOPATHOLOGY

Defective immunological protection can leave the host organism suceptible to opportunistic infections by foreign substances; in addition, healthy cells caught up within the local battle can hardly proceed with normal body function, or without some damage to themselves. A disease process (pathology) can also result from the normally protective immune system providing either a too little or too vigorous immunological response, thus (in Figure 7.23):

- if an unusually severe reaction against an invading antigen is aroused, healthy cells or body systems may become hyperactive and damaging e.g. mast cell responses;
- infection results if sufficient action against an invading antigen is not aroused (immunodeficiency). This deficiency may be congential (present from birth) or acquired later in life;
- the body may inadvertently produce antibodies against itself and destroy its own tissues (autoantibodies);

HYPERSENSITIVITY

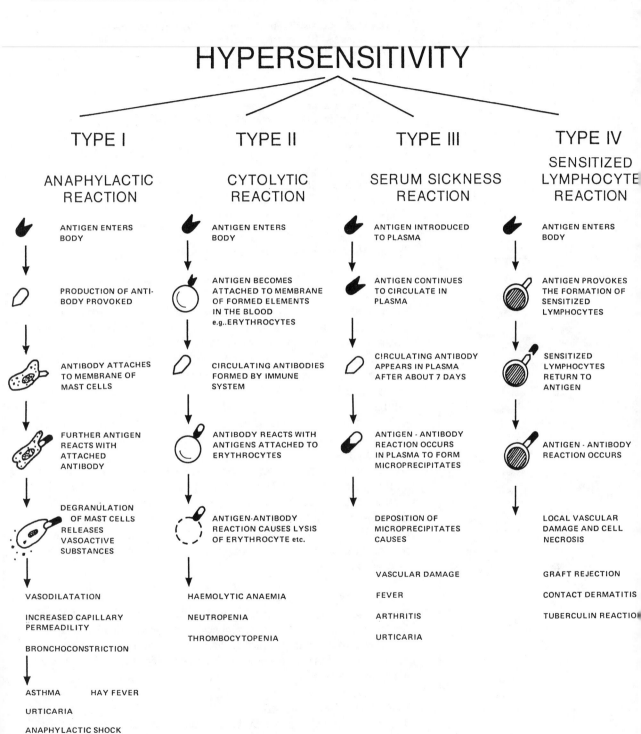

TYPE I	TYPE II	TYPE III	TYPE IV
ANAPHYLACTIC REACTION	CYTOLYTIC REACTION	SERUM SICKNESS REACTION	SENSITIZED LYMPHOCYTE REACTION

TYPE I — ANAPHYLACTIC REACTION

ANTIGEN ENTERS BODY

PRODUCTION OF ANTIBODY PROVOKED

ANTIBODY ATTACHES TO MEMBRANE OF MAST CELLS

FURTHER ANTIGEN REACTS WITH ATTACHED ANTIBODY

DEGRANULATION OF MAST CELLS RELEASES VASOACTIVE SUBSTANCES

VASODILATATION

INCREASED CAPILLARY PERMEADILITY

BRONCHOCONSTRICTION

ASTHMA   HAY FEVER

URTICARIA

ANAPHYLACTIC SHOCK

TYPE II — CYTOLYTIC REACTION

ANTIGEN ENTERS BODY

ANTIGEN BECOMES ATTACHED TO MEMBRANE OF FORMED ELEMENTS IN THE BLOOD e.g..ERYTHROCYTES

CIRCULATING ANTIBODIES FORMED BY IMMUNE SYSTEM

ANTIBODY REACTS WITH ANTIGENS ATTACHED TO ERYTHROCYTES

ANTIGEN-ANTIBODY REACTION CAUSES LYSIS OF ERYTHROCYTE etc.

HAEMOLYTIC ANAEMIA

NEUTROPENIA

THROMBOCYTOPENIA

TYPE III — SERUM SICKNESS REACTION

ANTIGEN INTRODUCED TO PLASMA

ANTIGEN CONTINUES TO CIRCULATE IN PLASMA

CIRCULATING ANTIBODY APPEARS IN PLASMA AFTER ABOUT 7 DAYS

ANTIGEN - ANTIBODY REACTION OCCURS IN PLASMA TO FORM MICROPRECIPITATES

DEPOSITION OF MICROPRECIPITATES CAUSES

VASCULAR DAMAGE

FEVER

ARTHRITIS

URTICARIA

TYPE IV — SENSITIZED LYMPHOCYTE REACTION

ANTIGEN ENTERS BODY

ANTIGEN PROVOKES THE FORMATION OF SENSITIZED LYMPHOCYTES

SENSITIZED LYMPHOCYTES RETURN TO ANTIGEN

ANTIGEN - ANTIBODY REACTION OCCURS

LOCAL VASCULAR DAMAGE AND CELL NECROSIS

GRAFT REJECTION

CONTACT DERMATITIS

TUBERCULIN REACTION

Figure 7.23. Shows how hypersensitivity can lead to the normally protective immune system providing either a too little or, too vigorous immunological response. Reproduced from **The Physiology of Disease**, by I.C. Roddie and W.F.M. Wallace ©1975. Reprinted with permission of Year Book Medical Publishers Inc.

Table 7.6. A classification of immunopathologic mechanisms. Reproduced with permission from Perez-Tamayo, **Mechanisms of Disease: an Introduction to Pathology,** 2nd ed. Copyright © 1985 by Year Book Medical Publishers, Inc., Chicago.

Humoral mechanisms
  Inactivation of biologically active molecules
  Stimulation of biologically active molecules
  Anaphylaxis
  Cytotoxicity
  Immune complex reactions
Cellular mechanisms
  Cytotoxic T cells
  Natural killer cells
  Antibody-dependent cell-mediated cytotoxicity
  Lymphotoxin and other cytotoxic lymphokines
  Cytotoxic macrophages
Combined humoral and cellular mechanisms

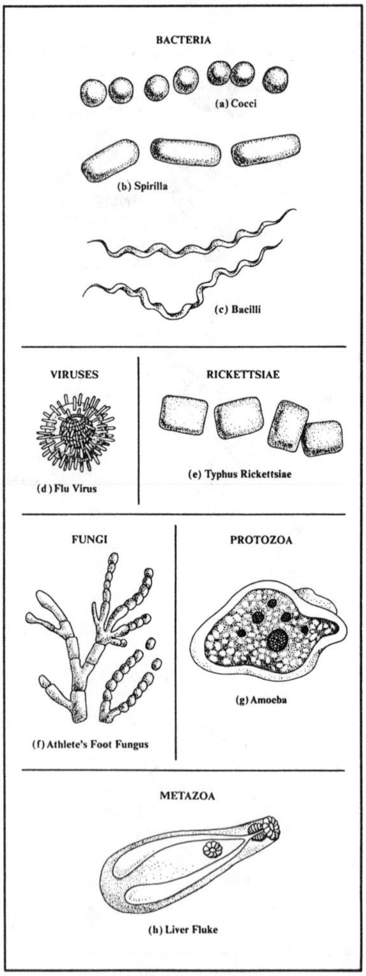

Figure 7.24. Classes of invasive organisms. Reproduced with permission from **Life and Health**, CRM Books, 1972.

- abnormal immune reactions from plasma cells can lead to excessive production of immunoglobulins—which is due to a cancerous growth of plasma cells called multiple myeloma;
- as indicated previously, tissue grafted from one person to another, in an attempted repair process (homo- or allografts), is rejected and dies by the action of transplantation antigens unless the latter are suppressed by drugs.

Increasingly, the lymphocytes of prospective recipient and donor, which carry the transplantation antigens (Human Leukocyte Antigens, HLA), are matched to ensure better graft acceptance. Immuno-suppressive techniques such as x-ray therapy, cytotoxic drugs for lymphocytes, antilymphocyte serum and glucocorticoid treatment are all used to aid in graft acceptance. These procedures however, increase the susceptibility of the recipient to disease from opportunistic infections. Care has to be taken to provide antibiotic treatment and a germ free environment for these patients. Table 7.6 summarizes common immunopathological disease mechanisms.

7.3.3 Extrinsic Factors

Regardless of inner predisposing conditions to illness from constitutional (genetic) or aberrant defensive (immunological) factors, many visible diseases derive directly from extrinsic factors in the form of infective agents or infestations from the external environment which temporarily or permanently overwhelm the body's resistance.

INFECTIVE ORGANISMS

These invasive organisms may be separated into classes (Figure 7.24) which include bacteria, viruses, rickettsia, fungi, single-celled organisms called protozoa, and multi-cellular organisms called metazoa, flukes, round worms and tapeworms. Insects like tics, lice and scabies (Figure 7.25) may also infest the skin and hair and produce disease-like symptoms.

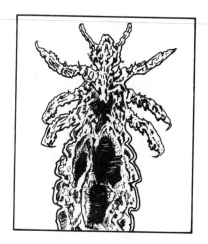 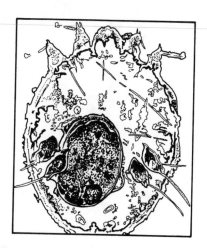

Figure 7.25. Infesting organisms lice (left) and scabies (right). Reproduced with permission from The Open University, **The Biology of Health and Disease,** ©1985. The Open University Press.

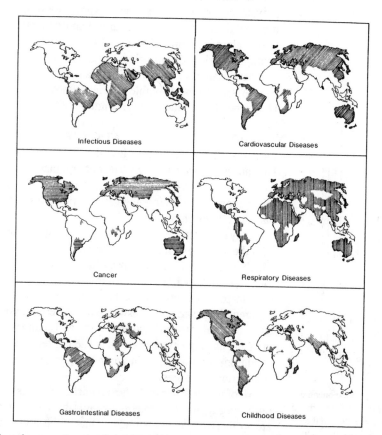

Figure 7.26. Showing the prevalence of some endemic disease throughout the world which have remained relatively unchanged for more than 25 years up to the present time. Reproduced with permission from **Life Health,** CRM Books, 1972.

Our understanding of the nature of individual disease processes, their prevalence, virulence, treatment and prevention has changed considerably during the course of the last century. Many endemic diseases—once highly prevalent in a particular area (Figure 7.26) have been eliminated e.g. smallpox worldwide, malaria in certain regions of Africa and the Panama Zone and Rabies in England. Simultaneously, other threatening diseases have arisen, the most notable in recent times being the Acquired Immune Deficiency Syndrome (AIDS) (Figure 7.27).

THE HOST-PARASITE RELATIONSHIP

Diseases usually result from invasion of the human by microorganisms. Humans play host to a large variety of organisms many of which may also live independent lives elsewhere, in soil, dead animals etc. Regardless of this independence, their human association may be thought of as a host—parasite relationship.

Many organisms may live in quite a symbiotic (agreeable) relationship with the host providing little aggression against the human in the area to which they are confined e.g. bacteria commonly found on the skin, teeth, tongue, throat, each slightly different since they live under the conditions peculiar to their environment. The millions of bacteria living in the gut are different from surface parasites. The bacterial colonization of this area changes in response to local environmental changes, such as with changes in diet. The majority of bacteria in the gut prefer anerobic (low oxygen) conditions with no sunlight and high humidity; quite different from the skin surface parasites.

All of the parasites in the host parasite relationship are capable of demonstrating aggressive behavior towards the host, or it to them if they invade areas otherwise "out of bounds". Thus, if the skin barrier is breached by a parasite so that tissues below the skin are contaminated, through a cut for instance, infection would result. At first this would be noticeable as inflammation resulting from the mobilization of counter agents by the host

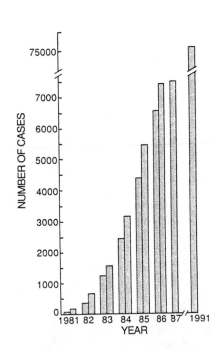

Figure 7.27. Showing the exponential rise in the incidence of AIDS by 6-month intervals every year since 1981 in the U.S.A. Data from U.S. Dept. of Health and Human Services, 1987 and the Coolfont Report, 1986, U.S. Public Health Service.

Table 7.7. Some defense mechansims of the host. Reproduced with permission from Perez-Tamayo, **Mechanisms of Disease: an Introduction to Pathology,** 2nd ed. Copyright © 1985 by Year Book Medical Publishers, Inc., Chicago.

I Local Defense Mechanisms
  A   Mechanical or physical—Dessication, temperature, cellular desquamation, organic secretions (tears, saliva, etc.), cough.
  B   Biochemical—Fatty acids, local pH
  C   Biologic—Lysozyme antibodies (IgA), phagocytosis
  D   Bacterial—Metabolic competition, antibiotic substances

II Systemic Defense Mechanisms
  A   Antibodies
  B   Nonspecific humoral substances—Complement B-lysin, interferon
  C   Phagocytosis—Oxygen-dependent and oxygen-independent microbicidal systems
  D   The immune response—Amplification, increased efficiency and increased specificity of inflammation

against the foreign invasion. The parasite is now termed a pathogen (disease producing). Several mechanisms designed to limit cell damage from aggressive pathogens are shown in Table 7.7. Immediate defense is offered initially at the site of invasion and secondarily by some of the systemic mechanisms already discussed.

LOCAL DEFENSE
Local protection is afforded by physical or mechanical means, biochemical action, biologic mechanisms and by bactericidal actions. In the first of these the physical character of the skin surface usually presents an effective barrier against surrounding pathogens. In addition, a general cleansing factor is effected by continuous desquamation and renewal of the skin surface. Additionally, mechanical filtration of respired gases provided respectively by the tortuosity of respiratory passages, the action of sticky mucous secretions in the pathways and the outward sweeping action of brush-like cilia of the mucosa in the upper respiratory tract protect against deep penetration of particles and bacteria which enter through the external openings of the respiratory system. An important enzyme, lysozyme, carried in the lacrimal fluid (tears) irrigating the eye and surrounding tissue is also carried to the upper respiratory tract through the lacrimal duct and exerts an important bactericidal action in the airways. Other important biochemical entities in the air passages are IgA antibody and complement proteins providing systemic digestive action and protection in these regions. Many bacteria which lack sialic acid in their structure activate what is called the alternative pathway of the complement system of defensive antibody-like protein. IgA is also an important defensive antibody in the respiratory tract because it is resistant to denaturation by the other enzymes and chemicals secreted there. Further on in the deep pulmonary air spaces (alveoli) pulmonary macrophages lie in wait to digest (phagotozise) any bacteria penetrating that far. They are helped in this by more complement and IgA antibodies. Macrophages are continually replaced from the lymphatic system every 20 to 30 days.

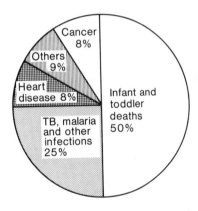

Figure 7.28. Showing the proportion of World deaths (60 million total per year currently) attributable to various causes. The predominant number of infant and toddler deaths are due to infectious diarrhea. From **Common Diseases**, 4th ed., by J. Fry ©1985. Reprinted with permission of MTP Press.

A major entrance to the body for many pathogenic parasites is the digestive tract, and both the number and efficiency of the latter's defenses are high. Nevertheless enteropathogenic (digestive tract—disease causing) bacteria are a serious threat to the immature defenses of infants. A majority of the current 30 million infant deaths per year (Figure 7.28) may be attributed to infectious diarrhea. The thick multistratified lining of the digestive tract is usually a solid defense. More thinly defended areas such as the tonsils are a particular site of infection as are cavities caused by the removal of teeth. The flow of saliva produces some bacteriostatic and bacteriocidal action in the pathway entrance at the mouth and foreign deposits are always moved towards the esophagus for digestion in the stomach, by saliva flow and continuous suction movements of the lips and tongue. Many bacteria penetrating the outer defenses of the digestive tract, e.g. **Salmonella,** are inhibited or destroyed by the acidity of the environment in the stomach. The incidence of **Salmonella** poisoning is nearly 3 1/2 times as high in patients with a total gasterectomy and when contracted is much more severe. During a small cholera outbreak in 1971, (Hornick et.al., 1971) 25% of the victims had had a gastric resection (removal of part of the stomach or intestines).

Some viruses are resistant to the acid environment of the digestive tract and may still flourish causing illness and continuing infection to others by being excreted in the feces (e.g. Hepatitus B virus). Peristalsis (muscular propelling movements of the intestinal wall) and the sweeping action of mucosal villae (filament-like projections from the mucosa) continually deposit bacteria in a thick mucus lining of the intestinal walls. The absence of peristalsis and villae movement will allow bacterial colonies of the digestive tract to flourish and overgrow disrupting fat absorption causing a fall in bile salt concentration and a rise in chemicals thought to be precursors to colon cancers. Paradoxically, some bacteria of the intestine, e.g. **E. coli,** are antagonistic to other enteric (bowel) pathogens and sometimes may be beneficial. The alternative pathway of **complement** activation (a digestive, antibody-like protein) and IgA activation also provide biologic defense against infection in the gut.

Table 7.8. The mononuclear phagocyte system. Reproduced with permission from van Furth, et al., **Mononuclear Phagocytes in Immunity, Infection and Pathology,** 1975.

Cells	Localization
Stem cell (committed)	
Monoblast	Bone marrow
Promonocyte	
Monocyte	Bone marrow
	Peripheral blood
Macrophage	Tissues
	Connective tissue (histiocytes)
	Liver (Kupffer cells)
	Lung (alveolar macrophages)
	Lymph nodes (free and fixed macrophages)
	Bone marrow (macrophages)
	Serous cavities (pleural and peritoneal macrophages)
	Bone tissue (osteoclasts)
	Nervous system (microglia cells)

In the genitourinary tract all the physical, mechanical, biochemical, biologic and bacteriocidal actions already discussed provide defense. Protection against retrograde infection of this system, from the outside is provided by the mechanical and pH effects of urine flow against bacteria ascending the urethra.

SYSTEMIC DEFENSES

General circulatory or systemic defense mechanisms are initiated when penetration of local defenses has been made by any parasite. The separation of systemic defenses into humoral and cellular components has been described previously under Immunopathology. In that context it is apparent during the course of any defensive action, inflammation, phagocytosis (ingestion and digestion of cells) and cellular death inevitably occurs. For the period that it lasts such an occurrence, regardless of outcome, represents a marked departure from normality, easily ranking as an illness or disease. This battle rages during the infective stage; actual development of disease in the host depends on whether the battle is won or lost.

Humoral defenses include the immune response, reacting specifically to particular antigens with specific antibodies to recognize and initiate lysis or phagocytosis of the invading cell. Non-specific substances of the system such as the complement proteins adopt a direct destructive role of their own against the invader forming the membrane attack complex (MAC) while the polypeptide interferons of the system enhance resistance of invaded cells, particularly to viral attack, by inhibiting viral replication.

Systemic cellular defense mechanisms are immediately initiated in response to an invader. This system operates solely for a short period during the time needed for the invader antigens to stimulate humoral antibodies and specific lymphoid cells (Killer T-cells). Phagocytosis continues at a greater rate after the induction of the immune response.

The cells mediating the immediate response, those of the mononuclear phagocyte system (Table 7.8) differentiate (develop) from a common stem cell in the bone marrow which is also the root of another phagocytic cell, the polymorphonuclear leukocyte, which is less specific and more local in action. After migration from the stem cell into the circulation monocytes of the mononuclear phagocytic system divide infrequently. Circulating monocytes are able to leave the blood for the peripheral tissue (where they are now called macrophages) either in response to local inflammatory responses there or to take up a fixed residence in a peripheral space (i.e. the lung) when they cease to divide.

When a parasite overcomes both local defenses and systemic defenses to any degree, a disease process will unfold depending on the parasite's pathogenicity—its capacity to generate disease (e.g. by its capacity to adapt to and multiply in the host) and by the virulence of the disease (measured either by the multiplying rate of the parasite or the powerfulness of any of its released toxins, or both). As noted previously the aggressive behavior of viruses towards a host is especially dangerous since viruses produce infection/disease by becoming incorporated into the genetic machinery of the host cells. It is little wonder that effective chemical treatment (drugs) has not yet been developed against viral infection in humans. It has remained for sensitization of the body's own immune response by vaccination—a preventive treatment, to provide the most effective resistance yet.

INFECTION AND DISEASE

The presence of biologic pathogenic agents in a host is called an infection regardless of whether it becomes manifest or whether it is transitory or permanent. If infection is harboured by a host this denotes a potentially hazardous condition for others whom the otherwise seemingly "healthy" host can infect. Focal infections are those contained by systemic defense mechanisms of the host to local areas such as septic dental caries. Normally these infections present little hazard except in cases where a secondary immune pathologic response is activated e.g. anaphylaxis. When the equilibrium between host and parasite tilts in favor of the parasite during any

Table 7.9. Age-adjusted death rates for selected causes of death, according to sex and race: United States, selected years 1950-84. Data are based on the National Vital Statistics System reported in U.S. Dept. of Health and Human Services, Public Health Service, Health United States, Maryland, 1985.

Sex, race, and cause of death	1950	1960	1970	1980	1981	1982	1983	1984
All races								
All causes			Deaths per 100,000 resident population					
All causes	841.5	760.9	714.3	585.8	568.2	553.8	550.5	547.
Diseases of heart	307.6	286.2	253.6	202.0	195.0	190.5	188.8	183.
Cerebrovascular disease	88.8	79.7	66.3	40.8	38.1	35.8	34.4	33.
Malignant neoplasms	125.4	125.8	129.9	132.8	131.6	132.5	132.6	133.
Respiratory system	12.8	19.2	28.4	36.4	36.6	37.5	37.9	38.
Colorectal	19.0	17.7	16.8	15.5	15.1	15.0	14.9	-
Stomach	14.1	9.3	5.9	4.3	4.2	4.1	4.0	-
Breast	22.2	22.3	23.1	22.7	22.7	22.8	22.7	23.
Chronic obstructive pulmonary diseases	4.4	8.2	13.2	15.9	16.3	16.2	17.4	18.
Pneumonia and influenza	26.2	28.0	22.1	12.9	12.3	10.9	11.8	12.
Chronic liver disease and cirrhosis	8.5	10.5	14.7	12.2	11.4	10.5	10.2	9.
Diabetes mellitus	14.3	13.6	14.1	10.1	9.8	9.6	9.9	9.9
Accidents and adverse effects	57.5	49.9	53.7	42.3	39.8	36.6	35.3	35.8
Motor vehicle accidents	23.3	22.5	27.4	22.9	21.8	19.3	18.5	19.2
Suicide	11.0	10.6	11.8	11.41	11.5	11.6	11.4	11.
Homicide and legal intervention	5.4	5.2	9.1	10.8	10.4	9.7	8.6	8.

infection, a disease state is apparent i.e. clinical features become manifest. Clinical symptoms include both the general and specific, thus fever and leukocytosis (an abnormal increase in the number of leukocytes in the blood) are common features of disease processes. The neurotoxic effect of tetanus toxin (characterized by spasmodic contraction of muscles especially those of the jaw) depends on specific tissue damage effected by the toxin released by the bacteria. Profound metabolic effects of infection include an increased energy requirement which, because it is primarily met from glycogen breakdown, induces a secondary protein catabolism as glycogen reserves are exhausted. This condition seems not to be supressible by serum glucose elevation, either by drinks or infusions, being included in the prescription for treatment. Infection also usually produces anorexia (lack of a desire to eat) and this compounds the problem. Not surprisingly recovered patients are often greeted with the comment "my haven't you lost weight". Some 60% of the protein lost during infections comes from muscle.

Individuals who are particularly susceptible to infection are those in whom the natural immunoresponse has been intentionally supressed as part of a clinical treatment e.g. during chemotherapy and homograft transplants. In the same way diabetes mellitus induces self-immuno suppression exposing the compromised host to continuing danger from opportunistic infection. Protein Energy Malnutrition (PEM) discussed in Chapter 8 also compromises immune system responses and probably accounts in some degree for the widespread infection accompanying this prevalent condition in underdeveloped countries. The epitomy of a compromised host today is the patient suffering from AIDS in whom the specific intent of the Human Immunodeficiency Virus is to destroy the cytotoxic stimulating action of T-Helper cells of the immune system.

7.4 MORBIDITY AND MORTALITY: THE FUTURE YEARS

The current profile of morbidity and mortality among Western nations is very similar. Morbidity in those who still retain some independence results

Table 7.11. Diseases which have a high incidence in poor countries or populations. From **Disease and the Environment,** by A.R. Rees and H.J. Purcell ©1982. Reprinted with permission of John Wiley and Sons Ltd.

Disease	Cause
Related to prevalence of specific infections	
Macronodular cirrhosis/hepatocellular carcinoma	Hepatitis B infection
Rheumatic heart disease	Streptococcal infection
Nephrotic syndrome/glomerulonephritis	Various infections
	P. *malariae*
	S. *Mansoni*
Iron deficiency anaemia	Hookworm infection
Tropical splenomegaly syndrome	Endemic malaria
Related to specific nutrional deficiency	Iodine deficiency
(excluding vitamin deficiency)	related to geography
Endemic goitre/cretinism	plus poor socio-economic conditions

Table 7.10. Diseases which have a high incidence in the Western world or a relatively high incidence in comparison with non-Western populations. From **Disease and the Environment,** by A.R. Rees and H.J. Purcell ©1982. Reprinted with permission of John Wiley and Sons Ltd.

Anatomical Site	Postulated Environmental* Factors
Gastrointestinal	
Hiatus hernia	Diet
Crohn's disease	Diet
Acute appendicitis	Diet
Ulcerative colitis	Diet
Diverticular disease	Diet
Adenomatous polyps	Diet
Carcinoma of the colon	Diet
Carcinoma of the rectum	Diet
Liver and gall bladder	
Cholelithiasis	Diet
Chronic cholecystitis	Diet
Carcinoma of the pancrease	Smoking
Cardiovascular	
Coronary heart disease	Diet. Smoking
Deep vein thrombosis	Diet
Varicose veins	Diet
Respiratory	
Chronic bronchitis and emphysema	Smoking
Carcinoma of the lung	Smoking
Female genital	
Endometriosis	Diet?
Endometrial carcinoma	Diet
Breast	
Fibrocystic disease	Diet?
Carcinoma of breast	Diet
Male genital	
Carcinoma of the prostate	Diet
Metabolic	
Diabetes mellitus Type 2	Diet

primarily from respiratory disfunction and then, in order, rheumatism, emotional problems, gastrointestinal disease and skin disorders. Increasingly in those older than 45 years both males and females suffer from osteoarthritis (a wearing out of joints), leading to arthritis, joint stiffness and pain. Those people committed to primary care have similar incapacities but the rank order changes to respiratory, emotional, gastrointestinal, skin and rheumatic afflictions.

Mortality in developed countries results primarily from cardiovascular disease, then, in order, cancer, respiratory disease, stroke and violence (including motor vehicle accidents). In underdeveloped countries death result, principally from infections, malnutrition and violence (Fry, 1985).

Age adjusted death rates in the U.S.A. for all age groups between 1950-84 from major disease (notably, these are all non-infectious diseases) are shown in Table 7.9. Diseases specifically prevalent in western and underdeveloped countries and their probable precipitating environmental stimuli are shown in Tables 7.10 and 7.11 respectively.

In recent years death from cardiovascular disease has declined remarkably in Western societies, a decline which peculiarly has not extended to the centrally planned economies of Eastern Europe. This decline and the distribution of cardiovascular diseases in some developed and developing countries of the world is shown in Figure 7.29.

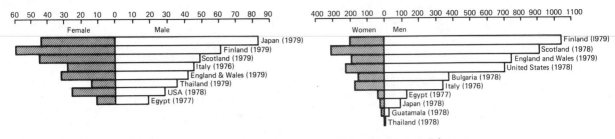

Cerebrovascular Disease

Coronary Artery Disease

Countries and areas	Period	Cardiovascular Diseases		Ischaemic Heart Disease		Cerebrovascular Disease		All Causes	
		Male	Female	Male	Female	Male	Female	Male	Female
Japan	1972-1982	-36.4	-41.8	-21.6	-34.5	-51.4	-50.9	-24.8	-32.0
Australia	1971-1981	-32.1	-39.2	-32.6	-35.6	-38.6	-47.3	-23.5	-27.1
United States of America	1970-1980	-28.4	-30.4	-35.8	-38.7	-44.7	-42.4	-20.4	-18.4
Canada	1972-1982	-25.8	-26.7	-27.8	-25.8	-37.8	-37.1	-15.7	-15.5
Belgium	1971-1981	-24.7	-26.8	-27.7	-29.8	-39.8	-37.7	-16.7	-17.6
New Zealand	1971-1981	-22.8	-22.5	-22.9	-17.1	-30.3	-34.7	-14.3	-10.5
France	1971-1981	-22.7	-35.1	-8.2	-24.6	-37.1	-42.3	-13.2	-21.0
Finland	1970-1980	-19.6	-40.2	-13.1	-23.1	-32.6	-47.1	-18.4	-27.8
England and Wales	1972-1982	-16.7	-19.6	-11.5	-7.1	-30.6	-28.1	-16.6	-11.4
Scotland	1973-1983	-16.2	-20.2	-9.9	-9.9	-32.9	-27.3	-13.0	-8.4
Netherlands	1972-1982	-16.1	-23.3	-20.0	-21.1	-25.8	-28.1	-13.0	-17.2
Germany, Federal Republic of	1972-1982	-11.2	-21.9	-5.8	-7.2	-28.8	-32.3	-14.7	-19.5
Switzerland	1971-1981	-11.2	-32.6	-0.2	-10.1	-31.6	-40.7	-15.1	-22.6
Norway	1972-1982	-10.1	-25.4	-5.2	-10.7	-40.3	-42.1	-6.3	-12.0
Italy	1970-1980	-8.9	-27.8	+1.0	-19.9	-20.0	-28.3	-8.6	-19.6
Denmark	1972-1982	-8.2	-17.4	-9.4	-10.9	-2.1	-30.8	-5.4	-5.7
Austria	1972-1982	-7.4	-20.6	-0.1	-17.2	-26.2	-29.7	-12.1	-16.3
Northern Ireland	1971-1981	-7.3	-12.3	-1.0	+12.8	-28.6	-37.6	-7.5	-5.5
Ireland	1970-1980	-2.5	-17.1	+6.8	-5.2	-31.8	-30.1	-8.0	-14.5
Sweden	1972-1982	-2.5	-20.1	+0.7	-19.4	-21.2	-24.3	-5.6	-12.3
Czechoslovakia	1972-1982	+12.0	+2.4	+8.8	+3.1	-1.2	-8.4	+6.0	-2.3
Romania	1972-1982	+15.7	-2.7	+53.1	+50.4	+5.3	-6.3	+11.0	-2.7
Yugoslavia	1971-1981	+23.5	+13.2	+34.8	+12.7	+6.6	-2.3	-1.6	-9.3
Poland	1970-1980	+31.3	+7.8	+58.0	+43.4	+62.2	+36.8	+15.8	-0.8
Hungary	1972-1982	+33.0	+3.0	+37.6	+5.7	+29.1	+23.2	+30.9	+9.5
Bulgaria	1972-1982	+34.1	+3.6	+20.4	-11.1	+23.6	+1.6	+13.0	-2.4

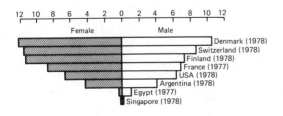

Venous Thrombosis and Embolism

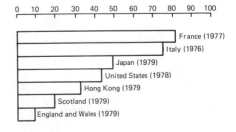

Cirrhosis

Figure 7.29. Showing the change in age standardized death rates in the 40-69 year age group during a recent ten year period for cardiovascular disease (middle) and the current comparative incidence of heart and liver diseases per 100,000 population in some developed and developing nations (surrounds). Pisa and Wamara, 1982 and 1985 and **WHO Expert Committee Technical Report**, 1986.

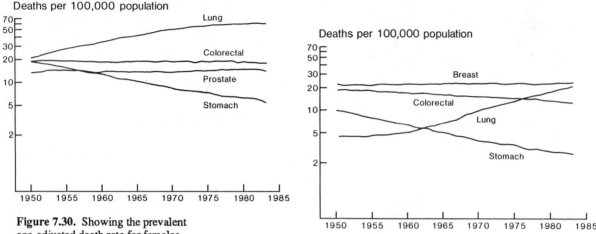

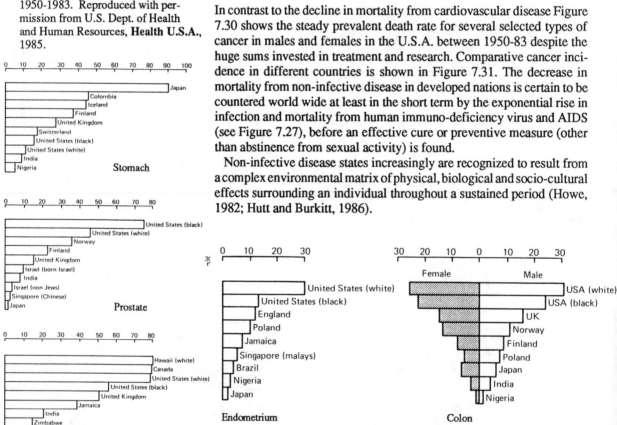

Figure 7.30. Showing the prevalent age-adjusted death rate for females (left) and males (right) for several types of cancer in the USA between 1950-1983. Reproduced with permission from U.S. Dept. of Health and Human Resources, **Health U.S.A.,** 1985.

In contrast to the decline in mortality from cardiovascular disease Figure 7.30 shows the steady prevalent death rate for several selected types of cancer in males and females in the U.S.A. between 1950-83 despite the huge sums invested in treatment and research. Comparative cancer incidence in different countries is shown in Figure 7.31. The decrease in mortality from non-infective disease in developed nations is certain to be countered world wide at least in the short term by the exponential rise in infection and mortality from human immuno-deficiency virus and AIDS (see Figure 7.27), before an effective cure or preventive measure (other than abstinence from sexual activity) is found.

Non-infective disease states increasingly are recognized to result from a complex environmental matrix of physical, biological and socio-cultural effects surrounding an individual throughout a sustained period (Howe, 1982; Hutt and Burkitt, 1986).

Figure 7.31. Comparative incidence of several types of cancer in some developed and developing countries per 100,000 population. From **Disease and the Environment,** by A.R. Rees and H.J. Purcell ©1982, adapted from Segi, 1977 and Waterhouse et. al., 1978. Reprinted with permission of John Wiley and Sons Ltd.

Although the primary stimuli in contraction of an infective disease are the pathogenicity and virulence of the invading antigen, predisposing factors which include individual susceptibility (constitutionality or genetic factors) (Egeland et. al. 1987; Hodgkinson et. al 1987), nutritional state (Wynder, 1977; Krehl, 1977), integrity of the host's local and systemic defenses, and environmental conditions (Howe, 1982), cannot be ignored. The diagnosis, cure and possible prevention of future infection by a particular disease process depends fundamentally on recognition of the role played by each of these factors.

Modern medicine is beginning to embrace the idea, particularly in regard to the treatment of non-infective disease, that an understanding of genetic and immunological predisposing factors in the etiology (the build up to) of a contracted disease state is fundamental to its management and eradication.

Nowhere is this better illustrated than in the contributions of molecular biology and immunopathology to an understanding of the pathogenesis of atherosclerosis (Olson, 1987). It is now recognized that cholesterol (lipid) traffic by low density lipoprotein (LDL) is proatherogenic whereas its transport by high density lipoprotein (HDL) is antiatherogenic. The protein component of LDL is apolipoprotein B (apoB) and the gene transcribing apoB resides on Chromosme 2. This gene will order the properties (phenotypical expression) of apoB protein, conferring its ability to attract and organize the protein-carbohydrate-lipid (cholesterol) complex, which is LDL-cholesterol, into a mature stable structure. Variation (mutations) in the apoB gene determined from a molecular engineering technique, using restriction endonucleases to identify specific sequences of DNA might identify aberrant DNA sequences of apoB, which may impair lipid carriage, in patients with recent coronary occlusion and myocardial infarction compared with normal DNA sequences in normal people and thus serve in early identification of those susceptible to atheroschlerosis. In addition the question, whether an aberrant lipoprotein condition is compounded by immune-complex formation stimulated by beef protein in the diet of such a patient is also important. Immuno-complex formation would aid deposition of cholesterol in blood vessels by producing arterial endothelial (wall) damage and LDL cholesterol entrapment in the vessel wall, an early stage of plaque formation (Crouch, 1982; Gallagher et al., 1982). If such a scenario were correct obvious management of a patient, potentially susceptible to coronary artery disease (i.e. one with high LDL cholesterol and aberrant DNA sequencing determined from apoB restriction endonuclease measurements) would be by strictly preventive treatment eliminating ingestion of both bovine protein and excess fat or calories from his diet. Similarly, it may be quite possible to harness and stimulate more completely and specifically systemic immune responses to viral antigens. Already a genetic susceptibility to the HIV-I virus has been described by a group of British scientists in St. Mary's Hospital, London by techniques which would have made such identification impossible only a few years ago (**The Economist**, May, 1987).

Thus a disease state is no longer a simple, one-cause and effect event, but an interactive physical, biological, socio-cultural and life-style complex of factors each playing a significant role in the etiology and manifestation of clinical symptoms. Several other chapters in this book focus specifically on some of the predisposing and alleviating conditions of the disease process in our environment. Burgeoning knowledge about the fundamental character of such processes and both our own and our progeny's potential degree of susceptibility or resistance to them, together with better co-ordination of health initiatives in the third World by developed countries hold out steady hope that disease will become eminently preventable in societies of the future.

7.5 REFERENCES

Barrett, M.J., Hurwitz, E.S., Schonberger, L.B. and Rogers, M.F. Changing epidemiology of Reye Syndrome in United States. **Pediatrics**, 77(4): 598-602, April, 1986.

Cameron, G.R. **Pathology of the Cell**. London, Oliver and Boyd, 1952.

Coolfont Report. Public Health Reports, U.S. Public Health Service, 101(4): 341-348, 1986.

Crouch, T.H. Is bovine protein involved in atherosclerosis? In: Rees, A.R. and Purcell, H.J., eds., **Disease and the Environment**. New York, John Wiley and Sons, 1982.

Doll, R.R. and Peto, R. British Doctors. **Br. Med. J.** 2: 1525, 1976.

Egeland, J.A., Gerhard, D.W., Paul, D.L. Bipolar affective disorders linked to DNA Markers on Chromosome II. **Nature**, 325: 783-787, 1987.

Fry, J. **Common Diseases: Their Nature, Incidence and Care**, 4th ed. Boston, MTP Press, 1985.

Gallagher, P.J., Goulding, N.J., and Gibney, M.J. Immunological aspects of atherosclerosis. In: Rees, A.R. and Purcell, H.J., eds., **Disease and the Environment**. New York, John Wiley and Sons, 1982.

Glass, R.I. New prospects for epidemiology. **Science**, 234: 951, 1986.

Gray's Anatomy, 36th ed. Oxford, Oxford University Press, 1980.

Henderson, R.H. EPI: Shots that save lives. **World Health**, Jan./Feb., 4-7, 1987.

Hodgkinson, S., Sherrington, R., Gurling, H. Mol. Gen. Evidence for Heterogeneity in Manic Depression. **Nature**, 325: 805-806, 1987.

Howe, G.M. Disease and the environment. In: Rees, A.R. and Purcell, H.J., eds., **Disease and the Environment**. New York, John Wiley and Sons, 1982.

Hornick, R.B., Music, S.I., Wenzel, R. The Broad Street Pump Revisited: Response of volunteers to ingested cholera vibrius. **Bulletin New York Academy of Medicine**, 47: 1181-1191, 1971.

Hutt, M.S.R. and Burkitt, D.P. **The Geography of Non-infective Diseases**. Oxford, Oxford University Press, 1986.

Kozel, N.J., and Adams, E.H. Epidemiology of drug abuse: an overview. **Science**, 234: 970, 1986.

Krehl, W.A. The nutritional epidemiology of cardiovascular disease. In Moss, P. and Mayer, J. (eds.) **Food and Nutrition in Health and Disease**. Annals New York Academy of Sciences, New York. **NYAS, 335**, 1977.

Life and Health. CRM Books, California, 1972.

Muench, K.H. **The Genetic Basis for Human Disease**. New York, Elsevier, North-Holland Inc., 1979.

Olson, R.E. Editor Nutritional Reviews. Molecular biology of coronary heart disease. **Nutritional Revue**, 45: 109, 1987.

Perez-Tamayo, R. **Mechanisms of Disease**. Chicago, Year Book Medical Publishers Inc., 1985.

Pisa, Z. and Wamara, K. Trends in mortality for I.H.D. and other cardiovascular diseases in 27 countries, 1968-77. **World Health Statistics Quarterly**, 35: 11-48, 1982.

Pisa, Z. and Warmara, K. Recent trends in cardiovascular disease mortality in 27 industrialized countries, 1970-80. **World Health Statistics Quarterly**, 38: 142-162, 1985.

Rees, A.R. and Purcell, H.J. **Disease and the Environment**. New York. John Wiley and Sons, 1982.

Remington, P.L., Rowley, D., McGee, H., Hall, W.N. and Monto, A.S. Decreasing trends in Reye Syndrome and aspirin use in Michigan, 1979 to 1984. **Pediatrics**, 77(1): 93-98, Jan. 1986.

Roddie, I.C. and Wallace, W.F.M. **The Physiology of Disease.** Chicago, Year Book Medical Publishers Inc., 1975.

Segi, M. **Graphic Presentation of Cancer Incidence by Site and by Area and Population.** Nagoya. Segi Institute of Cancer Epidemiology, 1977.

Shands, K.N. Toxic Shock. **New England Journal of Medicine,** 303: 1436, 1980.

Snow, J. Snow on cholera. In: May, J.M. (ed.). **Studies in Disease Ecology.** Hafner, New York, 1961.

Stern, C. **Principles of Human Genetics,** 3rd. ed. San Francisco, W.H. Freeman and Co., 1973.

St. George-Hyslop, P.H., Tanz, R.E. and Polinsky. The genetic defect causing familial Alzheimer's disease maps on chromosome 21. **Science,** 237: 885-890, 1987.

The Economist. Why some people get AIDS and others don't. May 23-29, 1987.

The Economist. Schools Brief: Medicine's home front. June 6-12, 1987.

The Open University, **The Biology of Health and Disease.** Milton Keynes, The Open University Press, 1985.

Truett, J., Cornfield, J., and Kannel, W. A multivariate analysis of the risk of coronary heart disease in Framingham. **Journal of Chronic Disease,** 20: 511-524, 1967.

U.S. Dept. of Health and Human Services, Public Health Service, Health United States, Maryland, 1987.

Van Firth, R., Langevoort, L., Schaberg, A. Mononuclear Phagocytes in Human Pathology: Proposal for an Approach to Improved Classification. In van Furth (ed.), **Mononuclear Phagocytes in Immunity, Infection and Pathology.** Oxford. Blackwell Scientific, 1975.

Virchow, R. **Cellular Pathology.** 2nd ed. (Translated by Chance, F., 1860). New York, Dover Publications Inc.

von Pirquet, C.F.R.H. and Schick, B. **Die serum krankheit.** Leipzig. Franz Deuticke, 1906.

Waterhouse, J.A.H. Muir, C.S., Correa, P., and Powell, J. (Eds.) **Cancer Incidence in Five Continents** Vol. III, VICC. Springer, Geneva, 1978.

Waterhouse, J.A.H., Shanmugarataun, K., Muir, C.S., and Powell, J.S. (Eds.) Cancer Incidence in Five Continents Vol. IV, IARC Pub. No. 142, Lyon, 1978.

World Health Organization. Community Prevention and Control of Cardiovascular Diseases. **Report of WHO Expert Committee Technical Report Service,** 732, Geneva, W.H.O., 1986.

Wynder, E.L. Nutritional carcinogenesis. In Moss, H. and Mayers, J. (eds.). **Food and Nutrition in Health and Disease,** Annals New York Academy of Sciences. New York, New York Academy of Sciences, 360, 1975.

Years of productive life. **Centers for Disease Control Morbidity, Mortality Weekly Report,** 35, 457, 1986.

7.6 STUDY QUESTIONS

1. Review some of the historical contributions to the study disease.
2. Define your own concept of disease and compare it with the definition given in Chapter 2.
3. Discuss exogenous and endogenous forces which contribute to development of a disease.
4. Discuss the prevalence of different diseases in three different age groups.
5. Write briefly on the contribution the study of genetics has made to an understanding of disease.
6. Draw a diagram to illustrate any autosomal single gene-defect, disease.
7. What is Down's Syndrome? How does it arise?
8. Name some types of therapy for alleviating genetic disease states.
9. Explain anaphylactic shock.
10. Describe the important elements of the immune system and how they are formed.
11. Name the successive defense mechanism the body can bring into play against invading micro-organisms e.g. bacteria and viruses.
12. Explain how the interaction of the socio-cultural, environmental and life-style factors affect the contraction and clinical progress of a disease.
13. Research other chapters of this book to compare and contrast the role of modern medicine in bioengineering and molecular engineering (recombinent DNA).
14. What role do you think preventive measures will play in future health care schemes of modern societies.

Part III

Fitness & Health in the 80s

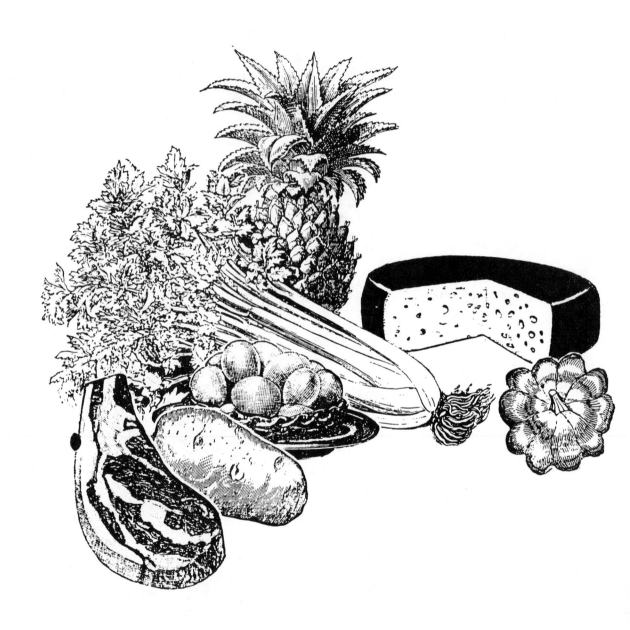

8

Nutrition

Water is the primary nutrient; its sufficiency in the body vitally affects every cellular function, particularly the body's heat regulating ability.

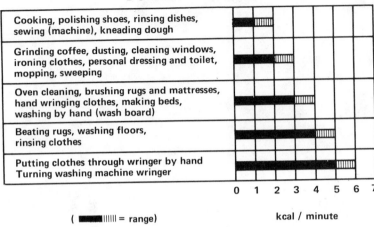

Figure 8.1. The average kilocalorie expenditure per minute in domestic work. Reproduced with permission from Banister, E.W. and Brown, S.R. In **Exercise Physiology**, Academic Press, 1968.

OBJECTIVES

When you have completed this chapter you should be able to:

- **Estimate** the energy cost of ordinary everyday activity.
- **Discuss** the interconversion of energy in the cycle from the sun to plants and animals and then to human energy expenditure in work and play and the degradation of metabolic energy to heat.
- **To distinguish** the separate contributions of the nutrients to adequate nourishment.
- **Identify** the elements of good nutrition and weigh the benefits of vegetarian versus meat diets.
- **Discuss** the hazards to health of various current components of the diet in developed countries.
- **Appreciate** the problems attending the development of a sufficiency of the food supply in the world today besides ensuring its continuance into the future.
- **Plan** your own nutritional health care.

KEY TERMS

carbohydrate
complex carbohydrate
energy
essential amino acids
essential minerals
fat
food distribution
food-energy balance sheets
horse power
human efficiency
improvement
malnourishment
metabolic energy

minerals
polyunsaturated fat
population explosion
potential dietary diseases
power
protein
recommended dietary allowances
saturated fat
soil erosion
vitamins
water
work

INDUSTRIAL OCCUPATIONS

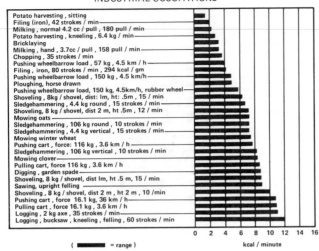

Figure 8.2. The average kilocalorie energy expenditure per minute in some industrial occupations. Reproduced with permission from Banister, E.W. and Brown, S.R. In **Exercise Physiology**, Academic Press, 1968.

8.0 INTRODUCTION

Good nutrition in the plant and animal kingdoms is a key element in converting primary forms of energy available on earth, such as sunlight and fossil fuels, into vital energy forms sustaining life, growth and all human activity. Without adequate nourishment plants, animals, and humans wither and die. Couched in human terms, work (activity of all kinds) or the rate of working (power output) requires energy; for us, running a mile, cycling to work, hoeing a field, playing pool, even just sitting, sleeping, and existing means using energy. The energy is extracted from the food we eat, which is itself stored in the body in forms of fat, carbohydrate, and protein. These stores, principally carbohydrate and fat, are released on demand, when energy requirements are elevated, and oxidized by oxygen from respired air (21% oxygen).

The efficiency of the human machine in this conversion process is approximately 25%. Thus four times the needed physical energy demand has to be produced metabolically to complete the work task set. Three quarters of the metabolic energy is always degraded as heat, causing the body to become warm, even to sweat if the energetic requirement is high enough. Figures 8.1, 8.2, and 8.3 show the energetic demands of some common tasks and sporting events.

8.1 ENERGY

8.1.1 Work

The quantity of physical and metabolic energy generated may be expressed in a variety of units which are readily interconvertible with one another. The commonest units used in measuring work rate are kilogram-meters per minute or joules per second (a Watt). Metabolic energy is usually expressed in kilocalories.

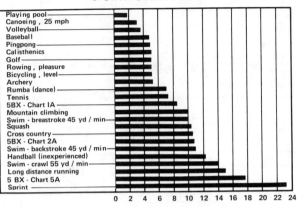

Figure 8.3. The kilocalorie energy expenditure per minute for typical sporting activities. Reproduced with permission from Banister, E.W. and Brown, S.R. In **Exercise Physiology**, Academic Press, 1968.

| Work done (WD) | = Force exerted (Newtons) | x Distance over which the Force is exerted (metres) | Newton·metres (N·m) |

| WD | = Weight (kg) x 9.81 (Newtons) | x Distance over which Force is exerted (metres) | N·m |

where $9.81 \, m \cdot sec^{-2}$ = acceleration due to gravity

Since 1 N·m = 1 Joule

| W.D. | = Weight moved x 9.81 (Newtons) | x Distance (metres) | Joules (J) |

The unit of a Joule is quite small so the kilojoule (KJ) or megajoule (MJ) is used:

(1,000 J = 1 KJ)
(10^6 J = 1 MJ)

$$WD = \frac{\text{Weight moved (kg) x 9.81 x Distance(M)}}{1,000} \quad \text{kilojoule (KJ)}$$

Also 4.18 KJ = 1 Kcalorie

$$WD = \frac{KJ}{4.18} \quad \text{kilocalories (kcal)}$$

8.1.2 Power

Energy output (Power Output) = Work performed per unit of time.

The units of horsepower and watts or kilowatts (kw) are used in nutritional science and their interrelationships ought to be understood. These units express the rate of doing work as noted above and:

1 watt (w) $= 1$ Joule·sec^{-1}
1 kilowatt (KW) $= 1$ KJ·sec^{-1}
1 Horsepower $= 0.736$ KW
  (HP) $= 0.736$ KJ·sec^{-1}
                  $= 0.176$ kcal·sec^{-1} since 4.18 J $= 1$ calorie
or
1HP $= 0.736$ KW $= 736$W x $\dfrac{1}{9.81}$ since 1 kg-wt·m·sec^{-1} $= 9.81$ W
                  $= 75$ kg-wt·m·sec^{-1}

8.1.3 Metabolic (Food) Energy

The body needs six principal nutrients for adequate energy and growth. They are:

- **Carbohydrate & Fat**: Primarily for energy
- **Protein**: Primarily for growth and tissue repair
- **Vitamins**: Primarily for maintanence of tissue integrity, growth and efficient hormonal and enzyme action
- **Minerals**: Primarily for cell function, nervous transmission, red blood cell function and enzyme activity
- **Water**: Primarily for fluid balance in the cell, pH regulation, thermoregulation, secretions, lubrication, etc.

Recommended intake of these nutrients were published by the Food and Agricultural Organization (FAO) in cooperation with the World Health Organization (WHO) in 1974 for world wide application (Table 8.1). These values were modified by the National Research Council, National Academy of Sciences in 1980 (9th ed.) for use in the U.S.A. and a new revision, although due in 1986 is not yet published. Table 8.2 shows the 1980 revisions. Differences may be noted principally in the level of protein intake recommended, in the fat soluble vitamins and in some minerals such as calcium. It may be expected that further supplementation of calcium intake will be recommended in the new revision, taken as a preventive measure against osteoporosis, an increasingly prevalent condition of old age.

Table 8.1. Reproduced with permission from FAO/WHO Expert Group Committee recommended intake of nutrients, 1974.

Age	Body Weight	Energy		Pro-tein	Vita-min A	Vita-min D	Thia-mine	Ribo-flavine	Niacin	Folic acid	Vita-min B$_{12}$	Ascorbic acid	Cal-cium	Iron
		(1)		(1,2)	(3,4)	(5,6)	(3)	(3)	(3)	(5)	(5)	(5)	(7)	(5,8)
	kg	kcal	mj	g	µg	µg	mg	mg	mg	µg	µg	mg	g	mg
Children														
<1	7.3	820	3.4	14	300	10.0	0.3	0.5	5.4	60	0.3	20	0..5-0.6	5-10
1-3	13.4	1360	5.7	16	250	10.0	0.5	0.8	9.0	100	0.9	20	0.4-0.5	5-10
4-6	20.2	1830	7.6	20	300	10.0	0.7	1.1	12.1	100	1.5	20	0.4-0.5	5-10
7-9	28.1	2190	9.2	25	400	2.5	0.9	1.3	14.5	100	1.5	20	0.4-0.5	5-10
Male adolescents														
10-12	36.9	2600	10.9	30	575	2.5	1.0	1.6	17.2	100	2.0	20	0.6-0.7	5-10
13-15	51.3	2900	12.1	37	725	2.5	1.2	1.7	19.1	200	2.0	30	0.6-0.7	9-18
16-19	62.9	3070	12.8	38	750	2.5	1.2	1.8	20.3	200	2.0	30	0.5-0.6	5-9
Female adolescents														
10-12	38.0	2350	9.8	29	575	2.5	0.9	1.4	15.5	100	2.0	20	0.6-0.7	5-10
13-15	49.9	2490	10.4	31	725	2.5	1.0	1.5	16.4	200	2.0	30	0.6-0.7	12-24
16-19	54.4	2310	9.7	30	750	2.5	0.9	1.4	15.2	200	2.0	30	0.5-0.6	14-28
Adult man (moderately active)														
	65.0	3000	12.6	37	750	2.5	1.2	1.8	19.8	200	2.0	30	0.4-0.5	5-9
Adult woman (moderately active)														
	55.0	2200	9.2	29	750	2.5	0.9	1.3	14.5	200	2.0	30	0.4-0.5	14-28
Pregnancy (later half)		+350	+1.5	38	750	10.0	+0.1	+0.2	+2.3	400	3.0	30	1.0-1.2	(9)
Lactation (first 6 months)		+550	+2.3	46	1200	10.0	+0.2	+0.4	+3.7	300	2.5	30	1.0-1.2	(9)

Three of these foodstuffs, carbohydrate, fat, and protein, can furnish energy for all bodily functions. Their physiological energy density per gram of substance is 7-10% less than the chemical energy released on their complete oxidation to ash and gaseous products with pure oxygen in a bomb calorimeter. Their physiological energy density is:

carbohydrate	4 kcal per gram (4 kcal·g^{-1})
fat	9 kcal/g (9 kcal·g^{-1})
protein	4 kcal/g (4kcal·g^{-1})

Table 8.2. Recommended Daily Dietary Allowances, U.S.A. 1980.

	Age (years)	Weight (kg)	Weight (lbs)	Height (cm)	Height (in)	Protein (g)	Fat-Soluble Vitamins			Water-Soluble Vitamins							Minerals					
							Vitamin A (µg RE) b	Vitamin D (µg) c	Vitamin E (mg ∂ TE) d	Vitamin C (mg)	Thiamin (mg)	Riboflavin (mg)	Niacin (mg NE) e	Vitamin B6 (mg)	Folacin (µg) f	Vitamin B12 (µg)	Calcium (mg)	Phosphorus (mg)	Magnesium (mg)	Iron (mg)	Zinc (mg)	Iodine (µg)
Infants	0.0-0.5	6	13	60	24	kg × 2.2	420	10	3	35	0.3	0.4	6	0.3	30	0.5[g]	360	240	50	10	3	40
	0.5-1.0	9	20	71	28	kg × 2.0	400	10	4	35	0.5	0.6	8	0.6	45	1.5	540	360	70	15	5	50
Children	1-3	13	29	90	35	23	400	10	5	45	0.7	0.8	9	0.9	100	2.0	800	800	150	15	10	70
	4-6	20	44	112	44	30	500	10	6	45	0.9	1.0	11	1.3	200	2.5	800	800	200	10	10	90
	7-10	28	62	132	52	34	700	10	7	45	1.2	1.4	16	1.6	300	3.0	800	800	250	10	10	120
Males	11-14	45	99	157	62	45	1000	10	8	50	1.4	1.6	18	1.8	400	3.0	1200	1200	350	18	15	150
	15-18	66	145	176	69	56	1000	10	10	60	1.4	1.7	18	2.0	400	3.0	1200	1200	400	18	15	150
	19-22	70	154	177	70	56	1000	7.5	10	60	1.5	1.7	19	2.2	400	3.0	800	800	350	10	15	150
	23-50	70	154	178	70	56	1000	5	10	60	1.4	1.6	18	2.2	400	3.0	800	800	350	10	15	150
	51+	70	154	178	70	56	1000	5	10	60	1.2	1.4	16	2.2	400	3.0	800	800	350	10	15	150
Females	11-14	46	101	157	62	46	800	10	8	50	1.1	1.3	15	1.8	400	3.0	1200	1200	300	18	15	150
	15-18	55	120	163	64	46	800	10	8	60	1.1	1.3	14	2.0	400	3.0	1200	1200	300	18	15	150
	19-22	55	120	163	64	44	800	7.5	8	60	1.1	1.3	14	2.0	400	3.0	800	800	300	18	15	150
	23-50	55	120	163	64	44	800	5	8	60	1.0	1.2	13	2.0	400	3.0	800	800	300	18	15	150
	51+	55	120	163	64	44	800	5	8	60	1.0	1.2	13	2.0	400	3.0	800	800	300	10	15	150
Pregnant						+30	+200	+5	+2	+20	+0.4	+0.3	+2	+0.6	+400	+1.0	+400	+400	+150	h	+5	+25
Lactating						+20	+400	+5	+3	+40	+0.5	+0.5	+5	+0.5	+100	+1.0	+400	+400	+150	h	+10	+50

The allowances are intended to provide for individual variations among most normal persons as they live in the United States under usual environmental stresses. Diets should be based on a variety of common foods in order to provide other nutrients for which human requirements have been less well defined. See p. 23 for heights, weights and recommended intake.

• Retinol equivalents 1 Retinol equivalent = 1µg retinol or 6 µg ß carotene. See text for calculation of vitamin A activity of diets as retinol equivalents

c As cholecalciterol 10µg cholecalciterol = 400 I.U. vitamin D.

d ∂-tocopherol equivalents 1 mg of ∂-tocopherol 1 ∂-TE. See text for variation in allowances and calculation of vitamin E activity of the diet as ∂-tocopherol equivalents.

e 1 NE (niacin equivalent) is equal to 1 mg of niacin or 60 mg of dietary tryptophan.

f The folacin allowances refer to dietary sources as determined by *Lactobacillus casei* assay after treatment with enzymes ('conjugases') to make polyglutamyl forms of the vitamin available to the test organism.

g The RDA for vitamin B12 in infants is based on average concentration of the vitamin in human milk. The allowances after weaning are based on energy intake (as recommended by the American Academy of Pediatrics) and consideration of other factors such as intestinal absorption, see text.

h The increased requirement during pregnancy cannot be met by the iron content of habitual American diets nor by the existing iron stores of many women. Therefore the use of 30-60 mg of supplemental iron is recommended. Iron needs during lactation are not substantially different from those of non-pregnant women but continued supplementation of the mother for 2 - 3 months after parturition is advisable in order to replenish stores depleted by pregnancy.

Table 8.3. Recommended energy intakes. Reproduced with permission from The National Research Council. **Recommended Dietary Allowances** (9th ed.). Washington, D.C.: National Academy of Sciences, 1980.

Category	Age (years)	Weight (kg) (mean)	(lb)	Height (cm) (mean)	(in)	Energy Needs (with range)a (kcal)	(MJ) kg x .48
Infants	0.0 - 0.5	6	13	60	24	kg x 115 (95 - 145)	kg x .48
	0.5 - 1.0	9	20	71	28	kg x 105 (80 - 135)	kg x .44
Children	1 - 3	13	29	90	35	1300 (900 - 1800)	5.5
	4 - 6	20	44	112	44	1700 (1300 - 2300)	7.1
	7 - 10	28	62	132	52	2400 (1650 - 3300)	10.1
Males	11 - 14	45	99	157	62	2700 (2000 - 3700)	11.3
	15 - 18	66	145	176	69	2800 (2100 - 3900)	11.8
	19 - 22	70	154	177	70	2900 (2500 - 3300)	12.2
	23 - 50	70	154	178	70	2700 (2300 - 3100)	11.3
	51 - 75	70	154	178	70	2400 (2000 - 2800)	10.1
	76+	70	154	178	70	2050 (1650 - 2450)	8.6
Females	11 - 14	46	101	157	62	2200 (1500 - 3000)	9.2
	15 - 18	55	120	163	64	2100 (1200 - 3000)	8.8
	19 - 22	55	120	163	64	2100 (1700 - 2500)	8.8
	23 - 50	55	120	163	64	2000 (1600 - 2400)	8.4
	51 - 75	55	120	163	64	1800 (1400 - 2200)	7.6
	76+	55	120	163	64	1600 (1200 - 2000)	6.7
Pregnancy						+300	
Lactation						+500	

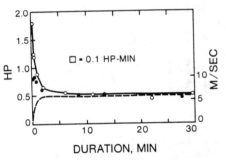

Figure 8.4. Left-hand ordinate: circles, maximal external mechanical power produced by champion athletes. Right-hand ordinate: dots, running speed, world records (Guinness, 1956). Abscissa: total duration of exercise (not time elapsed since the beginning of exercise). The broken line shows the energy available from oxidative processes. To this is added 0.58 hp · min⁻¹ of work from anaerobic (hydrolytic) sources, to give the theoretical curve, full line. Note: 1 hp = 0.746 kg-wt · meter · sec⁻¹. Reprinted with permission from Wilkie, **Ergonomics**, I: 1960.

Table 8.4. Average per capita daily supply of energy and protein (1970). Reproduced with permission from "The State of Food and Agriculture, 1974." FAO, Rome, 1975.

Country	Energy kilocal	Energy as % of Rqurm'ts	Proteins (grams)	Protein/ Energy Ratio %
Japan	2,470	106	76.2	12.3
Sweden	2,800	104	83.8	11.9
Brazil	2,600	109	63.8	9.8
Chile	2,460	101	70.9	11.5
Costa Rica	2,470	110	63.0	10.2
Mexico	2,560	110	65.1	10.1
Nicaragua	2,380	106	70.1	11.7

Normal energy requirements at different stages of life in average males and females is shown in Table 8.3. Requirement for athletes training heavily range 2-4 times these values.

The average energetic output of athletic adults able to be sustained for longer than 30 minutes reaches about 1/2 HP (Figure 8.4). This rate of working, approximately 5 kcal·min⁻¹, is higher than the 1/10 to 1/3 HP which may be maintained without rest pauses by manual labor in field work during an 8-10 hour working day (Figure 8.2). It is much higher than the rather sedentary type of work carried on by much of a developed nation's work force. If 1/10 HP = 66 kcal·hour⁻¹, 660 kcal are needed for a 10 hour day.

Although protein is an energy source, carbohydrates and fats are the important energy producing foods. Protein energy density of the diet forms only some 9-12% of the necessary nutrient energy in several developed and developing countries (Table 8.4). Carbohydrate and fat, on oxidation in the metabolic, biochemical pathways, furnish the high energy intermediate adenosine triphosphate (ATP). Together with adenosine diphosphate (ADP) and creatine phosphate (PCr) ATP is the immediate energy source for all cellular action. Carbohydrate is stored as glycogen in the body prior to oxidation while excess carbohydrate intake above on-going metabolic requirements is stored as fat, together with fat in the fat depots. Oxidation of these stored energy sources during the formation of high energy intermediates (ATP) is carried out with approximately 60% efficiency. The energy-producing hydrolysis and reformation of ATP process has approximately a 40% efficiency. Overall, therefore, the efficiency of the human machine is approximately:

Efficiency = 60% x 40% = 24%

Practical measurements range between 24 and 30%.

Table 8.6. Biological measurements of protein quality. Reproduced with permission from Hensley, E.S. **Basic Concepts of World Nutrition.** Springfield, Charles C. Thomas, 1981.

1. **Biological value (BV):** proportion of absorbed nitrogen (N) that is retained in the body for maintenance and/or growth.

$$\frac{\text{N intake - (fecal N - metabolic N) - (urinary N - endogenous N)}}{\text{N intake - (fecal N - metabolic N)}} \times 100 = BV$$

2. **Net protein utilization (NPU):** proportion of nitrogen (N) intake that is retained in the body for maintenance and/or growth.

$$\frac{\text{N intake - (fecal N - metabolic N) - (urinary N - endogenous N)}}{\text{N intake}} \times 100 = NPU$$

3. **Protein efficiency ratio (PER):** weight gain of a growing animal (or human infant) divided by its protein intake.

$$\frac{\text{Weight gain}}{\text{Protein intake}} = PER$$

Fecal Nitrogen—nitrogenous compounds excreted in the feces, made up of both undigested (or unabsorbed) food nitrogen and metabolic nitrogen. **Metabolic nitrogen**—generally refers to fecal endogenous nitrogen; comprises substances originating in the body, such as residues of bile and other digestive juices, epithelial cells from alimentary tract taken by food passing through it, and bacterial residues. **Urinary nitrogen**—protein catabolism representing metabolic processes of living cells; represented by excretion of creatine,

8.2 NUTRIENTS

8.2.1 Protein

Protein forms part of every living cell, playing a vital role in the integrity of every structure as well as in several regulatory functions. These regulatory functions include neurotransmission, acid-base balance, osmolarity, and fluid exchange between cellular, vascular, and interstitial spaces.

The basic unit of protein is the amino acid. Of the 20 amino acids needed by the body, nine cannot be manufactured sufficiently, or at all by it, and are termed "essential amino acids" of the diet. It is not essential that the remaining eleven form part of the diet, since the body manufactures them in sufficient degree if needed. Optimal growth, development, repair, and function of vital structures depends, however, upon the quantity and quality of dietary protein. Optimal provision of all needed protein in the diet is obviously desirable. The essential and non-essential amino acids used in the body are shown in Table 8.5.

Biological definition of the effectiveness of dietary protein uptake is measured from the degree of nitrogen retention from ingested protein. Actual chemical measurement of the amino acid composition of ingested food may also be made for comparison against an ideal standard food. Foods such as egg and milk are defined as making optimal provision of sufficient amino acid, both in number and in the correct proportion of essential to non-essential amino acids (usually 1:2). Poor quality protein might lack essential amino acids and contain 1/4 rather than the 1/3 portion of essential amino acids defined above.

Table 8.6 shows formulae for calculation of the biological definitions of dietary protein sufficiency. The Chemical Score definition expresses the milligram concentration of essential amino acids present in 1 gram of food protein as a proportion of essential amino acids in 1 gram of a criterion food protein, such as egg or milk or indeed any arbitrary criterion food decided upon (FAO/WHO, 1973).

Table 8.5. Essential and non-essential amino acids of the diet.

Essential Amino Acids (non-dispensable)	Non-essential Amino Acids (dispensable)
Threonine	Glycine
Leucine	Alanine
Isoleucine	Aspartic acid
Valine	Glutamic acid
Lysine	Proline
Methionine	Cysteine(Cystine)
Phenylalanine	Tyrosine
Tryptophan	Serine
Histidine	Arginine
	Asparagine
	Glutamine

Table 8.7. Protein quality values of common foods. Adapted and reproduced with permission from FAO/WHO ad hoc Expert Committee. **Energy and Protein Requirements**. Rome: FAO, 1973, p. 67; Hegstad, D. **Assessment of Protein Quality.** Improvement of Protein Nutriture. Washington, D.C.: National Acadamey of Sciences, page 70, 1974.

Protein Source	BV	NPU	PER	Chemical Score[1]
Whole egg	94	94	3.92	100
Human milk	95	95		100
Cow's milk	85	82	3.09	95, 60[2]
Fish	76	80	3.55	71[2]
Beef	74	67	2.30	69[2]
Soybeans	73	61	2.32	47[2]
Soybean flour		54		74
Wholewheat	65	40	1.53	53, 43[2]
Maize	59	51	1.12	49, 51[2]
Rice, polished	64	57	2.18	67, 56[2]
Sunflower seed	70	58	2.10	61[2]
Peanuts	54	48	1.65	65
Cottonseed meal	67	53	2.25	81,47[2]
Sesame	62	53	1.77	50, 42[2]
Potatoes, white	67	60		34[2]
Cassava				41[2]

[1] Based upon FAO 1973 provisional pattern
[2] Based upon egg pattern

$$\text{Chemical score (CS)} = \frac{\text{mg essential amino acids in 1g food protein x 100}}{\text{mg essential amino acids in 1g criterion protein or reference protein}}$$

Table 8.7 shows the indices of protein quality measured in various foods compared with egg and milk products. Both biological measurements, such as BV (biological value), NPU (net protein utilization), and chemical indices such as (CS), are expressed as percentage values. Specifically, these are the percentage of nitrogen uptake, weight gain as a proportion of ingested nitrogen (biological measurements), or the proportion of essential amino acid in the food protein relative to a criterion protein food (chemical score).

Overall, protein intake is measured in terms of grams of protein per kilogram of body weight per day (g prot.kg^{-1}·day^{-1}). This requirement has been determined from careful balance studies measuring both the amount and quality (individual amino acid profile) of nitrogen intake and loss during extended periods. These studies have served to determine mineral requirements, too. Such studies take into account nitrogen loss from excretion (feces, urine) and from other means (e.g., through hair, skin, nails, menstruation, etc.). They also consider the effectiveness of dietary uptake and utilization of protein in growth and repair of tissue (particularly in children). The method determines the lowest protein intake necessary to maintain nitrogen equilibrium in adults and a positive nitrogen balance (thus allowing for growth) in children (Table 8.8). The latest authoritative tables published in 1973 by the Food and Agriculture Organization of the World Health Organization (FAO/WHO) are based on balance studies. These studies upgrade previous estimates based on older factorial studies, which measured nitrogen loss from individuals without consideration of protein intake. New tables specifying protein requirements incorporate the following.

Table 8.8. Amino acid requirement patterns compared with egg and milk protein (mg per g of protein). Adapted and reproduced with permission from FAO/WHO ad hoc Expert Committee. **Energy and Protein Requirements.** Rome: FAO, p.58, p.63, 1973.

Amino Acid	Suggested Patterns of Requirement			1957 FAO Reference Pattern (all ages)	1973 FAO Provisional Pattern (all ages)	Reported Composition		
	Infant	Schoolchild 10-12 years	Adult			Human Milk (mean)	Cow's Milk	Egg
Histidine*	14	-	-	-	-	26	27	22
Isoleucine	35	37	18	42	40	46	47	54
Leucine	80	56	25	48	70	93	95	86
Lysine	52	75	22	42	55	66	78	70
Methionine +cystine	29	34	24	42	35	42	33	57
Phenylalanine +tyrosine	63	34	25	56	60	72	102	93
Threonine	44	44	13	28	40	43	44	47
Tryptophan	8.5	4.6	6.5	14	10	17	14	17
Valine	47	41	18	42	50	55	64	66
TOTAL								
+histidine	373	-	-	-	-	460	504	512
-histidine	-	326	152	314	360	434	477	490

* needed for growth in infants

1. A base protein requirement calculated from balance studies or from previous factorial requirements multiplied by 1.3. (1.3 is a figure by which balance studies found factorial studies in error.) Since only a few balance studies have been performed due to their cost and complexity, evidence from factorial studies is still used.
2. A 30% additional cushion is added to this base, compensating for individual differences and ensuring a universal "safe level" standard.
3. An additional intake compensates for the quality of ingested protein rated as high (80%), medium (70%), or low (60%) by the chemical score (CS). Below a 60% quality rating, increased intake will not compensate for quality.

Table 8.8 shows FAO/WHO 1973 safe level recommendations of protein intake by age and gender. Adjustments to intake can be made (Table 8.9) in order to compensate for the quality of ingested protein, based upon its essential amino acid content (referenced to the FAO 1973 pattern in Table 8.8). Such adjustments are calculated by multiplying the number of grams of protein per day (calculated for body weight) by 1.25, 1.42, or 1.66 respectively. The choice of these three numbers is made depending on whether the essential amino acid content is rated high (from a mixed full diet of meat, eggs, fish, vegetables and cereals), medium (1.42, with limited animal protein), or low (1.62, lacking meat and high quality cereal).

It is noteworthy that protein is more efficiently used if energy needs are also adequately met. As shown previously (Table 8.4), the percentage of protein energy in the diet of several nations ranges from 9% to 12%. It has been suggested that in adequately fed, moderately active adults, this ratio need only be approximately 5. It will be higher, as reflected in the national figures shown in Table 8.4, when less food is eaten, either due to lower energy needs or due to inadequate food availability.

8.2.2 Carbohydrate

Carbohydrate forms 50% of the diet of developed countries and up to 80% of the diet of underdeveloped countries. Cereals of every kind, fruit, roots, leaves, and pulses (seeds) are sources of carbohydrate. Carbohydrates are characterized as either simple or complex (Table 8.10). Besides acting as a prime source for the energy needs of the body, an increasingly recognized role for certain carbohydrates is to provide bulk, or roughage, in the diet. Roughage aids in the elimination of waste products and in suppression of cancer-inducing chemicals formed in the digestive process (Wynder, 1977). Structural polysaccharides, cellulose, hemicellulose, lignins, pectins, and gums make up dietary fiber when eaten. Fiber foods are cereals, whole grain flour, legumes, and dried potato peel. Because fiber is not digested, it provides bulk in the intestinal tract. It is reported to be helpful in decreasing transit time of potentially harmful residues (bile and neutral steroids) in the tract, thus inhibiting their cancer-inducing effects (Kritchevsky, 1977).

These fibers also bind bile acids, aiding compensatory conversion of cholesterol to bile salts, thus potentially reducing the circulating cholesterol level. Abnormal plasma glucose and lipids have been observed to decrease dramatically on a high soluble fiber diet regimen. Non-urban African populations dependant on lightly milled cereals and leguminous foods have low serum cholesterol and little heart disease.

8.2.3 Fats

Fats form approximately 40% of North American diets. They are not a major component of diets in less developed countries. In areas where oil seeds are not produced, less than 10% of dietary energy comes from this source. Besides forming an energy source, fats function as components of cell walls and hormones, transport fat soluble vitamins, and provide insulation to the body.

Dietary fat comprises molecules of glycerol, to which are attached

Table 8.9. Safe levels of protein in diets of protein quality ranging from 60 to 80% relative to milk or eggs. Reproduced with permission from FAO/WHO ad hoc Expert Committee. **Energy and Protein Requirements**. Rome: FAO, p. 74, 1973

Age	Body Weight (kg)	Safe Level of Protein Intake		Protein Intake Adjusted for Quality g per person per day		
		g protein per kg per day	g protein per person per day	Score 80	Score 70	Score 60
Infants						
6-11 months	9.0	1.53	14	17	20	23
Children						
1-3 years	13.4	1.19	16	20	23	27
4-6 years	20.2	1.01	20	26	29	34
7-9 years	28.1	0.88	25	31	35	41
Male adolescents						
10-12 years	36.9	0.81	30	37	43	50
13-15 years	51.3	0.72	37	46	53	62
16-19 years	62.9	0.60	38	47	54	63
Female adolescents						
10-12 years	38.0	0.76	29	36	41	48
13-15 years	49.9	0.63	31	39	45	52
16-19 years	54.4	0.55	30	37	43	50
Adult man	65.0	0.57	37	46	53	62
Adult woman	55.0	0.52	29	36	41	48
Pregnant woman, latter half of pregnancy			Add 9	Add 11	Add 13	Add 15
Lactating woman, first 6 months			Add 17	Add 21	Add 24	Add 28

Table 8.10. Carbohydrate forms in food.

Type	Name	Source
Simple	**Monosaccharides** glucose, fructose, mannose galactose alcohol sugars, mannitol, sorbitol	fruit, vegetables, honey
	Disaccharides sucrose lactose maltose	sugar cane, sugar beet milk germinating cereals
Complex	**Polysaccharides** complex repeating glucose units glycogen—animal storage form starch—plant storage form cellulose-plant structural form	muscle, liver plant body stems, leaves, grain seeds, hulls

Table 8.11. Some common fatty acids. Reproduced with permission from Hensley, E.S. **Basic Concepts of World Nutrition**. Charles C. Thomas Publisher, Springfield, Illinois, 1981.

Name	Length of Carbon Chain[1]	Food Source
Saturated		
Butyric	Short	Butter
Caproic	Short	Butter
Caprylic	Short	Coconut oil
Capric	Short	Palm oil
Lauric	Long	Coconut oil
Myristic	Long	Butter, nutmeg, coconut oil
Palmitic	Long	Lard, palm oil
Stearic	Long	Beef tallow
Arachidic	Extra long	Peanut oil
Monounsaturated		
Oleic	Long	Animal and vegetable fats
Polyunsaturated		
Linoleic	Long	Vegetable oils (corn, cottonseed, peanut, soybean)
Linolenic	Long	Soybean oil, linseed oil
Arachidonic	Extra Long	Animal fat

[1] Short-chain fatty acids contain 10 or fewer carbon atoms; long-chain fatty acids contain 12 to 18 carbon atoms; extra-long chain fatty acids contain 20 or more carbon atoms.

combinations of fatty acids, varying in chain length. One fatty acid combination is attached to each hydroxyl (OH) group of the 3 carbon alcohol, glycerol. In this form fat is known as a triglyceride. Properties of the triglycerides depend on the different side chain fatty acids attached to the glycerol unit and the number of double bonds representing unsaturated carbon atoms in these chains (i.e. carbon atoms capable of combining with more hydrogen atoms during "hydrogenation" to produce "saturated" fatty acid side chains). Monounsaturated fatty acids have only 2 positions available on the carbon atoms of the fatty acid side chains for hydrogen. Polyunsaturated fatty acids have 4 or more positions available for hydrogen in the side chain carbons of the fatty acids. Common fatty acids in food are shown in Table 8.11. Only linoleic acid may be considered an essential one, in the same sense as the essential amino acids, in that it is not able to be synthesized in the body. The polyunsaturated fatty acids increase the body's requirement for Vitamin E, an antioxidant, to protect their structures from non productive (energetically speaking) oxidation. Free fatty acids enter specific metabolic pathways after hydrolysis releases them from their glycerol spine. They finally enter the same metabolic pathway (the Krebs Cycle) as carbohydrate and protein to form the ATP high energy storage molecule common to all the energy producing pathways.

The solid fats available in animal foods contain more saturated fatty acid in the glycerol side chain than do vegetable oils except for coconut oil (90% saturated) and palm oil (50% saturated).

Unsaturated fatty acids seem to play a lesser role in the complex etiology (originating causes) of degenerative heart disease (the formation of fatty plaques originating in blood vessel walls, which eventually extend to block the whole artery) than do saturated fats. Cholesterol, another type of fat (a sterol) component of animal tissue has been intimately linked with the development of heart disease in humans (Krehl, 1977). Cholesterol is also synthesized by the body. Thus, the combined effect of overeating (where excess protein, carbohydrate, and fat are stored as fat), consuming

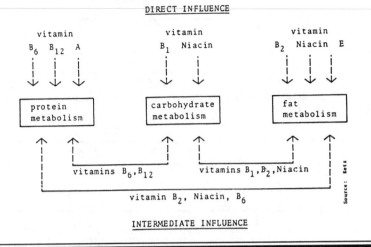

VITAMIN REQUIREMENT FOR METABOLISM

Figure 8.5. Vitamin requirement for metabolism. Reproduced with permission from Konopka, P., Wander Ltd., 1982.

cholesterol and animal fat (which may contribute to additional synthesis of cholesterol by the body), and lack of exercise (which might have utilized the energy density of the excesses) may all constitute cardiac risk factors if unalleviated.

Cholesterol and absorbed fat are transported in the blood attached to protein molecules. The combination is termed "lipoprotein". Various fractions of lipoproteins exist, being termed high density (HDL), low density (LDL) and very low density lipoprotein (VLDL). It appears more beneficial to transport dietary cholesterol in the HDL form to the liver for degradation than in the LDL form, since the latter seems able to infiltrate arterial walls to begin plaque formation and ultimate blockage of an artery. Regular exercise seems to increase the proportion of cholesterol carried safely as HDL.

8.2.4 Vitamins

Vitamins are essential components of protein, fat, and carbohydrate metabolism. In small quantities they become part of enzyme systems and accessories in hormonal effects, and in red blood cell and calcium metabolism. Table 8.12 shows fat soluble and water soluble vitamins. Figure 8.5 shows the direct and secondary influence of various enzymes on energy metabolism. Recommended daily intake of vitamins for normally active individuals is shown again in Table 8.13. The fat soluble vitamins may be stored in various body sites and may become toxic if taken in excess, due to this solubility factor. Water soluble vitamins are not stored and must be replenished daily, but do not usually become toxic, since they do not accumulate in the body. Exceptions are vitamins C and B_6 when taken in excessive megadoses.

Most foods are sources of vitamins; deficiencies occur wherever plant growth is impaired by water scarcity, poor soil and long dry periods. Recommended daily allowances for protein, are also shown in Table 8.13, but these values are probably inadequate for both protein and vitamins for heavily training athletes. Protein ingestion in the amount of 2g.kg⁻¹ is

Table 8.12. Vitamin nutrients.

Fat-soluble Vitamins
    Vitamin A
    Vitamin D
    Vitamin E
    Vitamin K

Water-soluble Vitamins
    Vitamin B complex
      Thiamine (B_1)
      Riboflavin (B_2)
      Niacin
      Pyridoxine (B_6)
      Pantothenic acid
      Biotin
      Folacin
      Cobalamin (B_{12})
      Choline (need is undetermined
      in human nutrition)
    Vitamin C

Table 8.13. Recommended daily dietary allowances. Reproduced with permission from the National Research Council, **Recommended Dietary Allowances**, (9th ed.), Washington, D.C., National Academy of Sciences, 1980.

	Age (years)	Weight (Kg)	(lbs)	Height (cm)	(in)	Protein (g)	Vitamin A (µg RE)b	Vitamin D (µg)c	Vitamin E (mg a TE)d	Vitamin C (mg)	Thiamin (mg)	Riboflavin (mg)	Niacin (mg NE)e	Vitamin B6 (mg)	Folacin (µg)f	Vitamin B12 (µg)g	Calcium (mg)	Phosphorus (mg)	Magnesium (mg)	Iron (mg)	Zinc (mg)	Iodine (µg)
Infants	0.0-0.5	6	13	60	24	kg × 2.2	420	10	3	35	0.3	0.4	6	0.3	30	0.59	360	240	50	10	3	40
	0.5-1.0	9	20	71	28	kg × 2.0	400	10	4	35	0.5	0.6	8	0.6	45	1.5	540	360	70	15	5	50
Children	1-3	13	29	90	35	23	400	10	5	45	0.7	0.8	9	0.9	100	2.0	800	800	150	15	10	70
	4-6	20	44	112	44	30	500	10	6	45	0.9	1.0	11	1.3	200	2.5	800	800	200	10	10	90
	7-10	28	62	132	52	34	700	10	7	45	1.2	1.4	16	1.6	300	3.0	800	800	250	10	10	120
Males	11-14	45	99	157	62	45	1000	10	8	50	1.4	1.6	18	1.8	400	3.0	1200	1200	350	18	15	150
	15-18	66	145	176	69	56	1000	10	10	60	1.4	1.7	18	2.0	400	3.0	1200	1200	400	18	15	150
	19-22	70	154	177	70	56	1000	7.5	10	60	1.5	1.7	19	2.2	400	3.0	800	800	350	10	15	150
	23-50	70	154	178	70	56	1000	5	10	60	1.4	1.6	18	2.2	400	3.0	800	800	350	10	15	150
	51+	70	154	178	70	56	1000	5	10	60	1.2	1.4	16	2.2	400	3.0	800	800	350	10	15	150
Females	11-14	46	101	157	62	46	800	10	8	50	1.1	1.3	15	1.8	400	3.0	1200	1200	300	18	15	150
	15-18	55	120	163	64	46	800	10	8	60	1.1	1.3	14	2.0	400	3.0	1200	1200	300	18	15	150
	19-22	55	120	163	64	44	800	7.5	8	60	1.1	1.3	14	2.0	400	3.0	800	800	300	18	15	150
	23-50	55	120	163	64	44	800	5	8	60	1.0	1.2	13	2.0	400	3.0	800	800	300	18	15	150
	51+	55	120	163	64	44	800	5	8	60	1.0	1.2	13	2.0	400	3.0	800	800	300	10	15	150
Pregnant						+30	+200	+5	+2	+20	+0.4	+0.3	+2	+0.6	+400	+1.0	+400	+400	+150	h	+5	+25
Lactating						+20	+400	+5	+3	+40	+0.5	+0.5	+5	+0.5	+100	+1.0	+400	+400	+150	h	+10	+50

a The allowances are intended to provide for individual variations among most normal persons as they live in the United States under usual environmental stresses. Diets should be based on a variety of common foods in order to provide other nutrients for which human requirements have been less well defined. See p. 23 for heights, weights and recommended intake.

b Retinol equivalents 1 Retinol equivalent = 1µg retinol or 6 µg ß carotene. See text for calculation

c As cholecalciterol 10µg cholecalciterol = 400 I.U. vitamin D.

d ð-tocopherol equivalents 1 mg of ð-tocopherol 1 ð-TE. See text for variation in allowances and calculation of vitamin E activity of the diet as ð-tocopherol equivalents.

e 1 NE (niacin equivalent) is equal to 1 mg of niacin or 60 mg of dietary tryptophan.

f The folacin allowances refer to dietary sources of vitamin A activity of diets as retinol equivalents

as determined by *Lactobacillus casei* assay after treatment with enzymes ("conjugases") to make polyglutamyl forms of the vitamin available to the test organism.

g The RDA for vitamin B12 in infants is based on average concentration of the vitamin in human milk. The allowances after weaning are based on energy intake (as recommended by the American Academy of Pediatrics) and consideration of other factors such as intestinal absorption, see text.

h The increased requirement during pregnancy cannot be met by the iron content of habitual American diets nor by the existing iron stores of many women. Therefore the use of 30-60 mg of supplemental iron is recommended. Iron needs during lactation are not substantially different from those of non-pregnant women but continued supplementation of the mother for 2 - 3 months after parturition is advisable in order to replenish stores depleted by pregnancy.

Table 8.14. Vitamin needs versus intake in endurance athletes. Reproduced with permission from Konopke, P., Wander Ltd., 1982.

Vitamin	Need	Intake
A	13,000 iu	13,700 iu
B1	4-8 mg	1.9 mg
B2	4 mg	2.9 mg
Niacin	30 mg	18 mg
C	500 mg	244 mg

recommended for athletes in training. Table 8.14 shows the estimated need for some vitamins in endurance athletes, together with their usual intake (already higher than the USA recommended daily allowance).

8.2.5 Minerals

Table 8.13 shows the recommended daily allowance for 6 of the 21 elements (minerals) needed in human nutrition. Major element involvement in neurotransmission, cell depolarization, bone mineralization, blood clotting and anemia is well known. Increasingly, roles in protein metabolism, growth, and protein energy malnutrition have been determined for several trace elements (e.g., zinc, chromium, copper, magnesium, and potassium). Toxic minerals (e.g., lead) may enter the body by ingestion, respiration, or through the skin. Increased regular physical activity causes progressive mineral loss, principally from sweating (in the case of sodium, magnesium, potassium, iron, etc.) and sometimes by suppression of absorption (in the case of iron). These losses may result in deficiency and impairment of performance if left uncompensated. Symptoms of Kwashiorkor and Marasmus or protein energy malnutrition diseases (PEM) are attendant upon mineral deficiencies of potassium, chromium, magnesium, copper, and zinc induced by protein malnutrition.

Table 8.15. Daily water balance of an average male.

Water Loss		Water Intake	
Urine	1,100 ml	Fluids	1,000 ml
Feces	100 ml	Food	700 ml
Lungs	200 ml	Metabolic water	300 ml*
Skin	600 ml		
Total	2,000 ml	Total	2,000 ml

* In breaking down stored carbohydrate and fat to release the required fuels for energy production, water is released.

8.2.6 Water

Water is the primary nutrient; its sufficiency in the body vitally affects every cellular function, particularly the body's heat regulating ability (thermoregulation). It constitutes 60-70% of an adult's body weight (4 litres in males, 3 litres in females), and loss of a mere 3-5% of it will elicit early symptoms of dehydration and heat fatigue. A 10% loss of water will result in heat stroke and circulatory collapse. Water becomes an important dietary concern during all increased working conditions, especially those carried out in hot and/or humid, ambient conditions. Individuals at particular risk include those unaccustomed to heat, the unfit and overweight, the malnourished, the elderly, and those experiencing illness or lack of sleep. Women and children are also particularly vulnerable to dehydration because of their small total body water content, compared with adult males. Prolonged air travel may contribute to dehydration due to insensible sweat loss in the pressurized airplane, as may the consumption of dehydrating fluids, such as coffee, tea and alcohol, and a high-protein diet.

The average adult needs to replace approximately 2 litres of fluid per day (see Table 8.15). At a maximum rate of working (athletically) 2-4 litres of fluid per hour may be lost and thus the need to replace fluids should not be overlooked.

8.3 FOOD GROUPINGS

Systematic arrangement of foods into major categories (e.g., cereals, milk, meat, etc.) together with identification of the major nutrients they contain has facilitated analysis of the nutritional effectiveness of dietary patterns in many parts of the world. In developed countries, this serves to identify the substantial nutritional deficiencies existing in the midst of relative abundance. It also demonstrates eating patterns likely to minimize the health risks arising from the wrong food (e.g., saturated fats; refined, nutrient-deficient foods) abusive eating (e.g., alcohol; junk foods), and overeating (gross inequality between energy intake as food versus physical energy expenditure). In underdeveloped and developing countries, such analyses serve to identify combinations of foods and their quantity needed to provide essential amino acids from the lower quality cereal protein mostly available to rural populations. The problem here is often one of minimizing the health risks from subsistence on the meager nutrient energy supplies available.

Table 8.16 shows six food groupings which allow a well-balanced daily diet at various kilocalorie levels by choosing several portions from each group according to Table 8.17. Weight losses attainable by calorie restriction are shown in Table 8.18. Table 8.19 shows a more extensive list of the nutrient value of foods in 4 groups. Both listings follow the comprehensive listing of food values published by the United States Department of Agriculture Handbook, No. 8 and 8-1.

Table 8.16. Food groupings, showing approximate kilocalorie (calorie) values for defined proportions. Reproduced with permission from Strasenburgh Co. Canada, 1970.

Group 1. Milk
Each Portion = 170 Calories
(12 gm. Carbohydrate, 8 gm. Protein, 10 gm. Fat)

Milk	Portion
Whole	1 cup
Skim*	1 cup
Evaporated	½ cup
Powdered, whole	¼ cup
Powdered, skim (non-fat dried milk*)	¼ cup
Buttermilk	
From whole milk	1 cup
From skim milk*	1 cup

*Add 2 Fat portions to your meal for each cup you use of skim milk or buttermilk made from skim milk.

The following foods may be used as desired:

Coffee*	Rennet tablets	Gelatin, unsweetened
Tea*	Pickles, sour	Cranberries
Clear broth	Pickles, unsweetened dill	
Bouillon (without fat)		

*Use with milk from daily allowance and artificial sweeteners, if desired.

Group 2. Vegetables
A. These vegetables may be used as desired in ordinary amounts. Carbohydrates and Calories are negligible.

Asparagus	Rhubarb
Broccoli	Sauerkraut
Brussels Sprouts	String Beans, young
Cabbage	Summer Squash
Cauliflower	Tomatoes
Celery	"GREENS"
Chicory	Beet
Cucumbers	Chard
Eggplant	Collard
Escarole	Dandelion
Lettuce	Kale
Mushrooms	Mustard
Okra	Spinach
Pepper	Turnip
Radishes	

B.—Vegetables: 1 serving equals ½ cup equals 100 grams (about 3 ounces)

Each Portion = 36 Calories
(7 gm. Carbohydrate, 2 gm. Protein)

Beets	Pumpkin
Carrots	Rutabaga
Onions	Squash, winter
Peas, green	Turnips

Remember that snacks can add many extra Calories to the daily total. Budget between meal snacks from your daily food portions.

Group 3. Fruit
Each Portion = 40 Calories
(10 gm. Carbohydrate)

	Portion
Apple (2" diam.)	1 small
Applesauce	½ cup
Apricots, fresh	2 medium
Apricots, dried	4 halves
Banana	½ small
Berries: Straw., Rasp., Black.	1 cup
Blueberries	⅔ cup
Cantaloupe (6" diam.)	¼
Cherries	10 large
Dates	2
Figs, fresh	2 large
Figs, dried	1 small
Grapefruit	½ small
Grapefruit Juice	½ cup
Grapes	12
Grape Juice	¼ cup
Honeydew Melon (7" diam.)	⅛
Mango	½ small
Orange	1 small
Orange Juice	½ cup
Papaya	⅓ medium
Peach	1 medium
Pear	1 small
Pineapple	½ cup
Pineapple Juice	⅓ cup
Plums	2 medium
Prunes, dried	2 tbsp.
Raisins	2 tbsp.
Tangerine	1 large
Watermelon	1 cup

Group 4. Bread
Each Portion = 68 Calories
(15 gm. Carbohydrate, 2 gm. Protein)

	Portion
Bread	1 slice
Biscuit or Roll (2" diam.)	1
Muffin (2" diam.)	1
Corn bread (1½" cube)	1
Flour	2½ tbsp.
Cereal, cooked	½ cup
Cereal, dry (flake or puffed)	¾ cup
Rice or Grits, cooked	½ cup
Spaghetti, Noodles, etc., cooked	½ cup
Crackers	
Graham (2½" square)	2
Oyster	20 (½ cup)
Saltines (2" square)	5
Soda (2½" square)	3
Round, thin (1½" diam.)	6-8
Vegetables	
Beans or Peas, dried, cooked (lima, navy, split peas, cowpeas, etc.)	½ cup
Baked beans, no pork	¼ cup
Corn	⅓ cup
Parsnips	⅔ cup
Potatoes, white baked, boiled	1
mashed	½ cup
Sweet or Yams	¼ cup
Sponge Cake, plain (1½" cube)	1
Ice Cream (Omit 2 Fat Portions)	½ cup

Group 5. Meat
Each Portion = 73 Calories
(7 gm. Protein, 5 gm. Fat)

	Portion
Meat or Poultry (med. fat)	1 oz.
beef, lamb, pork, liver, chicken, etc.	
Cold cuts (4½" x ⅛" thick): salami, bologna, liverwurst, luncheon loaf, minced ham	1 slice
Frankfurter (8-9 per pound)	1
Fish	
Cod, Haddock, Mackerel, Trout, etc.	1 oz.
Salmon, Tuna, Crab, Lobster	¼ cup
Oysters, Shrimp, Clams	5 small
Sardines	3 medium
Cheese	
Cheddar, American	1 oz.
Cottage	¼ cup
Egg	1
Peanut Butter	2 tbsp.

The following seasonings may be used as desired:

Chopped parsley	Pepper and other spices	Nutmeg	Mustard
Garlic	Lemon	Cinnamon	Onion
Celery	Mint	Saccharin	
	Vinegar		

Group 6. Fat
Each Portion = 45 Calories
(5 gm. Fat)

	Portion
Butter or margarine	1 tsp.
Bacon, crisp	1 slice
Cream, light	2 tbsp.
Cream, heavy	1 tbsp.
Cream cheese	1 tbsp.
French dressing	1 tbsp.
Mayonnaise	1 tsp.
Oil or cooking fat	1 tsp.
Nuts	6 small
Olives	5 small
Avocado (4" diam.)	⅛

Table 8.17. Proportions from each food group providing the daily kilocalorie allowance shown in column 1.

Daily Calorie Allowance	Group 1. Milk Group (portions)	Group 2. Vegetable Group (portions)	Group 3. Fruit Group (portions)	Group 4. Bread Group (portions)	Group 5. Meat Group (portions)	Group 6. Fat Group (portions)
2100	2.5	2	6	7.5	8	6
2000	2.5	2	5	7.5	8	5
1900	2.5	2	5	7	7	5
1800	2.5	2	4	6	7	5
1700	2.5	1	4	6	6	5
1600	2	1	4	6	6	5
1500	2	1	4	5	6	4
1400	2	1	3	5	6	3
1300	2	1	4	4	5	3
1200	2	1	4	4	5	1
1100	2	1	4	3	5	0
1000	2	1	3	2	5	0
900	1.5	1	3	2	5	0
800	1.5	1	2	1	5	0

Locate your Daily Calorie Allowance level on the chart above and read across to obtain your Daily Portion Prescription for each of the six main food groups.

Table 8.18. Weight loss able to be attained by daily kilocalorie food restriction. Reproduced with permission from Strasenburgh Co., Canada, 1970.

Cut Your Daily Intake of Calories By*	1 lb	2 lb	3 lb	4 lb	5 lb	6 lb	7 lb	8 lb	9 lb	10 lb
100	40	80	120	160	200	240	280	320	360	400
200	20	40	60	80	100	120	140	160	180	200
300	13.3	26.6	40	53.3	66.6	80	93.3	106.6	120	133.3
400	10	20	30	40	50	60	70	80	90	100
500	8	16	24	32	40	48	56	64	72	80
600	6.4	13.2	20	26.4	33.3	40	46.6	53.3	60	66.6
700	5.7	11.4	17	22.8	28.6	34.3	40	45.7	51.4	57.1
800	5	10	15	20	25	30	35	40	45	50
900	4.4	8.8	13.3	17.7	22.2	26.6	31.1	35.5	40	44.4
1000	4	8	12	16	20	24	28	32	36	40
1100	3.6	7.3	10.9	14.5	18.1	21.8	25.4	29.1	32.7	36.4
1200	3.3	6.6	10	13.3	16.6	20	23.3	26.6	30	33.3
1300	3.1	6.1	9.2	12.3	15.3	18.4	21.5	24.6	27.7	30.8
1400	2.8	5.7	8.6	11.4	14.3	17.1	20	22.8	25.7	28.6

*Your weight x 15 = Your daily Calorie intake which maintains your present weight.

Table 8.19. Comprehensive list of food. Reproduced with permission from The National Dairy Council, 1984; and the U.S.A. Department of Agriculture Composition of foods Agricultural Handbook No. 8. Washington, D.C. Revised 1963.

MILK GROUP

	Calories	Protein g	Carbohydrate g	Fat g	Vitamin A IU	Vitamin C mg	Thiamin (B₁) mg	Riboflavin (B₂) mg	Niacin mg	Calcium mg	Iron mg
Buttermilk, 1 cup	99	8	12	2	81	2	0.08	0.38	0.1	285	0.1
Cheese, American, 1 oz, 1 slice	106	6	—	9	343	0	0.01	0.10	Trace	174	0.1
Cheese, Cheddar, 1 oz, 1 slice	114	7	—	9	300	0	0.01	0.11	Trace	204	0.2
Cheese, Cottage, ½ cup	109	13	3	5	171	Trace	0.02	0.17	0.1	63	0.2
Cheese, Swiss, 1 oz, 1 slice	107	8	1	8	240	0	0.01	0.10	Trace	272	0.1
Cocoa, ¾ cup	164	7	19	7	239	2	0.08	0.33	0.3	224	0.6
Ice Cream, Vanilla, ½ cup, ¼ pint	135	2	16	7	272	—	0.03	0.17	0.1	88	0.1
Milk, 1 cup	150	8	11	8	307	2	0.09	0.40	0.2	291	0.1
Milk, Chocolate, 1 cup	208	8	26	8	302	2	0.09	0.41	0.3	280	0.6
Milk, Lowfat (2%), 1 cup fortified with vitamin A	121	8	12	5	500	2	0.10	0.40	0.2	297	0.1
Milk, Skim, 1 cup fortified with vitamin A	86	8	12	—	500	2	0.09	0.34	0.2	302	0.1
Milkshake, Chocolate, 10.6 oz container	356	9	63	8	258	0	0.14	0.67	0.4	396	0.9
Pudding, Chocolate, ½ cup	161	4	30	4	169	Trace	0.03	0.20	0.1	133	0.4
Yogurt, Strawberry, 1 cup	225	9	42	3	111	1	0.08	0.37	0.2	314	0.1

MEAT GROUP

	Calories	Protein g	Carbohydrate g	Fat g	Vitamin A IU	Vitamin C mg	Thiamin (B₁) mg	Riboflavin (B₂) mg	Niacin mg	Calcium mg	Iron mg
Bacon, 2 slices	92	5	1	8	0	—	0.08	0.05	0.8	2	0.5
Beans, Refried, ½ cup	142	9	26	1	—	—	—	—	—	5	—
Beef, Roast, 3 oz	182	26	0	8	17	—	0.04	0.20	3.9	11	3.2
Beef Liver, 3 oz	195	23	5	9	45,417	23	0.22	3.56	14.0	9	7.5
Bologna, 1 slice	86	3	—	8	0	—	0.05	0.06	0.7	2	0.5
Chicken, Fried, 3 oz	201	26	2	9	148	—	0.06	0.38	5.9	12	2.0
Egg, Fried, large	83	5	1	6	286	0	0.03	0.13	Trace	26	0.9
Egg, Hard-cooked, large	79	6	1	6	260	0	0.04	0.14	Trace	28	1.0
Egg, Scrambled, large	95	6	1	7	311	.13	0.04	0.16	Trace	47	0.9
Frankfurter, 2 oz	172	7	1	15	—	—	0.09	0.11	1.4	3	0.9
Ham, Baked, 3 oz	179	26	0	8	0	—	0.56	0.26	4.9	11	3.2
Meat Loaf, 3 oz	230	15	13	12	106	Trace	0.27	0.24	3.4	68	2.4
Meat Patty, 3 oz	186	23	0	10	17	—	0.08	0.20	5.1	10	3.0
Peanut Butter, 2 tbsp	186	9	6	16	—	0	0.04	0.04	5.0	20	0.6
Peanuts, Salted, ¼ cup	211	9	7	18	—	0	0.12	0.05	6.2	27	0.8
Peas, Blackeye (immature), ½ cup	134	10	22	1	434	21	0.37	0.14	1.7	30	2.6
Peas, Blackeye (mature), ½ cup	94	6	17	—	12	—	0.20	0.05	0.5	21	1.6
Perch, Fried, Breaded, 3 oz	193	16	6	11	—	—	0.09	0.09	1.5	28	1.1
Pork Chop, 3 oz	308	21	0	24	0	—	0.82	0.24	4.9	9	2.7
Sausage, 2 links	135	5	—	13	0	—	0.22	0.10	1.1	2	0.7
T-Bone Steak, 3⅓ oz	212	29	0	10	19	—	0.08	0.22	5.6	11	3.5
Tuna, 3 oz	168	25	0	7	68	—	0.04	0.10	10.1	7	1.6

*In most cases food values were calculated from the amounts given for 100 gram portions in Composition of Foods, Agriculture Handbook No.8. Dairy products and eggs are from Agricultural Handbook No. 8-1.

Table 8.19. (continued).

FRUIT-VEGETABLE GROUP

	Calories	Protein g	Carbohydrate g	Fat g	Vitamin A IU	Vitamin C mg	Thiamin (B₁) mg	Riboflavin (B₂) mg	Niacin mg	Calcium mg	Iron mg
Apple, medium	80	—	20	1	124	6	0.04	0.03	0.1	10	0.4
Applesauce, ½ cup	116	—	30	—	51	1	0.03	0.01	Trace	5	0.6
Apricots, Dried, 4 halves	39	1	10	—	1635	2	Trace	0.02	0.5	10	0.8
Asparagus, 4 spears, ½ cup	12	1	2	—	540	16	0.10	0.11	0.8	13	0.4
Banana, medium	101	1	26	—	226	12	0.06	0.07	0.8	10	0.8
Beans, Green, ½ cup	16	1	3	—	338	8	0.04	0.06	0.3	31	0.4
Beans, Lima, ½ cup	94	7	17	—	238	14	0.15	0.09	1.1	40	2.1
Broccoli, stalk, ½ cup	20	2	4	—	1938	70	0.07	0.16	0.6	68	0.6
Cabbage, ⅙ head, ½ cup	13	1	3	—	87	17	0.01	0.01	0.1	30	0.2
Cantaloupe, ¼ medium	29	1	7	—	3273	32	0.04	0.03	0.6	13	0.4
Carrots, ½ cup	22	1	5	—	7613	4	0.04	0.04	0.4	24	0.4
Carrot Sticks, 5″ carrot	21	1	5	—	5500	4	0.03	0.03	0.3	19	0.4
Cauliflower, ½ cup	13	1	3	—	36	33	0.05	0.05	0.4	13	0.4
Celery Sticks, 8″ stalk	10	1	2	—	136	5	0.02	0.02	0.2	22	0.2
Coleslaw, ½ cup	82	1	3	8	91	16	0.03	0.03	0.2	25	0.2
Corn, ½ cup	70	2	16	1	291	3	0.02	0.04	0.8	4	0.4
Corn, 5″ ear	114	4	26	1	500	11	0.15	0.13	1.8	4	0.8
Fruit Salad, ½ cup apple, orange, banana, lettuce	99	2	25	1	530	44	0.11	0.08	0.7	45	0.9
Grapefruit, Pink, ½ medium	48	1	13	—	94	45	0.05	0.02	0.2	19	0.5
Grapes, ½ cup	48	—	12	—	71	3	0.04	0.02	0.2	9	0.3
Greens, ½ cup mustard greens, kale, turnip greens	17	2	3	—	5306	36	0.08	0.13	0.4	104	1.4
Lettuce, ⅙ head, ½ cup	10	1	2	—	250	5	0.05	0.05	0.2	15	0.4
Okra, 4 pods, ½ cup	12	1	3	—	208	9	0.06	0.08	0.4	39	0.2
Orange, medium	65	1	16	—	263	66	0.13	0.05	0.5	54	0.5
Orange Juice, ½ cup	56	1	13	—	249	56	0.11	0.01	0.4	11	0.1
Peaches, ½ cup	100	1	26	—	550	4	0.01	0.03	0.8	5	0.4
Pear, medium	101	1	25	1	33	7	0.03	0.07	0.2	13	0.5
Peas, Green, ½ cup	54	4	9	—	480	10	0.22	0.07	1.4	15	1.5
Pineapple, large slice	90	—	24	—	61	9	0.10	0.02	0.2	13	0.4
Potato, Baked, large	132	4	30	—	Trace	28	0.14	0.06	2.4	13	1.0
Potatoes, Boiled, 2 small	79	2	18	—	Trace	20	0.11	0.04	1.5	7	0.6
Potatoes, French-Fried, 20 pieces	233	4	31	11	Trace	18	0.11	0.07	2.6	13	1.1
Potatoes, Mashed, ½ cup	63	2	13	1	20	10	0.08	0.05	1.0	23	0.4
Potato, Sweet, ½ medium	78	1	18	—	4455	12	0.05	0.04	0.4	22	0.5
Raisins, 4½ tbsp	123	1	33	—	9	Trace	0.05	0.03	0.2	26	1.5
Squash, Summer, ½ cup	16	1	3	—	462	12	0.05	0.08	0.8	26	0.4
Squash, Winter, ½ medium, ½ cup	56	2	14	—	1435	13	0.05	0.13	0.7	40	1.1
Strawberries, ½ cup	28	1	6	—	45	44	0.02	0.05	0.4	16	0.7
Tomato, ½ medium	22	1	5	—	900	23	0.06	0.04	0.7	13	0.5
Tomato Juice, ½ cup	26	1	5	—	972	19	0.06	0.04	1.0	9	1.1
Tossed Salad, ¾ cup lettuce, green pepper, radish, carrot	13	1	3	—	1380	26	0.03	0.04	0.3	26	0.6
Watermelon, 1 cup	52	1	13	—	1180	14	0.06	0.06	0.4	14	1.0

Table 8.19. (continued).

GRAIN GROUP

	Calories	Protein g	Carbohydrate g	Fat g	Vitamin A IU	Vitamin C mg	Thiamin (B₁) mg	Riboflavin (B₂) mg	Niacin mg	Calcium mg	Iron mg
Bagel	165	6	28	2	30	0	0.14	0.10	1.2	9	1.2
Biscuit, Baking Powder, enriched	103	2	13	5	Trace	Trace	0.08	0.08	0.8	34	0.4
Bread, White, slice, enriched	61	2	12	1	Trace	Trace	0.09	0.06	0.8	19	0.6
Bread, Whole Wheat, slice	55	2	11	1	Trace	Trace	0.06	0.03	0.6	22	0.5
Cornbread, 2½" x 3", enriched	191	6	30	5	264	1	0.14	0.20	0.9	93	1.2
Cornflakes, ¾ cup	72	2	16	—	0	0	0.08	0.02	0.4	3	0.3
Crackers, Graham, 2	54	1	10	1	0	0	0.01	0.03	0.2	6	0.2
Crackers, Saltines, 5	60	1	10	2	0	0	Trace	0.01	0.1	3	0.2
Hominy Grits, ½ cup, enriched	62	2	14	—	74	0	0.05	0.04	0.5	1	0.4
Noodles, Egg, ½ cup, enriched	100	3	19	1	56	0	0.11	0.06	1.0	8	0.7
Oatmeal, ½ cup	66	2	12	1	0	0	0.10	0.02	0.1	11	0.7
Pancake, 4" diameter, enriched	61	2	9	2	68	Trace	0.06	0.08	0.3	58	0.3
Rice, ½ cup	112	2	25	—	0	0	0.11	0.07	1.0	10	0.9
Roll, Frankfurter, enriched	119	3	21	2	Trace	Trace	0.16	0.10	1.3	30	0.8
Roll, Hamburger, enriched	119	3	21	2	Trace	Trace	0.16	0.10	1.3	30	0.8
Roll, Hard, enriched	156	5	30	2	Trace	Trace	0.20	0.12	1.7	24	1.2
Toast, White, slice	61	2	12	1	Trace	Trace	0.09	0.06	0.8	19	0.6
Tortilla, Corn, 6" diameter, enriched	63	2	14	1	6	0	0.04	0.02	0.3	60	0.9
Waffles, 2, 3½" x 5½", enriched	130	4	17	5	109	Trace	0.09	0.14	0.6	113	0.6

COMBINATION FOODS (foods made with ingredients from more than one food group)

	Calories	Protein g	Carbohydrate g	Fat g	Vitamin A IU	Vitamin C mg	Thiamin (B₁) mg	Riboflavin (B₂) mg	Niacin mg	Calcium mg	Iron mg
Beans, Baked, Pork and Tomato Sauce, ½ cup	156	8	24	3	166	3	0.10	0.04	0.8	69	2.3
Beef and Vegetable Stew, 1 cup	209	15	15	10	2303	16	0.14	0.16	4.5	28	2.8
Chili Con Carne with Beans, 1 cup	333	19	31	15	150	—	0.08	0.18	3.3	80	4.3
Custard, Baked, ½ cup	152	7	15	7	464	Trace	0.05	0.25	0.1	148	0.5
Macaroni and Cheese, ½ cup	215	8	20	11	430	Trace	0.10	0.20	0.9	181	0.9
Pizza, Cheese, ¼ of 14" pie, enriched	354	18	43	13	945	12	0.38	0.49	3.8	332	2.7
Soup, Chicken Noodle, 1 cup	59	3	8	2	45	Trace	0.02	0.02	0.7	9	0.5
Soup, Cream of Tomato, 1 cup	173	7	23	7	1200	15	0.10	0.25	1.3	168	0.8
Spaghetti, Meat Balls and Tomato Sauce, 1 cup	332	19	39	12	1587	22	0.25	0.30	4.0	124	3.7
Taco, Beef	216	17	15	10	352	4	0.10	0.19	3.0	174	2.6

"OTHERS" Category (fats, sweets, alcohol)

	Calories	Protein g	Carbohydrate g	Fat g	Vitamin A IU	Vitamin C mg	Thiamin (B₁) mg	Riboflavin (B₂) mg	Niacin mg	Calcium mg	Iron mg
Bar, Milk Chocolate, 1 oz	147	2	16	9	77	Trace	0.02	0.10	0.1	65	0.3
Beer, 1½ cups	151	1	14	0	—	—	Trace	0.11	2.2	18	Trace
Butter, 1 tsp	36	—	—	4	153	0	Trace	Trace	Trace	1	Trace
Cake, Devil's Food, 1/16 of 9" cake	234	3	40	9	104	Trace	0.02	0.06	0.2	41	0.6
Cake, Sponge, 1/12 of 10" cake	196	5	36	4	297	Trace	0.03	0.09	0.1	20	0.8
Chocolate Syrup, 2 tbsp	93	1	24	1	Trace	0	0.01	0.03	0.2	6	0.6
Coffee, Black, ¾ cup	2	—	—	—	0	0	0	Trace	0.5	3	0.2
Cookie, Sugar, 3" diameter, enriched	89	1	14	3	22	Trace	0.04	0.04	0.4	16	0.3
Doughnut, Cake Type, enriched	125	2	17	6	26	Trace	0.07	0.07	0.5	13	0.4

8.4 NUTRITION AND DIET IN NORTH AMERICA

North Americans are probably more preoccupied with what they eat, when they eat, and with whom, than people in most other parts of the world. Their abundant supply of readily available foods and highly developed, affluent way of life makes their obsession with food paradoxical. This trait is more easily understood if one recognizes that food is regarded, not so much as a means of sustenance, but as a symbol of higher level needs: emotional security, social acceptance, and prestige. As a result, the decisions people make about diet are more often a reflection of cultural traditions or of what is currently in vogue than a response to bodily need. Certain foods, such as caviar and lobster (both high in cholesterol), are considered desirable because they symbolize wealth and extravagance; others (such as oatmeal porridge or baked beans) are generally regarded as foods consumed by the less affluent. Even though they may be more nutritious, they are less desirable.

Certain foods, associated with emotional security, are often consumed in excess during times of loneliness or unhappiness. Ironically, many of the foods offered as reward in our society (such as the cookie or candy) are low in nutritional value. Here again, nutritious foods are often considered less desirable to serve as "treats". An obsession with "time saving" and "fast food" is also prevalent. It is little wonder, therefore, that the food choices made daily by a majority often are not in the best interests of health, and many North Americans have lost touch with the essential meaning of good food (i.e., physical nourishment).

Fortunately, the past ten years has witnessed a resurgence of interest in eating for nutrition. The public has become increasingly concerned about the relationship between poor diet and several "diseases of affluence", about the growing numbers of chemical substances added to foods, and about the diminishing sensory quality of the food available on supermarket shelves. There is now a growing trend toward eating the "natural" foods consumed by our ancestors, such as fresh fruits and vegetables, with less

Table 8.20.
Energy inputs in corn production in Mexico using only manpower.
Reproduced with permission from Pimentel, D. In Nutrition in Health
and Disease, Moss, W.H. and Meyer, J., **Annals of the New York
Academy of Sciences**, 26: 32, 1977.

Input	Quantity/ha[†]	kcal/ha
Labor	1,144 hrs	-
Ax & hoe	16,500 kcal	16,500
Seeds	10.4 kg	36,608
Total	-	53,106
Corn yield	1,944 kg	6,842,880
kcal return/kcal input	-	128.8
Protein yield	175 kg	-

[†] hectare

reliance on highly refined foods (thus decreasing salt, sugar and fat intake).
Large numbers of people, however, still fail to make wise food choices,
either because they lack nutritional awareness or because they fail to
recognize the effect that food can have on one's general sense of well
being. Disease from nutritional causes occurs in modern developed
societies more from the malnutrition of excess (obesity, heart disease,
cancer) than from that of deficiency (rickets, osteomalacia, anemia).

8.5 GLOBAL PERSPECTIVES

8.5.1 Population
Global nutrition is dominated by several concerns whose interactions are
not easily understood. First among these is the exponential rise in the
number of people populating the earth. By most estimates, world population will reach 6-7 billion by the year 2000; in 1986 it was 5.4 billion, well
on target to the number projected. One may ask, therefore, can food
production indefinitely meet the demands for nourishment of so many
people?

8.5.2 Energy Balance Sheet
Food production in underdeveloped countries is a product of labor
intensive processes. Table 8.20 shows the kilocalorie return in food
products for kilocalorie input in labor in Mexico. This return depends upon
the patient, relatively uncompensated (according to developed nations
standards) labor of the farm worker. As estimated earlier in this chapter,
sustained physical effort over a 10 hour working period can reach approximately 64.0 kcalories per hour (1/10 HP), or 640 kcalories per 10-hour day.
Developed nations increase production, often on limited area or initially
on marginally fertile land, by massive conversion of other forms of energy
to the process of growing food. It has been estimated that a gallon of
gasoline (burned to drive a tractor, to produce pesticide, to irrigate, for

Table 8.21 Energy inputs in U.S. corn production in kcal/ha.* Reproduced with permission from Pimentel, D. In Food and Nutrition in Health and Disease, Moss, N.H. and Meyer, J. (eds), **Annals of NY Academy of Sciences**, 26-32, 1977.

Input	1945	1970
Machinery	539,000	1,078,000
Fuel	1,400,000	2,060,000
Nitrogen	121,440	1,897,500
Phosphorus	25,600	112,000
Potassium	13,200	147,400
Seeds for planting	77,440	147,840
Irrigation	103,740	187,000
Insecticides	0	82,790
Herbicides	0	82,790
Drying	9,880	296,400
Electricity	39,500	380,000
Transportation	49,400	172,900
Total inputs	2,379,200	6,644,220
kcal return/kcal input	3.15	2.69

* kcal/hectare

drying processes, etc.) provides 7200 kcalories of energy. This is equivalent to an 11 HP workrate carried on for 1 hour, or roughly 110 times the equivalent energy produced by a single person in a working day. A typical balance sheet for energy input (in the shape of fossil fuel burned) to energy output (in the kilocalorie value of food produced) in America is shown in Table 8.21 (Pimentel et al, 1977). The 2.69 ratio compares very unfavorably with the 128.8 ratio shown in Table 8.20 for a labor intensive process. An equally disturbing question must therefore be, how can depletion of the world's fossil fuel resources by developed and aspiring nations continue at such a rate without exhaustion?

Illustrating this dilemma is the growth in population and energy consumption in the world between 1600 and 1975 and their projections beyond (shown in Figure 8.6).

Indian scientists (Gopalan 1977) have predicted that her food requirements to 2000A.D. for self sufficiency, (shown in Table 8.22), are realizable if irrigation is increased from 17% to 57% and fertilizer output from 2 Megatonnes (Mt) to 14Mt.

Where will the fossil fuel for these obvious fuel intensive rather than human intensive energy expenditures come from in this long term?

8.5.3 Global Resources

CARBON

One limiting factor in food production is the supply of carbon in reduced form (Pirie, 1977). Table 8.23 shows estimates of this resource on earth. The major source of carbon for food is carbon dioxide reduced by photosynthesis in plants. Paradoxically, although this is currently a small resource, it is seemingly growing to excess as we pollute the air with it from humans, automobiles, waste burning, and razing the world's forests.

Carbon petroleum products are also a source of food, called single cell protein (SCP). This includes bacteria and yeast grown on petroleum and

Table 8.22. India's food needs in 2000 AD (Megatonnes). Reprinted with permission from Gopalan In **People and Food Tomorrow** Eds. D. Hollingsworth and E. Morse, Applied Science Ltd., 89-102, 1977.

	1971	2000
Food grains	100	180
Milk	23	65
Meat	0.7	2
Fish	2	7
Eggs (number)	6,000 m	28,000 m

Table 8.23. Mass of carbon in various forms on each square metre of total world surface, i.e. $5 \times 10^{14} m^2$. Reprinted with permission from Pirie, In **People and Food Tomorrow** Eds. D. Hollingsworth and E. Morse, Applied Science Ltd., 157-169, 1977.

Reduced carbon	
Methane	40.0 g
Petroleum	140.0 g
Oceanic sediment	1.9 kg
Soil organic matter	2.9 kg
Oceanic water	5.4 kg
Coal, lignite, etc.	10.0 kg
Kerogen in rock	5.0 t

Oxidised carbon	
Atmospheric CO_2	1.1 kg
Oceanic CO_2	70.0 kg
Limestone and dolomite	18.0 t

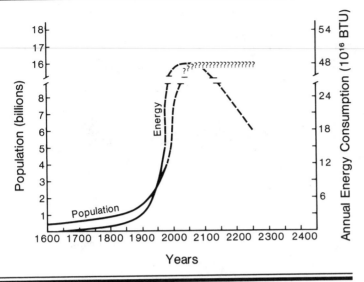

Figure 8.6. Estimated world population numbers (____) from 1600 to 1975 and projected numbers (- - -) (????) to the year 2250. Estimated fossil fuel consumption (____) from 1650 to 1975 and projected (- - -) to the year 2250. Reprinted with permission from Pimentel In **Nutrition in Health and Disease**, Eds. NH. Moss and J. Mayer, Annals of New York Academy of Sciences, 26-32, 1977.

gas oil with ammonium salts and air. A 15-20% diversion of the World's petroleum production to this new process would meet the entire yearly protein requirement of the current world population (some 5 billion people), but might detract from other food producing processes utilizing fossil fuel (Mauron, 1977).

In developed nations, plant protein resources are converted to higher level animal protein. In the U.S.A. alone more than 6 million metric tons of animal protein are produced from 26 million metric tons plant protein fed to animals. Feeding the world on America's high protein/kilocalorie diet would cost 6,250 Billion liters of fuel annually. Fuel used at this rate, to produce food will exhaust the world's reserves in 13 years (Pimentel, 1977). If only grass fed livestock were raised livestock protein production would decline to 2 million metric tons.

SCP protein is presently consumed by fish as plankton. An estimated 1,000 kcal of energy as algae reduces to 150 kcal as plankton protoplasm, and further to only 30kcal when eaten by fish (smelt). When humans eat smelt only 6 kcal of the original 1,000 kcal have been recovered. If another fish, such as a trout, intervenes in the food chain route, a human receives only 1.2 kcal of the original 1,000 kcal from the fish.

As we now know, judicious choice of both quality (essential amino acids) and quantity of plants eaten yields an adequate diet, especially if supplemented with the products of some foraging rather than grain fed livestock. One may therefore ask, would it not be better for us to become principally vegetarian? The reader should weigh the pros and cons of this statement for themself. What do you think?

LAND

Estimates of potential arable land in the world range from 1.4 billion (Pimentel, 1977) to 3.4 billion (Pirie, 1975) or 5.2 billion hectares (Gross, 1985). Twenty-seven million hectares are added annually to the 3.5 billion hectares of desert area in the world as a result of overgrazing, fuel wood gathering, agricultural expansion on marginal soil, erosion, and conversion to non-farm uses. Twenty-three billion tons of top soil are lost to the

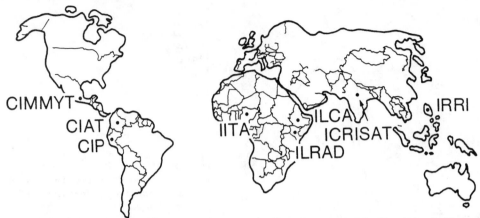

Figure 8.7. Locations of International Agricultural Research Centers pioneered by the Rockefeller Foundation, in Mexico in 1963, followed by the Ford Foundation in the U.S.A. Agency for International Development (AID). Reprinted with permission from Pereira In People and Food tomorrow. Eds. D. Hollingsworth and E. Morse, Applied Sciences Ltd., 94, 1977.

rivers and seas each year all over the world. It is calculated that by 2000 A.D. 64 countries will have critical land shortages. Arid lands are now home to 860 million people (Gross, 1985)-a total expected to increase to 1.2 billion by 2000 A.D. Solutions to these few of the many problems of providing adequate food supplies to the world's population lie in achieving a balance, in every nation, between the complex ecological, political, economic, social and technological forces at play.

TECHNOLOGY

Technological advances like the Green revolution (a package of newly developed, highly productive strains of wheat backed with intense fertilization, pesticides, dense planting, and irrigation techniques) with similar new advances from agricultural research centers around the world (Figure 8.7) have led to remarkable gains in food productivity world wide. These gains, however, have barely kept pace with population growth in underdeveloped countries (Figure 8.8). Currently, there seems to be adequate food in the world to feed everyone 3,000 kcalories per day with a defined protein (4 kcal·g^{-1}) energy/total kcal energy ratio of 10%, yet for whatever reasons of politics, profit or transport/distribution problems cited, few are fed adequately.

Importance of Breaking the Cycle of Poverty

The distinguishing characteristic of the malnourished in many parts of the world is their impoverishment (Joy, 1977). Growth and distribution of food has to be at a local level. Also, technological innovation has to be practically relevant at this level (i.e., smaller designed tractors) and has to proceed in step with social innovation, so that even the poor are productive. The welfare of the land is directly tied to those who work it and earn from it. To implement the suggestion made earlier to return to a vegetarian diet in North America would precipitate massive displacement of people from jobs (Lappe and Collins, 1979). This presents the potential for future impoverishment and malnourishment such as that currently existing in less affluent societies.

IRRI International Rice Institute, 1960

CIMMYT International Center for Improvement of Wheat and Maize, 1964

IITA International Institute for Tropical Agriculture, 1965

CIAT International Center for Tropical Agriculture, 1968

CIP International Potato Center

ICRISAT International Center for Research in the Semi Arid Tropics, 1972

ILRAD International Laboratory for Research into Animal Diseases, 1974

ILCA International Livestock Center for Africa, 1974

ICARDA International Center for Arid Regions Dryland Agriculture (not shown)

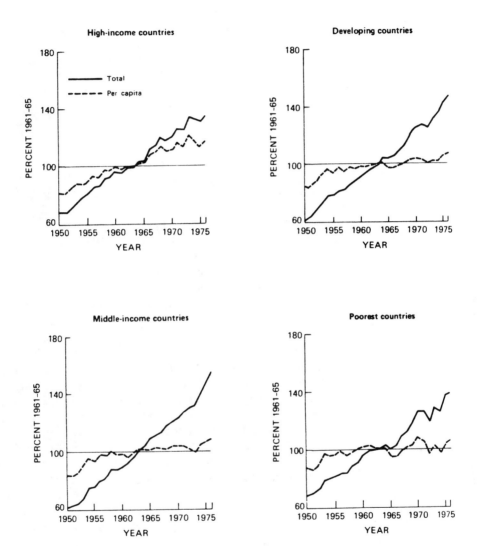

Figure 8.8. Food production indices: total and per capita, 1950-1976 (1961-65=100). Reproduced with permission from U.S. Department of Agriculture, Washington, D.C. Economic Research Service, 1977.

In Britain today one may witness the social effects of such precipitous, relative impoverishment in the demise of the industrial North amid the seeming continued affluence of the South. Such change in the social fabric of a society is dangerous, containing the seeds of violence or revolution and disintegration of the society.

Undoubtedly scientific knowledge and technological innovation will solve the food supply problem, but not without a political will in underdeveloped countries to: return the land to the small landholder and local control (easing distribution problems); restrict the ownership of land and the export of food for profit by foreign conglomerates (ensuring that its own people are fed); educate each farmer on good farming practice and thus allow the poor to be productive. Those countries implementing such procedures are solving their food supply problems: countries such as China, Cuba, and India. In India, in an area of rich agricultural resource, the Indian and Pakistani Punjab lie adjacent to each other. In the former, government support of irrigation and electrification schemes, support of relevant technological practice, establishment of local control by the small farmers, with provisions for their continuing education, has produced remarkable returns in food production (a tripling in production of wheat since the 1960's) and alleviation of malnourishment. Those policies contrast sharply with the old ways, followed in the Pakistani Punjab. Here, one finds large tract ownership, absentee landlords, and impoverishment of displaced farmers (without the resources to farm large tracts). The attendant poor local food production and malnourishment is not unexpected. (**Economist**, March 15, 1987).

8.6 SUMMARY

Any rational analysis of the sometimes conflicting data on worldwide resources, and the production of and need for food, seems to indicate that the world's current food production is adequate. Its equitable distribution, however, is frustrated by political mismanagement of agricultural policy, and vested, multinational, and corporate interests. These interests channel major proportions of crop away from the growing areas for export, without regard for first achieving food self-sufficiency in a region or the longterm welfare of the land. Safeguarding the long-term supply of food in the world depends on how well the nation-states can begin to think globally to solve their common problems. These problems concern the environment (principally pollution of every sort negative to the growth of life), the exhaustion of world resources (principally fossil fuels, carbon, nitrogen, phosphorus, and the top soil), the declining integrity of social structures (in part attributable to job displacement, impoverishment, and malnutrition), and a burgeoning world population.

8.7 ESSENTIAL FURTHER READING

Hensley, Elizabeth S. **Basic Concepts of World Nutrition.** Charles C. Thomas Publisher, Springfield, Illinois, 1981.

World Hunger: Ten Myths. The Institute for Food and Development Policy, 1885 Mission Street, San Francisco, California, 94110. 1 to 6 copies $2.25 each; 50 copies $1.35 each.

Publications of the U.S. Department of Agriculture. Human Nutrition Information Service, Hyattsville, MD, 20782.

8.8 REFERENCES

AH 8-1. Composition of Food: Dairy and Egg Products U.S.A. Department of Agriculture, Washington, D.C., Superintendent of Documents, US Government Printing Office.

Banister, E.W. and Brown, S.R. The relative energy requirements of Physical activity. In **Exercise Physiology.** Ed. H.B. Falls, New York Academic Press, pp. 267-322, 1968.

Behar, M. Protein-Calorie Deficits in Developing Countries, In **Food and Nutrition in Health and Disease,** Eds. N.H. Moss and J. Mayer, New York. **Annals of the New York Academy of Sciences,** 176-187, 1977.

FAO/WHO ad hoc Expert Committee **Energy and Protein Requirements,** Rome. FAO, 1973.

Food and Agricultural Organization of the United Nations. **Handbook on Human Nutritional Requirements.** Rome FAO, 1974.

Food and Agricultural Organization of the United Nations. **The States of Food and Agriculture,** Rome, 1975.

Food and Nutrition Board, National Academy of Sciences, **Recommended Dietary Allowances,** Washington D.C.: National Academy of Sciences, 1980.

Gopalan, C. Growing populations and rising aspirations. In **People and Food Tomorrow,** Eds. D. Hollinsworth and and E. Morse, London. Applied Science Ltd., 89-102, 1977.

Gross, M. Time running out on desert spread. United Nations Environmental Program Head Says. **Globe and Mail** (Canada), Dec. 24, 1985.

Hegsted D. **Assessment of Protein Quality. Improvement of Protein Nutritive.** Washington D.C. National Academy of Sciences, 64-88, 1974.

Hensley, E.S. **Basic Concepts of World Nutrition.** Springfield. Charles C. Thomas Publisher, 292, 1981.

Joy, L. Families who cannot afford to feed themselves. In **People and Food Tomorrow,** Eds. D. Hollingsworth and E. Morse, London. Applied Science Ltd., 157-165, 1977.

Konopka, P. **Correct Diet Means Better Performance.** Hertfordshire. Wander Sport Nutrition Division, Wander Ltd., p. 20, 1982.

Krehl, W.A. The Nutritional Epidemiology of Cardiovascular Disease. In **Food and Nutrition in Health and Disease** Eds. N.H. Moss, and J. Mayer New York, New York Academy of Sciences, 335-359, 1977.

Kritchevsky, D. Dietary Fiber: What it is and what it does. In Food and Nutrition in Health and Disease Eds. N.H. Moss and J. Mayer, New York. **Annals New York Academy of Sciences,** 283-289, 1977.

Lappe, F.M., and Collins, J. **World Hunger: Ten Myths.** Institute for Food and Development Policy San Francisco, p. 72, 1979.

Malmros, H. Prevention of a therosclerosis by a Fat-Modified Diet. In Food and Nutrition in Health and Disease, Eds. N.H. Moss and J. Mayer, New York. **Annals of the New York Academy of Sciences,** 379-382, 1977.

Mauron, J. Future Trends in the use of Protein Resources. In **People and Food Tomorrow**. Eds. D. Hollingsworth and E. Morse, London. Applied Sciences Ltd. 131, 1977.

Pereira, H.C. Scientific Progress in World Food Production In **People and Food Tomorrow**, Eds. D. Hollinsworth and E. Morse, London. Applied Science Ltd. 89-102, 1977.

Pimentel, D. Energy Resources and hand Constraints in Food Production. In Food and Nutrition in Health and Disease, Eds. N.H. Moss and J. Mayer, New York: **Annals of the New York Academy of Sciences**, 26-32, 1977.

Pimentel, D., Dritschilo, W., Krummel, J., and Kutzman, J. Energy and Land Constraints in Food-Protein production, **Science**, 190: 754-761, 1975.

Pirie, N.W. Physical Limitations on the Food Supply, In **People and Food Tomorrow** Eds. D. Hollingsworth and E. Morse, London, Applied Science Publishers Ltd., 157-165, 1977.

Reddy, B.S., and Wynder, E.L. Large bowel carcinogenesis: Fecal constituents of populations with diverse incidence rates of colon cancer. **Journal of National Cancer Institute**, 50: 1437-1442, 1973.

Steering Committee World Food and Nutrition Study, Commission on International Relations National Research Council, Washington. National Academy of Sciences, p. 192, 1977.

Strasenburgh Co. of Canada Ltd. **Are you really serious about losing weight**. pp. 68.

The National Dairy Council Food Power. **A Coache's Guide to Improving Performance**. Rosemount: The National Dairy Council, pp. 36, 1984.

Wilkie, D.R. Man as a Source of Mechanical Power. **Ergonomics**: 1: 1-8, 1960.

Wynder, E.L. Nutritional Carcinogenesis. In Food and Nutrition in Health and Disease Eds. N.H. Moss and J. Mayer, New York. **Annals of the New York Academy of Sciences**, 360-377, 1977.

8.3 STUDY QUESTIONS

1. What are the six major categories of nutrients?
2. What guidelines are presently available to help determine the amounts of nutrients required for optimal health? What are some of the limitations of these guidelines?
3. What are the consequences of failing to obtain adequate amounts of the essential nutrients?
4. Are vitamin supplements (generally) necessary? What is their role in the dietary needs of athletes?
5. Outline the dietary guidelines as summarized by the U.S. Department of Agriculture.
6. Outline some of the major hazards associated with excess consumption of meat.
7. Why must vegetarians pay particular attention to dietary planning?
8. Is brown bread better for you than white bread?
9. What are the normal requirements in terms of caloric intake for males and females who are moderately active?
10. Are carbohydrates essential nutrients? What value do they have in physical training programs?
11. What are the two major contributors to daily energy requirements?

12. What are the major food sources of the body's
    energy?
13. Discuss the contribution of food distribution once
    it is produced to the problem of malnutrition in
    the world.
14. How do politics and world food conglomerates
    contribute to the inequitable distribution of food
    in the world? (Research this).
15. Discuss the problem of soil erosion and agricul-
    tural production. (Research this).
16. Why are all the plants of the world disappearing
    (250,000 kinds in the next 30 years)?
    (Research this).

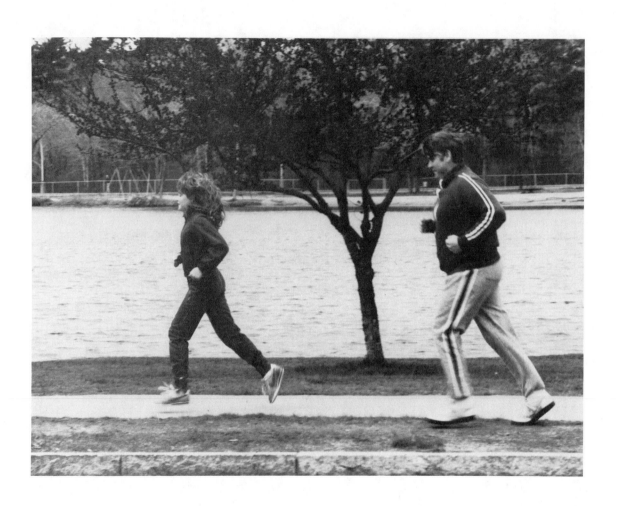

9

Fitness and Sports Medicine

Physical fitness is crucial for the attainment and maintenance
of optimal health—both physical and mental.

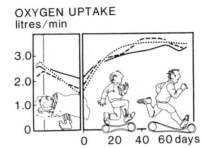

OXYGEN UPTAKE
litres/min

Figure 9.1. Showing changes in maximum oxygen uptake following bed rest and training as reported by Saltin et al., **Circulation**, supp. 7, 37-38, 1968. Reproduced with permission from Astrand, P.O. **Health and Fitness**. Ottawa: Fitness and Amateur Sport Canada, page 48, 1975.

OBJECTIVES

When you have completed this chapter, you should be able to:
- **Describe** the effects of exercise on normally healthy people, the young and the old.
- **Distinguish** between the prospective and retrospective studies that have attempted to identify the benefit of exercise for humans.
- **Evaluate** the role of exercise in ameliorating or preventing the development of clinically debilitating illnesses, and describe the latent threat of degenerative disease states.
- **Explain** the waning responsiveness of humans to exercise as they grow older and the necessity of commitment to regular exercise if they are to continue to benefit from the activity.
- **Describe** the national policies of various countries concerned with sport and fitness in the context of their ideological political systems.
- **Discuss** mass participation—benefits, costs, and how to achieve it.
- **Explain** the problem of injury in any mass participation of previous sedentary people in a program of exercise.
- **Outline** the effect exercise has upon various body systems (cardiovascular, respiratory, muscle); for this you will need some understanding of human physiology.
- **Describe** the forces at work in the body during exercise.
- **Discuss** appropriate preventive action against accidental injury, that is, trauma and those injuries resulting from so-called "over-use syndromes" (tennis elbow or shinsplints).
- **Understand** the broad activity and concerns of sports medicine and sport science.

KEY TERMS
cardio-respiratory fitness
compression

epiphysitis
inflammation

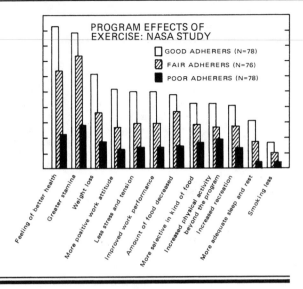

PROGRAM EFFECTS OF
EXERCISE: NASA STUDY

□ GOOD ADHERERS (N=78)
▨ FAIR ADHERERS (N=76)
■ POOR ADHERERS (N=78)

Feeling of better health
Greater stamina
Weight loss
More positive work attitude
Less stress and tension
Improved work performance
Amount of food decreased
More selective in kind of food
Increased physical activity beyond the program
Increased recreation
More adequate sleep and rest
Smoking less

Figure 9.2. Program effects of exercise: NASA study. Modified and reproduced with permission from Durbeck et al., **Am. J. of Cardiol.** page 30, 1972.

direct trauma
muscle contusion
over-use syndrome
rehabilitation
sedentary

ligament
spasticity
stress fracture
tendonitis

9.0 INTRODUCTION

Chapter Nine deals with an important area of preventive health care: Fitness and Sports Medicine. Physical fitness is crucial for the attainment and maintenance of optimal health—both physical and mental. However, in order to prevent exercise-related injuries, sports medicine must also be given equal attention in any complete fitness program.

9.1 EXERCISE IN MODERN SOCIETY

The ancient Athenians proposed a most enticing formula relating sport and health. This notion was to use sport as a means of harmonizing the human body, of establishing an ideal balance between body and soul, thus obtaining happiness and a greater awareness of life. Today more and more people are beginning to relate exercise, fitness, and health together in this way.

Normally healthy, but otherwise inactive, people often find their tolerance for extended physical effort reduced. However, such people are often surprised at how quickly the body responds to regular exercise of any type by adapting to the increasing physical demands. The cardiorespiratory (endurance) and musculo-skeletal (strength) systems are particularly responsive (Figure 9.1). This figure shows an obvious decline in oxygen uptake when activity is severely curtailed by enforced bed rest for 21 days. Fitness of the cardiorespiratory system may be reactivated, however, by progressive training so that previous levels of fitness reflected in maximum oxygen uptake measures may be recovered and even surpassed. Figure 9.2 shows that a physical training program produces changes in many more lifestyle attributes than just fitness. In the National Aeronautics and Space Administration's study, 242 employees

Table 9.1. Effect of exercise on primary and secondary risk factors for CHD.

	Factor	Exercise Effect
Primary	Age	no effect
	Sex	no effect
	Arterial Blood Pressure	decreases
	Serum Lipids (fat)	decreases
	Cigarette Smoking	decreases
	Inactivity	decreases
Secondary	Obesity	decreases
	Heredity	no effect
	Stress	decreases
Metabolic Abnormalities	Glucose intolerance	decreases
	Gout	no effect
	Hypothyroidism	no effect

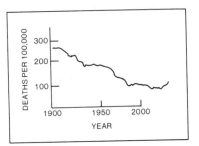

Figure 9.3. Declining death rate due to infectious diseases from 1900, projected until 2050. Modified and reproduced with permission from Glazier, W.H. **Scientific American,** 228: 1973.

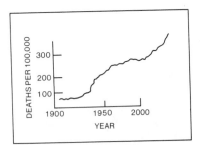

Figure 9.4. Increase in death rate in modern society from degenerative diseases such as heart and circulation disorders and lung disease. Modified and reproduced with permission from Glazier, W.H. **Scientific American,** 228: 1973.

participated voluntarily in a training program run 5 days per week. The good adherers (greater than 3 days per week attendance) had a more positive response on an attitudinal questionnaire than fair adherers (less than 3 days attendance) and poor adherers (once per week). Generally, these changes contribute significantly to an overall improvement in health, quality of life, and "joie de vivre."

In modern societies, death and incapacity, for the most part, are no longer caused by infectious disease but by the insidious onset of diseases caused by degeneration of the body's systems. Notice how the decline in deaths from infectious diseases (shown in Figure 9.3) in the Western World have been almost paralleled by the rise in deaths (shown in Figure 9.4) from degenerative disease states (heart and circulation disorders, emphysema, cancer, etc.) in the years since 1900. Fortunately, the systems particularly susceptible to degeneration, the heart, lungs, and circulation, are those on which regular exercise training seems to exert its most beneficial effect. Thus, the effects of training shown in Figure 9.5 are that it is usually accompanied by better circulation in body organs, particularly muscle, because an increased number of blood vessels serve them. The efficiency and even the size of the heart also increases so that more blood may be pumped by each beat of the heart and the heart rate is able to decrease. Fat is better used and the overall fat around the body, particularly around internal body organs, is reduced improving their operation. Table 9.1 shows the effects of training on the principle risk factors for coronary heart disease. Although death from cardiovascular disease is always more prevalent in older age groups, the fit older individual is likely to retain mobility and thus sociability and a better quality of life even if the evidence for a longer life accompanying fitness is not yet proved (Sidney and Shepherd, 1978). Inherited and sexual protection against degeneration of body systems seem unaffected by exercise, but an impressive list of human attributes positively affected remains (Figure 9.2). From a social point of view, this means that both the individual and society may contribute significantly

Coronary artery
↑ Capillary/fiber ratio
↑ Collateral blood flow
↑ Vessel diameter

Heart ↑ Cardiac output
↑ Heart rate
↑ Stroke volume
↓ Myocardial oxygen consumption

Adipose Tissue
↑ Free fatty acid mobilization

Exercise training

Coagulation system
↑ Fibrinolysis

Intestines

Pancreas
↑ Insulin secretion
↑ Glucagon secretion

Liver
↑ Triglyceride production (very-low-density lipoproteins)

↑ Chylomicron production

Figure 9.5. Cardiovascular and metabolic adaptations that occur with exercise training. Modified and reproduced with permission from Simonetti and Eaton, **Postgraduate Medicine**, 63: 71-77, 1978.

to alleviating the burgeoning cost of health care that we are now facing. Examples of current health care costs are shown both for the USA and Canada in Figures 9.6 and 9.7. Individuals can do this by making exercise a regular part of their leisure activity. Society as a whole can also contribute by providing facilities and programs to encourage mass participation in physical activity.

9.1.1 Beneficial Effects of Exercise on Health

Direct positive effects of exercise on longevity and health remain difficult to prove unequivocally. Health scientists and physicians have accumulated impressive evidence through retrospective studies (historical surveys), suggesting that generally exercise benefits cardiorespiratory fitness, while inactivity is deleterious to it (Table 9.2). Similarly, some prospective studies (i.e., studies that deliberately set out to follow the effect of some course of treatment or habit) show that exercise has demonstrated beneficial effects upon mortality (death) and morbidity (general incapacity). The incidence of any of the 3 disease states shown in these tables is always less in the active group.

The evidence for the benefits of a moderate lifestyle, incorporating some vigorous leisure activity daily, is now considerable, most people today believe that it is better:
1. to be active rather than sedentary;
2. not to smoke rather than to smoke; and
3. to be leaner rather than fatter (Lalonde, 1974).

Recently, the prestigious American College of Sports Medicine, with a membership of more than 10,000 practising physicians, exercise scientists, nutritionists, physiotherapists, and biochemists, issued a positive statement indicating that

both the QUALITY and QUANTITY of exercise is important for the development and long term maintenance of health and vigour in an otherwise presently healthy adult.

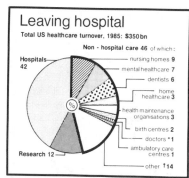

Leaving hospital
Total US healthcare turnover, 1985: $350 bn

Non - hospital care 46 of which :

Hospitals 42

Research 12

nursing homes 9
mental healthcare 7
dentists 6
home healthcare 3
health maintenance organisations 3
birth centres 2
doctors *1
ambulatory care centres 1
other †14

* Solo practices   † Includes group practices, pain centres & diagnosis centres
Source: Health Industry Manufacturers Association

Figure 9.6. Total U.S. healthcare turnover, 1985: $350 billion. Reproduced with permission from **The Economist**, p. 73, March 22, 1986.

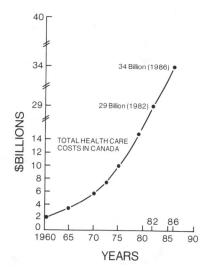

34 Billion (1986)

29 Billion (1982)

TOTAL HEALTH CARE COSTS IN CANADA

$BILLIONS

YEARS

Figure 9.7. Exponential growth of health care costs in Canada.

Table 9.2.
Epidemiological studies: ratio of incidence of coronary disease in groups of active and sedentary people.

$$R = \frac{\text{Incidence in active people}}{\text{Incidence among sedentary people}}$$

Author-year Place (reference)	Categories studied	Coronary Diseases	Infarction	Deaths
		R-Value		
Morris, 1953 London	31,000 urban transit employees Active conductors, sedentary drivers, 35-64 years	0.70	0.53	0.46
	180,000 man-years. Postal workers Active delivery staff/telephonists and sedentary employees 35-39 years	0.75	-	0.50
Brown, 1957 Birmingham	1,062 men aged between 60-69, including 89 coronary sufferers. 158 very active occupations/137 sedentary occupations	0.29	0.63	-
	766 fairly active/137 sedentary	0.53	0.60	-
Chapman, 1957	772 civil service employees 40-59 years 492 active/236 sedentary (differences not significant)	1.03	0.98	-
Zukel, 1959 North Dakota	1,886 controls and 288 cases of coronary diseases. Over age 35. Farmers/other occupations	0.70	0.48	-
Stamler, 1954-57 Chicago	740 public service employees, 50-59 years, blue collar/white collar	0.78	Difference not statistically significant	-
McDonough, 1964	3,102 agricultural workers, 15-74 yrs. Considerable/inconsiderable degree of physical activity.	0.17-0.50	-	-
Rose, 1969 London	9.777 civil servants, 40-64 years. Ratio of incidence of ECG lesions. 3,561 walkers/436 non-walkers	0.61	-	-
Brunner, 1949-59	4,500 (102 cases of infarction) 4,000 (9 cases of infarc.), age 30-55 yrs. Active occup./sedentary occup. Same kind of life in 58 kibbutzim.	-	0.33	0.33
Taylor, 1954-60 USA	Railway workers: switchmen/clerks (61,630 man-years)/(85,112 man-years)	-	-	0.63
	Section men (44,837 man-years)/clerks (sedentary employees fatter and more urbanized than manual workers)	-	0.49	-

Table 9.2. .....continued
Modified and reproduced with permission from Reville, **Sport for All**, Council of Europe, Strasbourg, 1970.

Author-year Place (reference)	Categories studied	R-Value		
		Coronary Diseases	Infarction	Deaths
Kahn, 1962 Washington	1,664 postal employees, Carriers/clerks	-	-	0.53-0.70
Hammond, 1955-62, USA	40-69 years highly active/inactive non-smokers/smokers	-	-	0.57 0.70
Kannel, 1961* Framingham study	4,469 persons 30-59 years; classified according to degree of activeness	-	-	0.28-0.47
Breslow, 1949-51, USA	45-64 years. Various occupations active/inactive	-	-	0.71
Franck, 1966* New York	110,000 persons (Health Ins. Plan) 301 cases of infarction, 25-64 years According to degree of occupational and/or non-occupational sport activeness	-	-	0.30-0.50
Morris, 1968 Indiana	10,520 farmers compared to 9,310 persons in sedentary occupations 35-75 years	0.68	-	0.59
Sarvotham, 1968 India	1,361 men and 669 women, over 30 years. Average degree of activeness/sedentariness	0.55	-	-
Paffenbargher* 1951-67 San Francisco	3,263 longshoremen, 291 infarct. deaths Highly active dockers/relatively inactive white collar workers	35-44 years 45-54 years 55-64 years	0.13 0.64 0.70	
Durbeck et al., 1972	988 NASA employees enrolled in fitness program 1, 2 or 3 or more days/week	Significant correlations between number of days exercised and reduction in risk factors. Greatest reduction with more days exercised.		
Chave et al., 1978	Study of British male civil servants, degree of leisure time activity related to death rate.	Direct correlations shown between degree of activity and death rate.		
Blair et al., 1983	Studied 753 men on treadmill fitness test after training.	Showed changes in coronary heart disease risk factors were associated with increased treadmill run time.		
Paffenbargher, R.S. et al., 1984	16,936 Harvard Alumni studied between 1962-1972.	Showed that habitual post college exercise not student sports play predicts low coronary heart disease risk.		

* Classic studies

Figure 9.8. Showing the decline in speed sit ups (maximum completed in 60 seconds) and push ups (maximum number) with age in a representative natural sample. Reproduced with permission from **Canada Fitness Survey**, Fitness Canada, 1981.

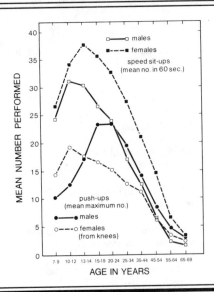

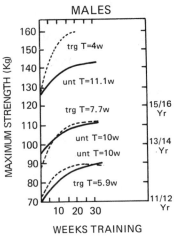

MALES

WEEKS TRAINING

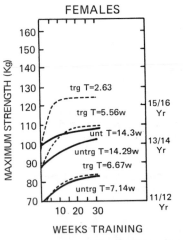

FEMALES

WEEKS TRAINING

Figure 9.9. Curves of strength gain in groups of male and female students accompany normal growth (thick lines) and when normal growth is supplemented with strength training (dashed lines). Modified and reproduced with permission from Banister, E.W. **National Strength Coaches Assoc. Journal 2**: 27-31, 1980.

Although few would claim that exercise will have ameliorating effects upon the pathology of chronic disease states, it is fair to say that the intolerance to effort, produced by a disease, may often be reversed by regular progressive training (Fentem and Bassey, 1982). There is evidence for this in the case of chronic respiratory diseases (Vyas et al., 1971; Paez, 1967); diabetes (Larsson, et al., 1962); aging generally (Sydney & Shephard,1978); and senility specifically (Schreuder, J.T.R., 1969).

Similar beneficial effects of exercise are to be noted in the course of pregnancy (Erkkola, 1976); childhood diseases (Fitch & Morton, 1971); the reversal of obesity, often in conjunction with psychological and nutritional counselling (Mayer, 1964); and depression and other psychological manifestations of stress (Donald, 1969; Doby,1967).

9.2 EFFECTS OF EXERCISE ON CHILDREN AND YOUTH

Children and young people are normally thought of as active and fit, but increasingly, in modern society, they are tending toward the role of being spectators—non-participants in even mildly vigorous activity.

Figure 9.8 shows the decline in muscular endurance in males and females measured recently in a substantial cross sectional sample of Canadian young adults (Canada Fitness Survey, 1982). Three Federally Funded standardized studies of fitness on children, completed in the USA in recent years, paint a discouraging picture. Although significant gains in the fitness of public school children were shown in the years between the first and second studies in 1957 and 1964, little or no improvement has been shown since, according to a later study in 1974. In another survey carried out in Michigan in 1974, it was found that 50% of a group of young people showed evidence of one or more of the triad of high cardiovascular risk symptoms: high blood pressure, high blood cholesterol, and low physical fitness (see Table 9.1). Neither should we be lulled into accepting mere improvement as encouraging if the level of accom-

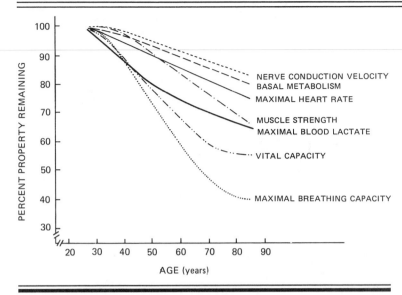

Figure 9.10. Decline in various physiological variables with age. Adapted and reproduced with permission from Skinner, in **Limiting Factors of Physical Performance**, G. Theime, Stuttgart, 1973.

plishment is still inferior, as it was found to be in another study recently of 4 million 6-17 year old USA children in Michigan. In 1979-80, 57% of them failed to achieve acceptable standards of fitness. In the USA also, 8,800 children in grades 5-12 taking part in a two year National Children and Youth Fitness Test were found to have too much body fat, and 50% of the sample received less than an appropriate amount of exercise each day (NCYFS, 1986). Figure 9.9, on the other hand, shows how a regular weight training regime increased muscle strength in experimental groups of boys and girls, beyond that normally expected simply by growing (Banister, 1980). In this figure, the full lines show normal gain in strength with age and the dotted curves show the enhanced gain resulting from strength training over the same period.

The time constant denoted by the Greek letter "Tau" (τ) describes the time it takes for a curve to grow from its lowest level to two-thirds of its steady state level. Short time constants indicate rapid growth.

9.3 EXERCISE AND THE ELDERLY

Aging is an inevitable process of natural decline in physical attributes. Figure 9.10 shows this decline with passing years in several vital physiological measures. The values shown have been normalized (expressed as a percentage of the mean 25-30 year value of each attribute). Figure 9.11 shows that participation for more than 5 hours per week declines and that those participating less than 1 hour per week increases with advancing age. Old people, especially, tend to become inactive and increasingly prone to morbidity and age-based deterioration induced by their lack of exercise (Figures 9.11 and 9.12). It may be noted that the life expectancy of Americans has increased in recent years from 69.7 in 1960 to 73.2 years in 1977 and to 74.1 years in 1981. Not all, if any, of this increase may be attributed to fitness training however, since surgical techniques, particularly the coronary bypass operation, have contributed and continue to contribute importantly to improving these figures.

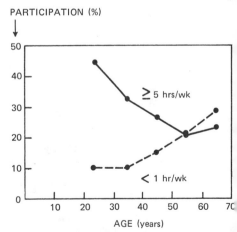

Figure 9.11. Decline in participation in active leisure with age shown as the relative amount of time spent in physical activity per week. Adapted and reproduced with permission from Skinner, in **Limiting Factors of Physical Performance**, G. Theime, Stuttgart, 1973.

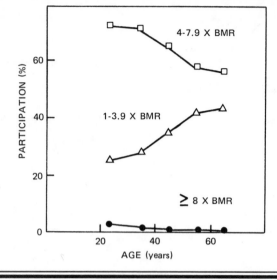

Figure 9.12. Percent participation according to age, of 1,695 men from Tecumseh, Mich., in leisure activities measured by the intensity of the most active 1.5 hours of the week. Modified and reproduced with permission from data of Cunningham et al., **J. Geront.** **23**: 551, 1968.

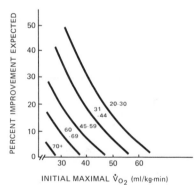

Figure 9.13. A hypothesized response to training showing that age (written on each line) and initial level of fitness (x axis) determine percent improvement (y axis). Modified and reproduced with permission from Skinner, In **Limiting Factors of Physical Performance,** G. Thieme, Stuttgart, 1973.

Although the body's sensitivity to a training stimulus declines with age, careful progressive training, carried out regularly, will bring about improvements in physical condition at almost any age (Figures 9.13, Table 9.3).

Institutionalization of elderly people is a private tragedy as well as a costly public expense. Maintenance of locomotor ability is an absolute prerequisite for elderly people in maintaining the social interaction and the independence of spirit so essential to the quality of their lives. Death and morbidity from hypothermia in the aged—a recently recognized phenomenon—may also be combatted with a well-organized regime of exercise. Studies show that there are detrimental effects on the health of older people when their control of their activities is restricted. In contrast, interventions (which must include mobility), that increased the range of options for their own control of their lives in nursing home patients promoted their health (Rodin, 1986).

It must be remembered that there is a progressive decline in the responsiveness to training as one grows older (peak responsiveness is probably around puberty). The diminished response accompanies the progressive decline in the body systems shown in Figure 9.10. This declining plasticity of response to a training stimulus suggests that careful training begun early in life will promote an optimal response throughout it and may even delay the rate of developing dysfunction shown by the untrained. Figure 9.13 shows how the extent of improvement in oxygen uptake ability, to be expected from training, declines with age and with the degree of a person's already attained fitness level. The results of some training studies in older subjects are shown in Table 9.3.

Table 9.3. Principal findings relating to physical exercise among elderly persons.
Modified and reproduced with permission from Reville, **Sport for All**, Council of Europe, Strasbourg, 1970.

Author-Year Place-Reference	Population Studied and Type of Training	Effects of Training
Barry, 1966 Philadelphia	8 persons between 55-78 years compared with 5 controls between 58-83 years, studied before and after 3 months' training (three 40-minute bicycle ergometer sessions per week).	• 76% increase in maximum work done with 50% increase in pulmonary ventilation (35-53 l·min⁻¹) and 38% increase in maximal oxygen intake on exertion. • Decline in tachycardia (126 to 106 beats per minute) and blood pressure (190 to 170 mm Hg) following exertion. • Improved results of psychological tests.
Bernestad, 1965 Oslo	13 men aged between 70-81 years, studied before and after 6 weeks with three weekly treadmill sessions.	• Decline in tachycardia on exertion from 131 to 117 beats per minute. • Improved heart work efficiency. • Decline in cholesterol level (2.70 to 2.57 grams per ml). • Feeling of improved well-being expressed spontaneously.
Fischer, 1965 Prague	84 men aged between 60-69 34 men aged between 70-79, one half of who trained on bicycle ergometer.	• Increased maximal oxygen consumption on exertion (+15%) and maximum breathing capacity (+22%) • Trained subjects equalled the performance of untrained subjects 10 years younger.
Saltin/Grimby, 1968, Sweden	Subjects between 50-67, five leading sedentary lives compared with 4 engaging in sport (skiing, cross-country running).	• Increase in maximum oxygen consumption (37 and 43 ml·kg·min⁻¹) and less heart acceleration (170 and 165 bpm) on exertion.
Hollmann, 1970 Cologne	133 subjects between 50-70, one half of whom have engaged in various sports for at least 2 hours per week without interruption.	• Improvement in breathing capacity tests on exertion, increase in maximum oxygen consumption, (25%). Performances comparable with those of untrained controls between 20 and 40 years younger.
Sidney and Shephard, 1978	42 elderly men and women, age 60-83 years, exercise training	• Significant correlations between increased fitness (VO_2) and training frequency.
Pell and Fayerweather, 1985	Morbidity and mortality in a large predominantly sedentary employed population between 1957-1983.	• Significant difference in mortality and morbidity found in those most sedentary in group.
Hossack, K.F. and Bruce, R.A. 1985	10 years study of 6,650 initially healthy people 20-84 years studied longitudinally for 10 years.	• Age over 55 years and exercise test evaluation improve detection of incipient disease.
Opiteck, et al., 1986.	15 healthy old men (74-93 years) trained for 6 weeks in a variety of low to moderate intensity exercise programs.	• Subjective improvement made in tolerance to exercise no quantitative changes. Longer periods of training probably needed to show effect in such fragile groups.

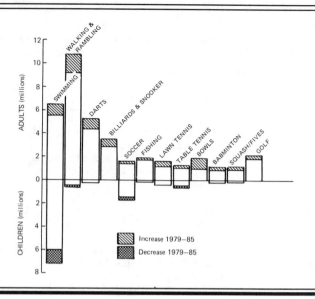

Figure 9.15. Projected increases in participation in sports and exercise from 1979-85. Modified and reproduced with permission from **Sport in the Community**, British Sports Council, 1982.

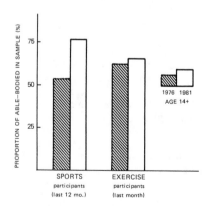

Figure 9.14. Surverys of participation in sport and exercise in Canada in 1976 and 1981. Reproduced with permission from **Canada Fitness Survey**, Fitness Canada, 1981.

9.4 MASS PARTICIPATION IN SPORT AND EXERCISE

Many countries have promoted exercise and several have set up special government departments to foster participation in sport and exercise, such as Fitness and Amateur Sport (Canada) (Figure 9.14, Table 9.4), the Sports Council (Britain) (Figure 9.15, Table 9.5 and 9.6), the German Gymnastics and Sports Federation (East Germany) (Table 9.7), and the President's Council on Physical Fitness and Sports in the U.S.A. The strategy adopted by Britain's Sports Council is to build an infrastructure for sport, to provide and manage facilities to promote participation, and to encourage excellence. The consequences of such government policies on health and fitness and the vigour of other national endeavors will be followed by social scientists with interest in future years.

Results from two surveys taken in 1976 and 1981 show that the degree of reported participation in sport and exercise in a Canadian population of adults has increased substantially. The proportion that reported participating in games or exercise at least once in the last 12 months and in the last month are shown in Figure 9.14.

This boom in fitness activity, however, may be illusory because of the low level of exercise required from those surveyed that characterized them as active. It is probable that these results are similar to a 1978 poll by Louis Harris in the U.S.A., sponsored by Perrier, in which 59% of adults surveyed reported that they exercised regularly. In fact, of this proportion, only 15% were active enough to achieve some increase in their fitness level.

Figure 9.15 shows projections by Britain's Sports Council on the increased number of participants in sports and exercise, which might be expected to result from Britain's extensive investment in training and playing facilities for the general population. The encouragement of people to use these facilities succeeded remarkably because of attractive programming and well-qualified staff.

Table 9.4. Growth in sports participation—Canada 1972-1976.
Modified and reproduced with permission from **Highlights of the 1976 Fitness and Sport Survey,** Fitness and Amateur Sport Canada, 1977.

Activity	Number of Participants—1972	Number of Participants—1976	% Growth in Participation
Tennis	732,000	2,175,000	197
Skiing (alpine, downhill, x-country)	1,001,000	2,534,000	153
Jogging	1,039,000	2,575,000	148
Golf	1,100,000	1,911,000	74
Swimming	4,191,000	7,117,000	70
Skating	2,155,000	2,930,000	36
Bicycling	1,743,000	2,225,000	28
Curling	643,000	826,000	28
Hockey	1,191,000	1,459,000	23
Walking for exercise	6,167,000	6,984,000	13

Table 9.5. Growth in number of facilities already built and those planned in Britain to 1993.
Modified and reproduced with permission from **Sport in the Community,** British Sports Council, 1982.

Facilities	Present	New
Sports Centers	500	800 (150 in areas of special need)
Swimming Pools	900	200 refurbished, 50 new
Playing Fields	35,000	3,000 new or refurbished (600 in areas of special need)
National Centers		7 new
PLUS Access to Coast & Country Programs with 20 selected sports		Improved Coaching Improved Administration

Table 9.6. Targets for increasing participation in sport 1983-93.
Modified and reproduced with permission from **Sport in the Community,** British Sports Council, 1982.

Mass Participation		Existing	Projected
Indoor Sport	Women	3.1 million	4.1 million
	Men	5.8 million	6.0 million
Outdoor Sport	Women	4.8 million	5.7 million
	Men	6.8 million	7.1 million

Table 9.7. Growth in membership of the DTSB of the German Democratic Republic. Modified and reproduced with permission from **Physical Culture in Sport in the GDR**, Panorama DDR Berlin. Zeit im Bild, 1978.

	1960	1965	1970	1975
Members (thousands)	1,439	1,813	2,156	2,595
Male	1,104	1,406	1,634	1,937
Female	335	407	552	658
Age Group: under 14	282	436	559	725
14-18 years	220	264	328	450
over 18	937	1,113	1,269	1,510
Proportion of the Population (%)	6.7	10.6	12.2	14.0

The growth in major facilities built in Britain since 1975 ("Present") and projected to 1993 ("New") is expected to produce the overall increase in participation, in adults of all ages, shown in Table 9.6.

The East German Democratic Republic posts impressive figures for participation, which actually reflect paid-up memberships by the participants in Sports Clubs (Table 9.7). The growth in membership of Sports Clubs, and thus the National Participation in Sport, marks a similar growth in strength of competition offered to the rest of the world by a small nation of only some 19 million people.

9.5 SPORTS MEDICINE

As seen by some, the national fervour for activity, promoted by governments, educators, sports organizations, commercial interests, and international associations, ignores the negative aspects of mass participation. The increasing morbidity engendered in every age group by sport and exercise related injury is a serious concern. In the last 20 years a whole new scientific and medical sub-interest called Sports Medicine has developed.

Sports Medicine is concerned with the **care and prevention of sport-related injury.** Lately, this interest has broadened to include exercise-related injury of every kind, in any age group, caused by a wide range of activities. Similar speciality groups have developed in Sport Science, Sport Psychology, Biomechanics, and Socio-cultural Aspects of Sports.

9.5.1 Injuries—Incidence

As an example of injury rate from a sport related activity, a 2 year survey of four Seattle high schools revealed that in 3,049 participants engaging in 19 different sports, there were 1,197 injuries—a rate of 39 injuries per 100 participants. The distribution of injuries among sports activities is shown in Figure 9.16. The preponderant ones were sprains (30%), strains (29%), and contusions (14%). At a national level (U.S.),

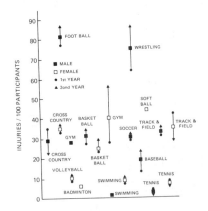

Figure 9.16. Injuries per 100 participants in various sports during a 2 year period in four American high schools. (Modified from **Sports Med. for Children and Youth,** Ross Laboratories, Columbus, Ohio 43216, 1979.

Figure 9.17. Showing the relationships between improvement in fitness (ΔVO_2 max) and the relative duration and intensity of exercise (expressed as the % of VO_2 max at which training is conducted) Modified and reproduced with permission from Davies and Knibbs, **Int. Z. angew. Physiol.**, 29: 299, 1971.

Figure 9.18. Showing the relationship between changes in fitness (ΔVO_2 max) and the frequency and intensity of training.

Table 9.8 shows the incidence of sprains and strains treated in hospital emergency departments through 1980. Table 9.9 shows the grouping of these injuries. Increasingly apparent are patterns of injury related to two major causes: **direct trauma** and the so-called **over-use syndrome**.

9.5.2 Exercise Stress

Exercise is essentially a debilitating process—a stressful activity from which respite (rest) is essential. Optimal levels of exercise for normal people involve no more than three or four 1-hour periods per week (Figures 9.17 and 9.18) of any activity that will keep the heart rate at 130-140 beats per minute throughout the period. This, of course, is the ideal. Very unfit people beginning to exercise would approach the 1-hour optimum in stages over a 3-6 month interval (see Table 9.10). Components of both strength and flexibility should be built in to any exercise regime (Johanessen et al., 1986).

Common sites of injury are those where limbs contact the ground (Figure 9.19). The joints must sustain large, weight bearing forces (up to 10 times the force of gravity) engendered by such apparently simple activities as jumping and jogging. During jogging the feet can strike the ground up to 5,000 times an hour, while in normal sedentary activity less than 1/50 of this number of steps might be taken.

It is likely that many of the lower extremity and back problems of the growing number of people who exercise stem from the incorrect gait of both young and old. The pronated foot (outward turning, duck footed plant), which in the very young gives stability and balance, seems to persist into youth and adulthood in modern society and is never corrected to a more forward pointing plant. When the strained musculature supporting this stance is subjected to more than sedentary activity overuse problems quickly appear. These problems include flat feet, sore knees, and a bad back.

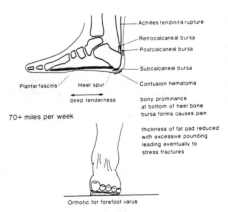

Figure 9.19. Points of particular susceptibility to over-use injury in the foot.

Table 9.8. Estimated numbers of hospital emergency department-treated strains and sprains.* Modified from **Sports Injuries: An Aid to Prevention and Treatment,** U.S. Tennis Association, American College of Sports Medicine and the American Orthopedic Association, 1980.

Sport	Number of Strains and Sprains, 1980
Track and Field	17,373
Squash, Racquetball and Paddleball	14,514
Tennis	15,187
Bicycling	47,633
Cross-Country Skiing	1,023
Football	159,388
Basketball	225,566

* From the Consumer Product Safety Commission, National Electronic Surveillance System, December, 1981. These figures do not include the number of sprains and strains treated at home or in doctor's offices.

Table 9.9. Injury Groupings. Modified and reproduced with permission from **Sports Injuries: An Aid to Prevention and Treatment,** U.S. Tennis Association, American College of Sports Medicine and the American Orthopedic Association, 1980.

I Tendinitis
    Achilles Tendinitis
    Iliotibial Band Syndrome
    Patellar Tendinitis
    Lateral Humeral Epicondylitis
    (tennis elbow)

II Strains
    Shoulder Girdle Muscles
    Quadriceps
    Hamstrings

III Sprains
    Knees
    Fingers
    Ankles
    Plantar Fasciae

IV Bursitis
    Elbow
    Shoulder
    Area Near Hips
    Knee

V Stress Fractures
    Foot
    Leg

Table 9.10. Suggested "easy" and "brisk" heart rates for initial 0-3 months and 3-6 months training (beats per 10 second interval). Modified and reproduced with permission from Duncan, Ross and Banister, **B.C. Medical Association Journal, 10:** 1-2, 1968.

Age	Max Heart Rate	0 - 3 Month Training		3 - 6 Month Training	
		Easy	Brisk	Easy	Brisk
15	35	23	28	25	30
25	34	22	27	24	29
35	32	21	26	22	27
40	30	20	24	21	26
45	28	19	23	20	24
50	27	18	22	19	23
55	26	17	21	18	22

9.6 SPORTS MEDICINE—SPORT SCIENCE IN PERSPECTIVE

The activities of Sport Medical Physicians and Sport Scientists are complementary and should integrate with the activities of several other specialty groups, such as biomechanists, nutritionists, physiotherapists, and psychologists, to study exercise performance and to develop better and safer ways to attain optimal health and fitness through activity. These groups are concerned with prevention of injury, rapid recognition of injury and sickness, rehabilitation from injury and sickness, and the return to full activity.

9.6.1 Prevention of Injury and Illness

There are three main ways of preventing injury: a pre-activity medical, correct conditioning, and the recognition of environmental hazards.

THE PRE-ACTIVITY MEDICAL
Your medical history must be checked, and a physical examination undergone, to screen for
• chronic problems;
• impaired vision;
• incipient asthma; and
• high blood pressure.

CORRECT CONDITIONING
Important points to remember in any training regime follow.
• Progressive loading is the basis for training.
• Time must be allowed for adequate adaptation at every stage.
• Overload training leads to overstress, causing recognizable symptoms of insomnia, irritability, appetite loss, infections.
• Rest and recovery is an important therapy.

RECOGNITION OF ENVIRONMENTAL HAZARDS

Watch out for:

- Heat exhaustion;
- Heat stroke—likely under exercise conditions of 72°C in high humidity; avoided by water repletion, head and neck protection, and training in the cool part of the day;
- Hypothermia and Frostbite—likely in wet, cold, windy conditions; avoided by wearing protective and breathable, but waterproof and windproof training clothes, and by protecting exposed parts and extremities;
- Training Surfaces and Obstructions—Games played on artificial surfaces require protection, principally against burns, and caution against twisting and turning injuries to knee and ankle joints. Be alert—avoid tripping over benches, fences, uneven track, meadow land, and so forth;
- Altitude—Decreased oxygen in the air at high altitudes causes some people respiratory distress during training or competition.

Acclimation takes 3 weeks or longer. Sleeplessness, headaches, and nausea are common problems, which are at their worst after one week's exposure. You may recall the difficulties in this regard that were experienced by some of the Olympic Competitors in the (1964) Summer Games in Mexico City, where the altitude is 7,500 feet above sea level.

9.6.2 Recognition of Injury and Illness due to Training

Knowing when one is injured or ill is half of the battle against real breakdown. Common injuries are traumatic injury and contusions.

TRAUMATIC INJURY

Abrasions and lacerations, for which the remedy is to:

- control bleeding by direct compression;
- use steristrips to close any wound;
- disinfect (wash in betadine);
- insure tetanus immunity is current, and,
- apply topical antibiotic (polysporin).

CONTUSIONS

Blows, knocks, etc., for which the remedy is:

- rest;
- ice;
- compression;
- elevation, and
- aspirin or buffered aspirin (e.g., Bufferin).

These five steps used as soon as possible after you become aware of an injury, but before you can see a physician, will ease your discomfort and make it easier to return more quickly to your sporting activity.

1. **REST:** As soon as you feel pain you should stop what you are doing and not continue to stress the injured part for at least one day. However, except in more severe strains, sprains, or fractures, complete and prolonged rest is not necessary unless prescribed by your physician. In fact, complete rest can often be the wrong course of action.

   Within a few days the tissues begin to repair themselves, but there are by-products of the injury such as clotted blood, that need to be cleared away. As soon as you feel comfortable after an injury has occurred, some form of proper rehabilitation exercises should be started to help remove injury by-products. Even if there is still some minor pain, the movement will help restore the muscle's ability to function properly, allowing you to return to your sports activity that much sooner.

2. **ICE:** Put ice on the injured area as soon as possible after an injury. Wrap the ice in a towel or plastic bag and apply it over a 30 minute period. However, move it every 5 minutes so as to avoid frostbite. This process can be continued several times. Ice is important because it reduces pain and swelling by constricting blood and lymph vessels. By reducing blood that collects around the injured area, there will be less inflammation and subsequent time required for recovery.

3. COMPRESSION: Compression also helps limit swelling which, if left uncontrolled, could lengthen healing time. Wrap an elastic bandage around the injured part. Be sure not to wrap too tightly as this could cut off the blood supply. You can tell the bandage is too tight if you feel numbness in the area, cramping, additional pain, or swelling beyond the edge of the bandage. Leave the bandage on for 30 minutes, then remove it for 15 minutes to ease circulation.

4. ELEVATION: Elevating the injured leg or arm to above the heart level helps drain excess fluid from the injured area. Both compression and elevation help limit muscular internal bleeding, decreasing the amount of injury by-products that need to be removed while the area is strengthening and repairing itself. You should continue to elevate the injured arm or leg even while sleeping.

MUSCLE STRAIN

This causes fatigue, irritability, and spasticity (floppiness). Treatment is the same as above.

LIGAMENTOUS SPRAIN

Stretched or torn ligaments often are associated with fractures. The rest, ice, and so forth regimen is followed immediately and elastic compression, splinting, and X-ray undertaken.

CONCUSSION

This is a serious problem. It requires immediate medical evaluation.

9.6.3 Overuse Injuries

TENDONITIS is attended by pain, swelling, and squeaking "crepitus." It is common in heel, shoulder, and forearm.

STRESS FRACTURES are indicated by pain and tenderness over a bone after exertion, present in a weight bearing area.

*It is too early to observe the effect that
mass participation will have on health
expenditures or on longevity.*

EPIPHYSITIS is a growth line irritation resulting from excessive muscular pull on bone. This is a particular problem in young people; it causes a painful knee and lower limb condition, termed Osgood Schlatter's disease.

INFECTION—Highly fit people, such as athletes, walk a fine line between excellence and breakdown because stress taxes the immune responses. Highly fit people are prone to suffer from furuncles and cellulitis, (e.g. boils) or staphylococcus infection. Basic hygiene should be good and polysporin is a useful medication. Tinea-Pedis (athlete's foot) fungal infection is another hazard. Tinactin and careful drying of infected areas is helpful.

Also, upper respiratory tract infections, for example colds and sore throats, can be a problem. Rest and appropriate medication is effective. With viral infections rest is mandatory.

9.7 SUMMARY
The exact role of sport and exercise in our society still remains to be defined. The full effect of promoting individual participation and physical vigor on the health and productivity of the nation is not yet determined. It is too early to observe the effect that mass participation will have on health expenditures or on longevity. The negative effects of exercise in terms of acute injury and morbidity from arthritis have not even begun to be considered as serious factors. Nevertheless, the idea of exercise as a worthwhile leisure pursuit is well established and will always remain compelling for many of us.

9.8 REFERENCES

Astrand, P.O. **Health and Fitness**. Ottawa: Fitness and Amateur Sport Canada, 1975.

Banister, E.W. Strength Gains from Muscle Training: Preparation for Competition, Part II. **National Strength Coaches Association Journal**, 2: 27-31, 1980.

Blair, S.N., Cooper, K.H., Gibbons, L.W., et al., Changes in coronary heart disease risk factors associated with increased treadmill time in 753 men. **American Journal of Epidemiology, 118**: 352-359, 1983.

Canada Fitness. Government of Canada Fitness and Amateur Sport, Canada Fitness Survey, #506-294 Albert Street, Ottawa, K1P 6E6, 1982 (Single copies free, multiple copies $2.00).

Chave, S.P.W., Morris, J.N., Moss, S. et al., Vigorous exercise in leisure time and death rate: a study of male civil servants. **Journal of Epidemiology and Community Health, 32**: 239-243, 1978.

Cunningham, D., Montoye, H., Metzner, H. and Keller, J. Active leisure time activities as related to age among males in a total population. **Journal of Gerontology, 23**: 551, 1968.

Davies, C.T.M. and Knibbs, A.V. The Training Stimulus. Int. **Z angew. Physiol. 29**: 299-305, 1971.

Doby, J.W., Pruett, E.D.R., Steinmetz, J.R., Page, H.F., Birhead, N.C. and Barry, A.J. Physical Activity and Psychic Stress/Strain. **Canadian Medical Association Journal, 96**: 848-857, 1967.

Donald, W.K. The effect of mental and physical stress on the cardiovascular system. **Proceedings Royal Society, 62**: 1180-1183, 1969.

Duncan, W.R., Ross, W.D. and Banister, E.W. Heart Rate Monitoring as a Guide to the Intensity of an Exercise Program. **B.C. Medical Association Journal, 10**: 1-2, 1968.

Durbeck, D.C., et al. The National Aeronautics and Space Administration—U.S. Public Health Service Health Evaluation and Enhancement Program. **American Journal of Cardiology, 30**: 784-79, 1972.

Erkkola, R. Correlation of Maternal Physical Fitness during Pregnancy. **Acta Obstetrica et Gynecoligia Scandinavica, 55**: 441-46, 1976.

Fentem, P.H. and Bassey, E.J. The Case for Exercise. **The Sports Council Britain: Publication #8**, 1982.

Fitch, K.O. and Morton, A.R. Specificity of exercise induced asthma. **British Medical Journal**, (ii): 577-88, 1971.

Glazier, W.H. The Task of Medicine. **Scientific American, 228**(4): 13-17, 1973.

Highlights of the 1976 Fitness and Sport Survey. Promotion and Communication Section, Fitness and Amateur Sport Branch, Health and Welfare Canada, The Journal Bldg., 365 Laurier Ave. W., Ottawa K1A 0T6, 1977.

Hossack, K.F. and Bruce, R.A. Prognostic value of exercise testing: the Seattle Heart Watch Experience. **Journal of Cardiac Rehabilitation, 5**: 9-19, 1985.

Johanessen, S., Holly, R.G., Lui, H., Amsterdam, E.A. High-frequency, moderate-intensity training in sedentary middle-aged women. **The Physician and Sports Medicine. 14**:99-102, 1986.

LaLonde. **A New Perspective on the Health of Canadians**. Ottawa: Information Canada, 1974.

Larsson, Y., Sterry, G., Ekengran, K., and Miller, T. Physical Fitness and the Influence of Training in Diabetic Adolescent Girls. **Diabetes, 11**: 109-117, 1962.

Leaving Hospital Total U.S. Healthcare Turnover 1985. **The Economist.** page 73, March 22, 1986.

Mayer, J. Physical Activity and Obesity. **Physical Therapy, 44**: 1102, 1964.

NCYFS, National Children and Youth Fitness Study Norms. **Journal of Physical Recreation & Dance,** January 1986.

Opiteck, J., Wrisley, D., Franklin, B., Zirkin, D., Burkhardt, C., Vander, T., Stepke, W., Solomon, W., Graham, D. and Rubenfire, M. Ineffectiveness of 6 weeks of low and moderate intensity physical training in extreme old age. **Medicine and Science in Sports & Exercise, 18(suppl.):** S84, 1987.

Organization of Sport in Fed. Republic of Germany. Deutscher Sportbund, Frankfurt am Main Germany, 1971.

Paez, P.N., Phillipson, E.A., Masangkay, M. and Sproule, B.J. The physiologic basis of training patients with emphysema. **American Review Respiratory Diseases,** 95(44):1967.

Paffenbargher, R.S. and Hale, W.E. Work Activity and Coronary Heart Mortality. **New England Journal of Medicine,** 292(545): 1975.

Paffenbargher, R.S., Hyde, M.A., Wing, A.L. and Steinmetz, C.H. A natural history of athleticism and cardiovascular health. **Journal of the American Medical Association, 252:** 491-495, 1984.

Pell, S. and Fayerweather, W.E. Trends in the incidence of myocardial infarction and in associated mortality in a large employed population, 1957-1983. **New England Journal of Medicine, 312:** 1005-10111, 1985.

Physical Culture and Sport in the GDR (East Germany) Panorama DDR, 1978.

Reville, P. **Sport For All: Council of Cultural Cooperation,** Strasbourg: Council of Europe, 1970.

Schreuder, J.T.R. (1969) Le maintien de la condition physique, measure therapeutique pour gens ages triangle, **Journal Sandoz des Sciences Medicales,** 9: 97-101, 1969.

Simonetti and Eaton. Cardiovascular and Metabolic Effects of Exercise. **Postgraduate Medicine,** 63: 71-77, 1979.

Skinner, J.S. Age and Performance. In **Limiting Factors of Physical Peformance.** Editor J. Keul. Stuttgart Georg Thieme, 1973. (Course Reader, Selection 14.1).

Sport in the Community. The Next 10 Years. The Sport Council 1982. The Sport Council, 16 Upper Wobum Place, London WC1H0QP, 1982.

Sports Injuries: An Aid to Prevention and Treatment. U.S. Tennis Association, American College of Sports Medicine, American Orthopedic Society, 1980.

Sports Medicine for Children and Youth. Ross Laboratories, Columbus Ohio 43216, 1979.

Sydney, K.H. and Shephard, R.J. Frequency and Intensity of Exercise Training for Elderly Subjects. **Medicine and Science in Sports,** 10:125-131, 1978.

Vyas, M.V., Banister, E.W., Morton, J.W., and Grzybowski, S. Response to Exercise in Patients with Chronic Airways Obstruction. **Amererican Review of Respiratory Diseases,** 103: 390-400, 1971.

9.9 STUDY QUESTIONS

1. What are some of the specific benefits, both physical and psychological, of exercise for the elderly? What are some of the concomitant dangers?
2. Name at least four ways in which physical activity can help prevent heart disease (CVD) or coronary artery disease.
3. What is "aerobic capacity"? Why is it a good idea to increase it?
4. Discuss the potential effect of the exercise "movement" on the cost of health care.
5. Discuss the effect exercise may have on the productivity of the work force in a country.

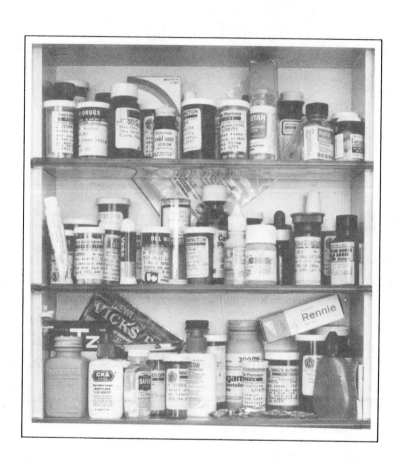

10

Drugs

Can we live better chemically?

OBJECTIVES

When you have completed this chapter, you should be able to:

- **List** the main kinds of drugs used in sports.
- **Explain** the uses and abuses of these drugs.
- **Discuss** the health hazards of smoking and the effectiveness of various ways of stopping smoking.

KEY TERMS

abstinence	narcotics
abuse	nicotine
anabolic	psychoactive
anti-depressants	prostaglandin inhibition
chemotherapy	sedative
dependency	stimulants
ergogenic	tranquilizers
hallucinogens	toxic effect withdrawal

KEY CONCEPTS/DEFINITIONS

- Chemotherapy is therapy with chemicals, i.e., drugs.
- Most drugs are purified derivatives of chemicals that occur in nature, either from animals or plants.
- A drug-oriented society is one that deems the value of drugs and chemicals to be high and perhaps even endowed with special powers.
- Drug abuse involves physical, emotional, social, legal, and health dimensions.
- Drug addiction is a dependency upon certain effects from a drug in order to maintain physical and mental stablility.
- Psychoactive drugs distort reality, a result which may not always be desirable.
- Smoking is the most serious, prevalent, and preventable cause of illness or disease in mankind.
- Drugs in sports medicine can serve as an example of the numerous drugs available to society.

*Smoking is the most serious, prevalent,
and preventable cause of illness
or disease in mankind.*

10.0 INTRODUCTION

*In the Garden of Eden, Adam's first intrigue with the apple turned to
curiosity about it's secret ingredient that made it so good to eat.*

Like Adam, mankind has continually sought those naturally occurring
substances that enrich and preserve life. When illness struck, early man ex-
perimented with the herbs and roots which aided recovery. Later sophis-
tication extended to attempts to discover the very essence of the "root"
cures and to extract and concentrate them for even better effect. In time,
we learned to synthesize them and to alter them chemically to enhance
their powers.

This route, from the discovery of natural occurrence to modern laboratory synthesis of useful chemicals, is the history of nearly every drug available today. Overall, the pharmaceutical industry is responsible for some
very useful products which do everything from killing bacteria, in order to
purify our water supply, right up to, in some cases, arresting cancer. We've
come a long way since Adam became curious about the contents of the first
apple.

In this chapter, the full gamut of drugs and chemicals in the pharma-
copeia cannot be covered; instead we will concentrate on those products
which are in common street use and those used in sports medicine. These
will serve as examples of some very useful drugs and some which do not
contribute to good health. Not all of the drugs used by society are used for
noble purpose.

10.1.1 Chemotherapy

The nobelest ideal for using a drug is to cure! Therapy with drugs is termed
"chemotherapy." The medical profession considers drugs as those substances containing chemicals intended for use in the diagnosis, cure, treatment, or prevention of disease, or in the relief of pain or discomfort. It
should be mentioned, however, that while all medicines contain drugs, not
all drugs are medicines; some are poisons.

Chemotherapy involves a great number of useful everyday products. Vaccines and toxoids are used to prevent communicable diseases such as smallpox, measles, polio, and tetanus. Antibiotics, such as penicillin, are used to combat bacterial infections. Insulin is for diabetes and anticonvulsant drugs are for epilepsy. Anaesthetics put us to sleep, stimulants keep us awake, tranquilizers calm us down, and analgesics numb us. Some drugs will tighten our bowels and yet others will loosen them. We know of drugs which will cause cancer, and others that can cure some cancers. If there is ever a new disease discovered, someone usually will soon find the drug to cure or modify it. Now that the virus causing AIDS disease has been identified, it is hoped that a cure for this recent (appearing only after 1981) mysterious disease is only 2-5 years away.

However, each of these drugs is a two-edged sword. One side cuts what you want, but the other side may cut what you don't want. This problem is called a **side-effect** of the drug. Such hazards must be considered carefully in choosing a remedy for any malady, and any decision on remedy must balance risk with the benefit. With care and attention however, we can live better and longer through judicious therapeutic chemical use.

10.1.2 Drug Misuse/Abuse

Drug misuse is the unintentional or unwise use of drugs, out of ignorance. Some individuals may overuse nose sprays, tranquilizers, analgesics, heart drugs, or drugs they thought were safe, even under a doctor's orders. Sometimes the instructions or communication between doctor, patient, and pharmacist become confused, but the one who suffers is the patient. These problems are unintentional and usually not serious. Most of the problems are resolved with cessation of use of the offending drug.

Drug abuse is another matter. It may be defined as the intentional misuse of drugs, including the use of illegal drugs or narcotics, the overuse of illegal drugs or narcotics, and the overuse of legal and prescribed drugs. Drug misuse may lead to the intentional misuse of drugs, even against the

Many persons are prescribed drugs that affect their moods. Using the drugs wisely can be important for physical and emotional health. But sometimes it is difficult to decide when, using drugs to handle stress, becomes inappropriate. It is important that adaptive use of drugs does not result in maladaption. Here are some "danger signals" that can help you evaluate your own way of using drugs.

1. Do those close to you often ask about your drug use? Have they noticed any changes in your moods or behavior?
2. Are you defensive if a friend or relative mentions your drug or alcohol use?
3. Are you sometimes embarrassed or frightened by your behavior under the influence of drugs or alcohol?
4. Have you ever gone to see a new doctor because your regular physician would not prescribe the drug you wanted?
5. When you are under pressure or feel anxious, do you automatically take a tranquilizer or drink or both?
6. Do you take drugs more often or for purposes other than those recommended by your doctor?
7. Do you mix drugs and alcohol?
8. Do you drink or take drugs regularly to help you sleep?
9. Do you have to take a pill to get going in the morning?
10. Do you think you have a drug problem?

If you have answered yes to a number of these questions, you may be misusing drugs or alcohol. There are places to go for help at the local level. One such place might be a drug abuse program in your community, listed in the Yellow Pages under Drug Abuse. Other resources include community crisis centers, telephone hotlines, and the Mental Health Association.

Figure 10.1. Danger signals of drug misuse. Reprinted with permission from National Institute on Drug Abuse, 1979.

wise counselling of friends, pharmacists, and doctors. The classic story is the injured person who starts with a "222" to relieve pain, then needs a "292," then more codeine, demerol, morphine and, finally, heroin. This story may be repeated with tranquilizers, sedatives, and hypnotics (sleeping pills).

Hallucinogenic drugs such as marijuana, LSD, and cocaine often are taken from the outset with the knowledge that they are mind-altering, dangerous, and illegal. These are known as recreational drugs. Apparently, there are enough people wishing to experience their effects to fuel a thriving illicit drug trade of major international proportions. Therapy and rehabilitation for such drug abusers is usually ineffective, and good rehabilitation programs are rare, especially considering the magnitude of the problem.

Consider the origins of our drug-oriented society. Which one of us, as a child suffering some illness or pain, did not have a parent offer a pill or medicine that tasted good, with the promise that soon everything would be better? Or, if the drug wasn't readily available, a doctor would probably have readily prescribed something to cure the discomfort. Modern societies learn quickly to rely on drugs.

10.1.3 Drugs in Sports

Drugs in sports often emphasize the principle of enhancing performance, and some athletes are prone to try anything in order to maximize their performance. The following discussion on drugs in sports will emphasize those drugs which are commonly used by athletes either to enhance their performance or to solve some of their maladies. Not all of the medications that athletes take achieve the desired result. Many of the drugs mentioned are just as applicable to ordinary people's ailments as they are to those of the athlete. As you read through this section, if you are not an athlete, imagine yourself as one in order to gain an understanding and perspective of drugs in sports.

*Every chemical substance has
a limit beyond which its toxic effects upon
the organism become evident.*

10.2 ERGOGENIC AIDS

Ergo means "work," **genic** means "to be produced by." Ergogenic aids are items used by athletes in the hope that they will enhance their performance. Some of these, which are referred to as natural aids, are such things as oxygen which, when taken in the normal amounts, allows athletic performance to proceed unhindered. However, when an athlete's oxygen supply is inadequate the performance suffers. This is a particular problem during some athletic events at high altitudes. We often don't realize how indispensible a particular substance is until we are required to go without it.

Many coaches and athletes alike, ponder the principle that, "if a little works, more may work better." However, to use the example of oxygen, excess amounts do not enhance performance. There is an optimum amount for each "drug" acting as an ergogenic aid. Excessive amounts will merely increase the hazards and risks of side effects. Even drinking excess water may cause bodily systems to malfunction, leading to death. Every chemical substance has a limit beyond which its toxic effects upon the organism become evident.

Another group of chemical substances used by athletes to try to enhance performance is known as **unnatural aids**. These are described below.

10.2.1 Stimulant Drugs: Amphetamines

Part of the group of potential ergogenic substances are drugs which lift the mood of an individual above a normal level. This mood-elevating effect may be associated with enhanced performance at work or at play. Stimulants are definitely abusive drugs, and natural or normal performances are not expected under their influences. In fact, these stimulants increase the death hazard during endurance work at a high level. Cocaine and dexedrine are examples which are nicknamed **speed**.

There are numerous types of central nervous system stimulants. Some of them are relatively mild, such as **ephedrin**. This is a mild stimulant to the sympathetic nervous system. It is a drug commonly found in some nasal decongestants and nose sprays. You may remember the last time you used a nose spray to clear up congestion and recall that your nasal lining felt stimulated. If this medication is taken internally, and in large enough doses, it can give a general stimulant effect to the entire body.

At the other end of the spectrum of stimulant drugs is **cocaine**, which is believed to work by blocking the breakdown of newly released adrenalin and noradrenalin. **Adrenalin** and **noradrenaline** are central nervous system catecholamines whose increased circulating levels effectively stimulate the central nervous system.

One of the more commonly used stimulants is **dexedrine**, a drug previously used by doctors to reduce appetite and thus aid in the management of obesity. However, it has since been banned for use in such circumstances due to its highly addictive nature. On ceasing use of dexedrine profound depression and suicide were noted in users. Today doctors steer away from the use of such medication. However, the stimulant effects of dexedrine led to its use and abuse among people seeking a chemical "high" or stimulation. Most good athletes are able to get themselves "up" quite naturally for a performance however some will always tend to rely on artificial means.

Research results concerning the effects of **amphetamines** (e.g. dexedrine) on performance have shown they increase the muscle strength able to be realized during activity, increase heart rate, increase ability to accommodate high levels of lactic acid and other products of muscle breakdown, and delay the onset of exhaustion produced by intense activity. There appears also to be an increase in alertness and attentiveness; an increased ability to do mental tasks without fatigue; and an increase in blood pressure, muscle tension, and pupil diameter under their effect. It seems that everything to do with performance ability is improved initially.

However, with prolonged use the beneficial or stimulant effect of these drugs seems to decrease gradually unless one takes greater and greater amounts of them to produce the same effect. New features of behavior

*What may start as a simple curiosity may build
into a dependency which ends in disaster.*

begin to appear. These include increased aggressiveness and hostility, paranoia, suspicion of others, and, occasionally, an unrealistic euphoric "head in the clouds" feeling. Most importantly, a definite chemical dependence upon the drug for ordinary day-to-day activities arises. Soon there is a disruption of thought processes, hallucinations, delusions of persecution, and overt schizophrenic thinking and behavior.

During withdrawal from such medications there is often profound depression, and suicide is a very real danger. In fact, it was the alarming rate of suicide among obese, diet pill (amphetamine) users which alerted the medical profession to the hazards of these stimulant drugs.

Increasing concern over the last decade has centered on **cocaine** abuse. In some parts of the United States the use of cocaine is widespread, and it is estimated that twenty-five billion dollars is spent yearly on this product alone. This is three times the business generated in the recording and movie industries put together. The euphoric high or "kick" that comes from cocaine is highly addictive, and those who are too curious about its effects often live to regret it. What may start as a simple curiosity may build into a dependency which ends in disaster. At present, the medical profession and drug rehabilitation programs are not organized to manage cocaine addiction, and, certainly, the cocaine industry itself does not seem disposed to care for victims of its business (Anderson, 1983). Can you imagine the likelihood of a drug rehabilitation program being sponsored by organized-crime for instance?

10.2.2 Anabolic Steroids

Anabolic steroids are "tissue-building" drugs used by athletes to promote rapid gains in muscular strength and body weight. Most of these drugs are C-17 alkylated derivatives of **testosterone** and possess significant androgenic (masculine) activity. This includes development of the male secondary sex characteristics as well as the development of the muscular system. It is the masculinizing effects of anabolic steroids that make the use of these drugs particularly undesirable, especially for women (Haynes, 1980), in addition to their other physiological effects noted below.

Studies on the effects of these drugs, however, have produced conflicting results and the subject remains controversial. Some suggest that anabolic steroids function by modifying protein metabolism in the cell, thus enhancing muscle building. Several other concomitant factors, however, are essential for the effective use of anabolic steroids. They include practice of an intense physical strength training program as well as an adequate protein intake. Some investigators suggest that it is these latter two factors alone that are important to muscle building. Most of the studies on anabolic steroids have used the normally prescribed dose level, and results have been conflicting. Most athletes who use these drugs, in fact, use anywhere from ten to twenty times the normally prescribed or legally allowable dose, and in these subjects there are reports of muscle building (Lamb, 1983).

Psychological influences may play a part in perceived increases in muscular strength. The **placebo effect** may be an important factor in the enhancement of human performance and, thus, caution must be used when crediting improved performance to the beneficial effect of anabolic steroids. These drugs also create aggressive behavior and personality in their users, and it is suggested that this aggressiveness, when applied to training, is what results in extra strength gains.

Several adverse reactions to anabolic steroids have been noted including: premature closure of epiphyseal plates; testicular atrophy; increased male pattern baldness; hirsutism (hairiness); edema; jaundice; gynecomastia (breast development in the male); decreased output of testosterones, sebaceous cysts, and reduced spermatogenesis. Unfortunately, not all of these effects are reversible upon cessation of taking the drug. The long term effect of large doses of anabolic steroids in humans is not yet known. A frightening incidence of hepatitis and hepatocellular carcinoma (liver cancer), which is usually fatal, accompanies long term use of the drugs. Several deaths have been attributed to abuse of the body from use of anabolic steroids (Lamb, 1983).

The use of anabolic steroids has been universally condemned by athletic associations such as the International Olympic Committee and the American College of Sports Medicine (ACSM) as well as Sports Canada. The organizers of most international calibre athletic meets have a drug-screening program designed to identify and disqualify those athletes using anabolic steroids or banned drugs of any kind. Despite this, their use continues to be widespread (ACSM, 1977).

10.2.3 Bronchodilators

Bronchodilators are drugs which function, as their name implies, to dilate the bronchioles. The bronchioles contain smooth muscle which, under some circumstances, may unduly constrict and, therefore, limit the movement of air in and out of the lungs. This problem is most commonly seen in asthmatics who often find that, during exercise, they may get the air in, but they cannot get it out as easily. Air tends to be trapped in their lungs, and the patient's overall ventilation is limited and their oxygen consumption is less, since the oxygen needed is contained in air breathed. Obviously, a subject's ability to work when the bronchioles are constricted is limited. Anything that would improve bronchial dilation would aid performance of any kind, even just walking.

There are two types of bronchodilators commonly in use, that is, **inhalants** (a spray) and **tablets**. The most common inhalant is called **Salbutamol** (Ventolin), whereas the most popular tablet is a preparation of **Aminophyllin** or **Theophylline**. For improved performance, the average asthmatic, whose affliction is exercise induced, takes a puff of Salbutamol about a half an hour before an exercise or competition and perhaps another puff about five minutes prior to exercise. This regime would reduce or prevent bronchiole constriction and enhance the air flow. Obviously, the expected performance would then be better. Tablets are usually taken regularly, three to four times per day.

Bronchodilators are categorized as stimulants and are still banned by official agencies which sponsor international athletic events. This is unfortunate, for the bronchodilator ergogenic aids have little value in non-asthmatics and their ergogenic effect in asthmatics is not to enhance activity, but to allow normal activity in the face of an otherwise debilitating pulmonary problem. A number of authorities in sports medicine are lobbying against the ban on bronchodilators in major international competitions.

10.2.4 Caffeine

Caffeine is widely available in such common foodstuffs as coffee, tea, and cola drinks, and it is also mixed with many analgesics (e.g., 292 tablets) to offset their sedative effects. Caffeine is a true stimulant for example, even one cup of coffee (100 mg caffeine) has an arousal effect upon the nervous system. At doses greater than 300 mg it can be uncomfortably stimulating, and by 10 gm it becomes an overdose leading to convulsions and death.

The initial overt effects of caffeine are an increased heart rate, elevated blood pressure, and increased respiratory rate. The drug also acts as a mild diuretic by directly decreasing renal tubular reabsorption of fluid in the kidneys. This means that the cup of coffee taken to replace fluid losses will, in actual fact, lead to enhanced fluid loss. Caffeine is also considered to be **mutagenic** (gene disturbing) and, therefore, is not recommended during pregnancy. Its potential to create cancer is still under investigation, and this topic is presently a very controversial one (Wilcox, 1982).

Although caffeine affects the heart rate and stroke volume (volume of blood pumped by the heart at each beat), it has not been linked to coronary heart disease, nor is it considered to be a primary cardiac risk factor. It may, however, be a disturbing factor in some patients with heart arrhythmias causing lowering of the irritability threshold at which arrhythmias begin in predisposed patients. However, as may be inferred, numerous other debilitating factors must be present before coffee may be be considered hazardous.

*Caffeine affects the brain stem
and is addictive.*

Caffeine affects the brain stem and is addictive. Upon withdrawal, uncomfortable feelings are initiated within the vegetative nervous system (autonomic area of the brain stem), the most common of these being a headache. Tolerance to caffeine may be developed after as little as four days of regular use, for instance, the uncomfortable effects of withdrawal are only minor, but dependence has been started. As an experiment, stop your own coffee intake for the next two days and you will notice a dull, frontal headache. If you drink too much coffee, on the other hand, you will become irritable and agitated, but with continued use these toxic effects subside as tolerance develops.

The stimulating effects of caffeine are associated with increased alertness. Increased performance in sports has not been credited to caffeine, perhaps because so many other stronger modulating factors influence athletic performance. One would expect that the arousal effects of caffeine would lead to enhanced athletic performance, but such findings have not been well established. Lately, caffeine has been reported to help endurance runners by stimulating the use of fat stores as a fuel (Costill, 1978).

Caffeine increases free-fatty acids (FFA) in the plasma, which are a source of energy for muscle. This lipolytic effect plus increased alertness are the ergogenic factors that would account for the increased work capacity and power demonstrated by subjects in some studies shortly after caffeine ingestion. As a corollary, athletes who habitually use caffeine, must continue their usual dose prior to athletic activity, otherwise withdrawal reactions might hamper performance.

10.2.5 Blood Doping

Blood is the great transport system of the body. It carries oxygen (attached to the red blood cell's hemoglobin) and nutrients into the cells of the body to nourish them with energy; and it removes cell wastes to be carried elsewhere for reprocessing or elimination. A lack of an adequate amount of blood within the circulating system is called anemia. An anemic athlete, or any anemic person for that matter, does not perform well. Basically, there is not enough oxygen-carrying capacity in blood lacking sufficient red blood cells (RBC) to provide working muscles with the oxygen that they require.

From the principle that with less blood we have impaired performance, we may deduce that the opposite must be true. Extra blood (providing more RBC to transport oxygen) leads to enhanced performance, and this principle has, in fact, been proven. To be successful, however, blood doping, as the process of adding blood to an already normal amount in the body has come to be called, should be performed only in those athletes who have adequate iron stores and normal nutrition, so that their hemopoetic (blood forming) system can replace any lost blood. This is because in this enhancing (doping) process, blood must first be removed from the subject's body and stored to be reinfused later.

Blood doping is performed by removing up to a litre of blood and preserving it by a special freezing technique. The blood is stored for several weeks during which time the athlete's natural restorative mechanisms return the blood hemoglobin level (contained in the RBC) to normal. At this point, which if timed correctly is about a week prior to an important competition, the stored blood is reinjected into the athlete whose blood volume and hemoglobin concentration then rise. (It is the hemoglobin molecule in blood which actually carries oxygen molecules). Normal levels of blood are around 15 mg per 100 cc of blood, but after blood doping, as described above, the hemoglobin can rise to as much as 18 or 19 grams per 100 cc of blood. As a result of this process, a much greater carrying capacity of oxygen within the blood occurs. In those athletic events, which require endurance and maximum transport of oxygen and nutrients to and from muscles, such an elevated blood level allows a greater performance capacity.

However, blood doping is not without its hazards. If the nutritional capacity of the athlete is abnormal, then the initial blood letting results in a weakened athlete. On the other hand, the elevated blood levels, after reinjection, cause a condition called polycythemia (excessive red blood cells). This thickened blood condition may lead to inadvertent clotting within small vessels and congestion within the circulation. Strokes, heart attacks, and high blood pressure are associated with polycythemia. Nevertheless, in the average athlete, induced polycythemia is of short duration and such hazards are unlikely. Contamination of blood during handling, storage, and reinjection is a remote possibility with good technique.

Blood doping is considered controversial and somewhat hazardous. Its practice is rare in North America, and athletic organizations on this continent have not relied upon it to aid the winning potential of their athletes. Blood doping, as described, also has little place in general medical practice (Williams, 1983).

10.2.6 The "Elixirs"

There are as many so-called aids to performance as there are those touted as cure-all medicines. At one time snake oil would cure everything, grow hair on bald heads, clean dentures, and, if ingested at the appropriate time, probably allow one's winning at the Olympics. The modern versions of such ancient elixirs, like their predecessors, tend to aim at certain small groups within society and tout their products by means of mystifying scientific jargon. In most cases these "wonder products" are ineffective but harmless. They are a marketeer's delight.

Bee pollen is a product advertised as a cure-all—"nature's food of the gods." It claims to have historical roots and to have been fed to royalty in ancient times. It is netted from the mesh traps through which bees must crawl to gain access to their hives; while going through the mesh the pollens that they have collected are rubbed off and collected. Bee pollen contains many minerals, amino acids, enzymes, and other chemicals in very minute quantities. In fact, the miniscule amounts of these ingredients contained in the pollen casts great doubt upon its possessing any ergogenic benefit at all.

Some athletes are so nervous and tense prior to a performance that they drain themselves of the energy necessary to win.

The outlandish claims for bee pollen or, for that matter, any other of the odd "elixers" which hope to lure gullible athletes or others into a purchase have not been substantiated. If you wish to purchase a placebo and believe the advertisements however, these products are probably harmless.

10.2.7 Hypnosis

As an ergogenic aid hypnosis is commonly used. It should be pointed out that although "ergogenic" means to enhance work performance, even those psychological maneuvers which allow the mind to get the most out of the body should be considered ergogenic and, in this case, a natural aid.

Mental practice, game rehearsal, positive mental attitude, Transcendental Meditation (TM), and hypnosis are all terms applied to the altered state of awareness used by many athletes and non-athletes to prepare for important events. Obviously, it is so simple a process that to use a mysterious word like hypnosis can be confusing. When elite athletes are observed, prior to performing an important maneuver, taking a few quiet deep breaths and seeming lost in thought, gazing off into space, one can be sure that they are practising in their mind the winning profile. Many coaches unknowingly practice hypnosis by giving pep talks and locker room coaching without realizing the technique they are using. At the same time, athletes use self-hypnosis without giving it a name.

Such mental ploys, utilized by many athletes to put their mind and body into the right state of preparedness, not too high or too low but just right, may make the difference between success or failure. Some athletes are so nervous and tense prior to a performance that they drain themselves of the energy necessary to win. Such athletes could use hypnosis to relax themselves, gaining strength and calmness at the same time. Others, such as weight lifters, use hypnosis to get themselves all **hyped up** with a sense of anger and hostility toward the weights and bars, and find this stimulatory effect gives them the winning profile.

*Among all the ergogenic aids proposed to assist
the athlete and non-athlete, alike,
the most important is a balanced lifestyle.*

Different techniques work for different individuals, and the greatest chance of winning goes to those who find and practice the method that works best for them. The above principles for improving performance may apply generally to everyday life too.

10.2.8 The Balanced Life

Among all the ergogenic aids proposed to assist the athlete and non-athlete, alike, the most important is a balanced lifestyle. This includes three balanced meals a day, a varied type of food intake with selection from each major food group, a balanced social life, seven to eight hours of sleep a night, and the avoidance of habituating drugs or chemicals. If such a life-style seems unexciting, consider that living it for a while trains the system for occasional lapses into excess which may then be enjoyed with ease and without qualm.

10.3 COMMON ABUSIVE DRUGS

Another group of drugs have no ergogenic potential but possess a powerful potential to alter mental processes, sometimes permanently. They are the common **street drugs;** they are highly abusive in the sense that they are either illegal, non-medicinal, and/or commonly misused intentionally. They also can be psychologically or physically addicting, or both.

10.3.1 Tetrahydrocannabinol (delta 9-THC)

Hashish, charas, bhang, ganja, and marijuana are terms used in various parts of the world to refer to cannabis. This not-so-innocuous psychoactive drug, whose use is very prevalent today, has recently been shown to have more dangerous side effects than originally thought. It is often used for its mild mind-bending euphoric relaxation and a general peace and mild humor which comes over the mind. It also causes a loss of short-term memory and a confusion of time, with a loss of distinction among past-present-future. Motor skills are definitely impaired in a manner which the user often does not realize at the time.

Studies of motor control under the influence of cannabis show an intermittent loss of gross and fine coordination skills, as if someone had turned a coordinating switch off and then back on again. There is a definite loss of strength, perhaps due to the loss of mental effort or drive usually experienced with the use of cannabis (National Institute on Drug Abuse, 1979).

A certain apathy often is noted by users of the drug, which is characterized by a loss of self-direction and motivation. The advocate of cannabis claims intrapersonal enhancement, characterized by an increased awareness of sights and sounds, which, previously ignored, are now perceived as amusing and novel. However, social exchanges are not enhanced due to the excessive, and often confusing, mental stimulation the individual undergoes.

Surprising and unpredictable toxic effects of cannabis are sometimes reported. They can occur in a first time user or they may suddenly appear in a long term user. These effects are characterized as bad trips. Some of the outcomes reported include psychosis, hallucinations, extreme depersonalization, paranoia, and an intense fear that the bad trip will never end. Long after the cessation of cannabis use there may be flashbacks or **bad trips**. It has even been suggested that the use of cannabis by latent schizophrenics may trigger a psychotic reaction which may become permanent (National Institute on Drug Abuse, 1979).

Withdrawal or abstinence symptoms have been noted after cessation of cannabis use by an addict. Such symptoms are said to include irritability, restlessness, nervousness, anorexia, insomnia, weight loss, tremor, chills, and hypothermia.

At one time proponents of cannabis use claimed it was non-addictive, but recent evidence suggests that it may, in fact, be addictive (WHO, 1974; National Institute on Drug Abuse, 1979).

Cannabis is usefully employed as an **antiemetic, antinauseant**, especially after cancer chemotherapy.

10.3.2 Benzodiazepines

Benzodiazepines (which include valium) are classified as mild tranquilizers. The initial information on this drug stressed its safety and use as a gentle, non-addicting tension reliever. Recently, however, drug manufacturers are finding it hard to sustain the image of benign safety in the face of many studies showing benzodiazepines to be addictive (el-Guebaly, 1973). Valium is gradually being replaced as the prime chemical tranquilizer by many similar new drugs. Most are benzodiazepines as well, but each has been advertised by the drug manufacturer as being safer than valium.

Mild tranquilization of a patient to ease anxiety does not solve the basic problem initiating the anxiety. It merely puts a gentle blanket of confusion over the issues, which, in fact, do not go away but tend to compound themselves through a lack of any attempt at solving the basic problems.

Benzodiazepines and many other similar drugs are prescribed as "safe sleeping pills." But there is no such thing as a "safe sleeping pill." They all alter normal sleep patterns; the user soon obtains a drug-type sleep which is not normal. Even then, the sleep-producing effect wears off quickly, thus requiring more and more of the drug. When one stops the use of dependency-producing sleeping pills, there is a period of several days to several weeks before normal sleep patterns are re-established.

10.3.3 Alcohol

Ancient man's valium-like preparation was said to have been made by Bacchus, the Greek god of wine. Alcohol is known to decrease inhibition and increase sociability. It also elevates high density lipoproteins and may exert a protective effect against arteriosclerosis. Such welcome benefits are quickly buried by the serious potential for dependency on, and abuse of, alcohol.

It is interesting to note that many Orientals lack two enzymes within the liver which break down the acetaldehyde, formed in the system when

The prolonged use of alcohol leads to many changes within the central and peripheral nervous systems, the cardiovascular system, and the liver.

alcohol is ingested. Acetaldehyde creates some very uncomfortable feelings immediately within the system and thus creates an aversion toward alcohol in many people of Oriental descent. For Caucasians this safety valve does not exist; they can consume large quantities of alcohol and still feel comfortable. The aversive physical reaction does not usually occur until the next morning when the hangover is present. Previous experience of the uncomfortable side-effects of drinking, delayed until the next morning, often does nothing to ensure moderation of behavior in face of the immediate gratification of the moment associated with drinking.

The prolonged use of alcohol leads to many changes within the central and peripheral nervous systems, the cardiovascular system, and the liver. Quite simply, alcohol either directly damages tissues or alters the way in which cells function.

The white matter that surrounds nerve fibers in the brain, spine, and peripherally is partially lost (demyelination). In essence this causes a short circuiting or dysfunction of many parts of the nervous system. This degeneration in the brain leads to Korsakoff's syndrome—a type of psychosis. Manifestation of the alcoholic personality is due, in part, to brain degeneration. Blindness may also result or the eye muscles become paralysed. Peripherally, muscles atrophy due to loss of nerve function and the limbs lose their sensation, but on the other hand, they may become painful to move.

Alcohol also attacks the liver. In an attempt to detoxify alcohol (break it down through metabolism) the normal balance of liver functions is distorted, and certain of its important metabolic pathways dysfunction. This can be damaging for other systems in the body which rely on the liver to modify various chemicals and nutrients into usable sustances. The liver normally functions much like a chemical filter which cleanses the system, but the alcoholic or cirrhotic liver allows toxic wastes to accumulate in the body. In addition, the scarring and blockage of circulation to the cirrhotic liver causes backpressure into the spleen. This can cause the spleen to enlarge, become fragile, and prone to rupture with minor trauma. The same backpressure in the hepatic (liver) circulation leads to large varicose veins at the junction of the esophagus and stomach. If these veins rupture from a coughing or a vomiting spell for example, the accompanying extensive bleeding could be fatal.

Alcoholics often vomit and sometimes aspirate vomitus into their lungs. When drunk, the normal co-ordination of vomiting is affected. This often leads to pneumonia and bronchitis.

Alcohol can be toxic to the heart muscle, leading to a type of cardiomyopathy—weak and degenerated heart muscle. It is regularly fatal if not quickly diagnosed.

Alcohol directly irritates the stomach lining causing gastric bleeding and vomiting. If this irritation should also include the varicose veins of the lower esophagus, fatal bleeding can easily occur.

Alcohol causes small blood vessels to dilate, an undesirable effect if one is trying to stay warm on a cold day. The shot of rum for the lost soul in the snow storm may be a fatal shot, for it will dilate the peripheral blood vessels and thus increase the body's heat loss. In addition, dilated blood vessels give the alcoholic a typical red nose and face. Their ruddy complexion is not a sign of health.

Alcohol interferes with blood production of the clotting factors in the bone marrow; alcoholics have prolonged bleeding even from simple cuts—compounded by the fact that their vessels are abnormally dilated. If they should have a major hemorrhage from their esophageal varices, the bleeding is very difficult to stop due to their poor coagulation factors. They are often anemic.

Alcoholics also often die from brain hemorrhages. They stumble and fall easily, knock their head which ruptures tiny dilated fragile blood vessels in their brain which cannot seal themselves due to poor coagulation.

Alcoholics typically develop small atrophic testicles.

*The most important step all of us can take
is to recognize that we, too, are potentially equally
vulnerable to being trapped and changed by alcohol.*

Everybody recognizes the alcoholic and thinks they know why a person drinks: Weak character. No self-control. Had a miserable childhood. Has a terrible marriage. Cannot face reality. Hates work. Is paranoid. Denials and rationalizations, self-pity and self-importance, guilt and anguish are all part of a predetermined type, the "alcoholic personality".

In actual fact, the well-recognized alcoholic personality is the result of alcoholism, not the cause. This is the startling and original conclusion of a notable report entitled The **Natural History of Alcoholism: Causes, Patterns, and Paths to Recovery** by Vaillant (1983). His studies have shown that what starts off as simple social grace turns into a habit which, carried on long enough, degenerates into dependency. This dependency in turn creates the multiple personality problems of the alcoholic. Even the most cautious social drinker must be aware that alcohol modifies the way the brain functions. One can be "soothed" into alcoholism quite easily. By the time problem drinking has been identified, it is usually impossible for the patient ever to return to social drinking. In the opinion of many experts in the field, "the alcohol-dependent or loss-of-control alcoholic is probably never again able to return to enjoy the luxury of a social drink without running the risk of a relapse" (O'Reilly, 1983). The most important step all of us can take is to recognize that we, too, are potentially equally vulnerable to being trapped and changed by alcohol. The successive steps toward dependency listed below serve to warn how insidious is the process no matter how little is consumed. The potentially dependent alcoholic:

• enjoys the taste of alcohol
• enjoys the feeling of one drink
• feels more sociable and less tense after a drink or two
• likes to celebrate with alcohol
• has wine with many meals
• enjoys a drink after work
• likes to get drunk occasionally
• drinks when bored

*The treatment of alcoholism is very complex
and is fraught with great frustration and failure.*

- now takes two drinks when one used to do
- deceives himself about how much was drunk at a party
- drinks more now than 5 years ago
- sneaks drinks, drinks before noon
- laughs or brags about getting "plastered"
- spends weekends around drinking friends
- denies it, or gets angry if a drinking problem is suggested
- misses work on Mondays
- experiences blackouts
- drinks to go to sleep, but awakes anyway around 3 a.m.
- drinks and drives
- impotent
- family and/or job problems likely related to alcohol, but denies the connection
- alcohol related separation, divorce, or job loss
- delirium tremens (DTs), sometimes with hallucinations
- cirrhosis and other medical problems
- death due to alcohol, directly or indirectly

The treatment of alcoholism is very complex and is fraught with great frustration and failure. Alcoholic foundations, Alcoholics Anonymous, physicians, and various self-help and other interested groups count many failures in the ranks of their enrolled. The best remedy for anyone is to recognize the incipient problem before it becomes chronic and to be aware that no one is invulnerable. Remember, it starts with an enjoyable drink!

10.3.4 Heroin

Papaver Somniferum is the Latin name for opium. Opium is derived from the juice of the poppy, and it was known by the ancient Sumerians. In 1803 an opium alkaloid (one of twenty) was isolated and named "morphine" after Morpheus, the Greek god of sleep. Heroin is the most potent of these naturally occuring opiate alkaloids and the one most sought after by those wishing to experience the "dreams of Morpheus."

Since 1975 and the discovery of **endorphin**, the endogenous morphine that is produced within our own body, many new synthetic analogs of the opiate have been developed which are much stronger even than heroin. Fortunately or unfortunately, as the case may be, they are not readily available except when obtained by researchers for use in scientific experiments.

Our interest here in the opiates or heroin lies not so much in their abuse, but rather in the physiology of their dependency. Recent research has shown that the endogenous (naturally occurring within the body) morphine—endorphin—has a parallel physiologic effect to morphine or heroin. Endorphin may be continuously secreted within our own brain and can be elevated during exercise. What this means is that after a 20-30 minute hard run or exercise, blood endorphins are elevated which seem to produce a mild opiate-like state. This feeling is one termed by some runners as the **Runner's High** (Appenzeller and Atkinson, 1981). This term, however, confuses many who do not feel "high," but rather merely "calmed" after running, a state which is actually more in keeping with the elevated endorphin level.

The body's response to opiates is well-documented, very complex, and far reaching. Opiates create **analgesia**, which is an elevated tolerance to pain, and **euphoria**, which is a sense of floating and elevated calm. They disturb thermoregulation, cause the pupils to become the size of pinpoints, and adversely affect the body's response to stress by reducing the secretion of ACTH (see chapter 6). They also modify numerous pituitary hormones, affect respiration, cause nausea and vomiting, slow down intestinal activity, lower blood pressure, and are associated with **amenorrhea** (a cessation of the menstrual period). Endorphins will cause all the above changes as well, except for the adverse reaction to stress. Naturally elevated endorphins are associated with an improvement in the management of stress rather than a deterioration.

The parallel physiological effect between heroin and endorphins is interesting in view of the opposite personalities represented by athletes on the one hand, with naturally elevated endorphins, and drug addicts on the other, with artificially elevated opiates. Athletes generally tend to be assertive, confident, unafraid of exploring new ideas, and unafraid of taking risks; they tend to be socially open and are not likely to suffer from neurosis, psychosis, or depression. With heroin addicts, all the positive traits of the athlete, noted above, are reversed. Proposed mechanisms of opiate abuse indicate that **exogenously** taken (from the outside) chemicals depress the **endogenously** produced (from within) chemical or its analog. This leads, ultimately, to a lack of sufficiently precise control of important regulatory processes in the body and, hence, a deterioration of integrated bodily functions.

Current evidence suggests that the so-called "runner's high," or "runner's calm," may be associated with elevated endorphins. This fits a model that may explain why over 15 million North Americans have taken up jogging. Many are obligatory runners; if they stop running or reduce their activity they develop withdrawal symptoms associated with depression, neurosis, feelings of persecution and paranoia, and a general ache and discomfort throughout the body. These symptoms are very similar to heroin withdrawal. It is, thus, possible to become dependent on physical activity (Allen, 1983).

In 1987 concern is not with these "almost now considered to be" innocuous drugs but with drugs many times stronger like cocaine in its pure smokable form called 'crack' (see chapter 16, page 528) and the even more threatening designer drugs flowing from entreprenurial chemists cutting, splicing or adding chemical groups from or to well known botanical drugs such as heroin (i.e. a synthetic analog fentanyl, and its analogs, 100 times stronger than morphine) and cocaine.

Many of these new synthetic drugs are first considered legal and as soon as they are declared illegal by law a small change in structure legalises a new analog. This is a never-ending legal chase after the skillfull "designer" chemist with literally a universe of analogs available to develop. In June 1986 the U.S. Drug Enforcement Organization held a nationwide conference to consider this most significant threat yet to the health of millions of potential addicts (Gallagher, 1986).

10.4 NON-ABUSIVE DRUGS

Not all drugs that are used are addictive and not all drug use is abusive. Although some emphasis has been placed on abusive drugs in medicine, it is well-recognized that the prudent use of drugs does allow us to live

*A little known side-effect of anti-inflammatory drugs
is that they disturb thermoregulation.*

better. It obviously is better to fight disease by the judicious use of
chemical agents than to allow rampant illness to develop. Nevertheless,
careful use of drugs, even those given as medication, must always be pre-
eminent in medicine.

10.4.1 Anti-inflammatory Drugs

The non-steroid, anti-inflammatory drugs (NSAID's) were first developed for use in rheumatic diseases. Their basic mechanism of action is that
of **prostaglandin inhibition**. During injury or inflammation of tissues, by
whatever means, there is release of prostaglandins within these tissues
which leads to greater swelling of the tissue. In turn, this irritates nerve
endings causing pain. The pain is due to swelling, and anything which
reduces swelling reduces both tissue damage and the pain.

Acetyl Salicylic Acid (ASA), sometimes known as aspirin, is the most
common of the anti-inflammatory drugs. More recently, the pharmaceutical industry has produced a host of newer, stronger anti-inflammatory
drugs, all of which work by reducing the synthesis of prostaglandins within
tissue. This does not mean that by taking these drugs there are no prostaglandins whatsoever produced but merely that there is a reduction in the
excess of prostaglandins produced during the period of the tissue injury.

For the athlete, this means that during extended physical activity where
tissue swelling might be expected, the use of anti-inflammatory drugs reduces the swelling, allowing faster healing and speedier recovery. The
side-effects or disadvantages of such medications are gastrointestinal irritation and occasional peptic ulcer formation. This problem is usually reduced by taking antacids or milk or, when necessary, by stopping the drug.
On rare occasions, some blood dyscrasias (abnormal blood cell formations) have been noted. Known offending drugs producing the most undesirable side effects have been removed from the market.

A little known side-effect of these medications is that they disturb
thermoregulation. This is an important consideration for the athlete who
is working hard on a hot day, producing a body temperature much higher
than normal. In such a case, the body's normal mechanism for ridding itself
of excess body heat will be reduced by the use of anti-inflammatory drugs.

Many arthritic patients who take anti-inflammatory drugs also use them prior to mild physical activity where they can expect to have some pain, discomfort, and swelling afterwards. Athletes are doing the same thing by taking anti-inflammatory drugs prior to long races or events where they would expect to be slightly injured. These drugs are non-addictive, do not cause emotional highs or lows, are not sedatives nor tranquilizers, and, when stopped, their absence does not produce withdrawal symptoms.

10.4.2 DMSO

Dimethylsulfoxide (DMSO) is an organic solvent which has been used widely in chemistry and, more recently, in the treatment of athletic injuries including sprains, bruises, acute and chronic bursitis, and arthritis for the alleviation of swelling and pain. Although it has been used in these conditions, its efficacy has not been firmly established, and some controversy exists about its value in sports medicine.

DMSO is a clear, colorless liquid. It was first synthesized more than a century ago in Germany. A by-product of the pulp and paper industry, it is relatively inexpensive. Because of its highly solvent nature, it is absorbed through the skin very quickly. For this reason, it is often applied to skin overlying the injured area, where it is absorbed into the system very quickly, causing a garlic type of odor and taste in the mouth.

Despite the fact that scientific studies have not validated its use in sports medicine, there continues to be widespread use of DMSO and testimonies by convinced users claim miraculous results (Percy, 1981). However, many of the claims for recovery produced by treatment with DMSO have been in patients where a spontaneous recovery might have been expected in any event. Nonetheless, some known cases of musculo-skeletal disorders have indeed shown surprising benefits from DMSO when other forms of therapy have been ineffective. The final position of DMSO as an adjunct in medicine has yet to be established.

10.4.3 Iron

Five hundred million people in the world are iron deficient. Despite the fact that iron loss in humans is only one-tenth that of other mammals, our

*It is worth noting that the use of vitamin C
will enhance the absorption of iron from all sources.*

iron intake is perhaps only 1/100th in comparison. The theory for this discrepancy is based on the fact that our ancient ancestors were raw meat eaters and, therefore, a major portion of their iron intake was from the blood of other animals. Modern human dietary intake of iron from this source is low, and although iron is available in several other food sources, it seems that in many people enough iron is never absorbed from the digestive system to fulfill all the body's needs.

Before you can absorb iron you must ingest it. Our dietary requirements for iron are fulfilled from: **(1) heme iron**, from animal sources which have 30% of their iron available for absorbtion, and **(2) non-heme iron** (plant sources), a major source of iron in our diet but which has only 5% availability. This means that, despite a large amount of iron ingested from plants, we only absorb 5% of it. It is worth noting that vitamin C will enhance the absorption of iron from all sources. The use of iron in the body is mainly for the production of hemoglobin for the red blood cell which serves to carry oxygen to all the functioning cells of the body. Important enzymes of the "oxygen-food" energy transducing system also contain iron. Low iron intake by the body means low hemoglobin because iron is continually lost through sweating, defecation, and menstruation. An adequate iron concentration in the body means normal hemoglobin concentrations which are approximately 15 gm per 100 ml of blood. Males have a slightly higher concentration than females. A low hemoglobin level is called anemia, but not all anemias are associated with a lack of iron. There are sophisticated tests to check for iron levels within the body and to determine if a case of anemia is or is not associated with iron deficiency.

Some athletes have been found to suffer from what is called **sports anemia** (Pate, 1983). This is due to the increased breakdown and the release of iron from red blood cells and insufficient recovery of iron for use in manufacturing new red blood cells, increased loss of iron in excessive sweating, and poorer than normal absorption of iron from the digestive system. Sports anemia may reduce the ability of an athlete to perform

*Placebos are perhaps among the most potent of all
the drugs in our medical armament.*

because of insufficient red blood cell hemoglobin and its associated oxygen carrying ability. A brief review of the paragraph on blood doping will remind you of this principle.

In women, the added loss of hemoglobin in menstrual flow each month may also speed the loss of blood and iron from the body. Women athletes, therefore, are more prone to sports anemia, and in almost all cases should be encouraged to take supplementary iron (Clement, 1981; Hamilton and Banister, 1984). It has also been noted that when iron stores are low in other body tissues (not just in blood), athletic performance is negatively affected.

10.4.4 Placebo

Placebos are perhaps among the most potent of all the drugs in our medical armament. Without doubt, this wonder "drug" is the safest of all and has wide application. At one time it was felt the placebo response was an imaginary one, but now it is considered a true and useful adjunct to therapy.

Basically, a placebo is a non-drug prescription, a pill that contains no chemically active substance. However, the consumer of such a pill is convinced that it will cure a problem. In cases where a cure is effected the mechanism remains totally unknown. Somehow, within the mind and body, certain natural mechanisms are induced which are beneficial and curative. The standard, beneficial response from the placebo is about 30%. The rather high benefit-risk ratio should not be discounted and is worthy of serious research. There is some suggestion that the placebo response is associated with the endogenous activation of endorphins. (A review of the section on heroin will reacquaint you with endorphins.)

Many high level athletes are desperate to find one simple, magical remedy which will give them a very tiny edge over their competitors. They are so keen to believe that something will help them that they will "grasp at straws" and believe anything. As you read this you might think that such athletes are gullible and, in fact, weak individuals. However, an undying

10.5 THE UBIQUITOUS CIGARETTE

In 1492 Columbus sailed to the new world and noted that the natives carried "rolls of dried leaves which they set afire and drank the smoke." By 1527 early Spanish settlers in Hispaniola (Haiti) were smoking cigars which, despite the anger of the church, they found "impossible to give up." In short order, members of the church were also smoking. But this was just the beginning; two 16th century sea captains persuaded three Indians to return to London with them. The Indians did, along with "their supply of tobacco, being unable to depart the habit." The sailors themselves soon succumbed to the habit, and spread cultivation of the weed throughout the world, ensuring their own personal supply at each port of call and unwittingly ensuring that each new local populace became exposed to nicotine (Brecher, 1972).

In 1604 King James I, in his celebrated condemnation of tobacco, referred to smoking as "a branch of the sin of drunkenness, which is the root of all sin." Perhaps it is some reflection of James' popularity that by 1614 over 7,000 tobacco shops flourished in London. James was not, of course, the only royalty to oppose the newly discovered sin (Russell, 1971).

Sultan Murad III, of Constantinople, in 1633 decreed the death penalty for smokers and was very zealous in carrying out his decree. Large numbers of the populace were tortured and beheaded, yet even fear of death was no deterrent to the passionate devotees of the practice. This may remind you of the modern-day doctors that threaten smokers with eventual death, and yet many continue to smoke until their demise.

Three out of four of these smokers wish,
or have tried unsuccessfully, to stop smoking,
but only one in four ever succeeds permanently.

In every country, from the most well-developed to the most primitive, tabbacism, or tobacco dependency, develops along well known drug dependency lines: curiosity, sampling, pleasure gratification, use, over-use, dependency. England showed a curious shift during the 18th century when the nobility found it fashionable to chew snuff. Shortly, many people followed the fashion, but the actual personal or total nicotine intake probably remained unchanged (Dunn, 1973).

Sigmund Freud (1856-1939) was himself the tragic archetypical smoker. His 20 cigars per day eventually led to cardiac arrhythmias, chronic chest disease, and cancer of the mouth and jaw requiring many debilitating and disfiguring operations. Freud's personal, psychological, jargonistic justification was a "constitutional intensification of the eroto-genic significance of the labial region." He resorted to extremes to control his labial libido by even having one testicle castrated! He died without it and without his jaw but with his cigars (Russell, 1971).

10.5.1 Profile of A Smoker

The patterns of smoking dependency are quite predictable. Less than 15% of those who have only one (1) cigarette escape dependency, and three or four casual cigarettes will ensure that even the most well adjusted individual probably will become dependent. Three out of four of these smokers wish to, or have tried unsuccessfully, to stop smoking, but only one in four ever succeeds permanently. Only 2% of smokers are casual or intermittent (Russell, 1971).

The natural discontinuance of smoking was reported in 1969 as about 15% overall for persons under 60 over a 10 year period (Todd, 1969). Yet the social and personality profile of the successful quitters do not seem to set them apart significantly from the average smoker or non-smoker and do not, therefore, stand as a model for those hoping to quit.

The efforts that smokers make to stop may be admirable, but the recidivism rate is over 75%, the same as for heroin addicts (Berstein,

1976). Among blue collar workers recidivism is very high, and it appears that other groups may succeed better. Twenty years ago in Britain, 50% of doctors smoked; now only 20% smoke. The frequency of smoking among teenage girls is increasing compared with the frequency in males. This is a recent phenomenon and perhaps due to the social trend toward equality between the sexes, but such a social equality in smoking is of dubious benefit. The incidence of smoking-related lung cancer is also rising among women, and if the trend continues, it will soon equal that of men. The interesting mass experiment in Greenfield, Iowa, on August 8, 1969, bears these figures out (Dunn, 1973). As a movie was then being filmed on "Cold Turkey," the whole town cooperated in a plan to stop smoking. However, in the final analysis only the upper socio-economic group succeeded partially.

With an iron-clad case against smoking for reasons of physical health, it becomes understandable that the health professions now work so actively in finding ways to curb the problem. To put it briefly, health hazards from smoking may be summarized as follows: A smoker shortens his life by five and one half minutes per cigarette smoked, which is about the time expended in smoking it (Todd, 1969; **Smoking or Health**, 1977).

On balance, the cigarette industry does not pay its way in society. Comparing the costs in morbidity and mortality that smoking creates to the industrial employment and taxable revenue it produces, the deficits far outweigh the benefits. Governments are loath to inflict a severe blow to the tobacco industry for fear of lost taxes at the corporate level as well as individually due to unemployment in that industry. So far, governments have been very short sighted and are likely fearful of antagonizing a large block of voters—the smokers.

Worse yet, in 1975 it was estimated that the 80 million pounds spent on promoting smoking in Great Britain was counteracted by only 1 million pounds spent on anti-smoking advertising, and most of that meagre amount was spent on confirming the already known harmful effects of smoking. Currently only 3.5 million dollars is appropriated by the U.S.A.

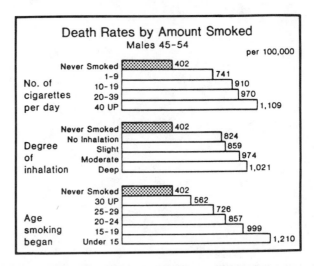

Figure 10.1. Mortality and smoking.
Reproduced with permission from
**National Clearinghouse for Smoking
and Health**, U.S. Public Health Service,
1973.

Congress each year to advertise against smoking while 2 billion dollars is spent on advertising by the industry. Each year there are 350,000 premature deaths from smoking in the U.S.A. and the health care cost of smoking to the economy is 65 billion dollars (The Economist, August, 1986). Few obstacles appear to be in the way of smokers for cigarettes now cost less in terms of real purchasing power than at any time since 1945 (Todd, 1969; **Smoking or Health**, 1977; WHO, 1974).

10.5.2 Physical and Psychodynamic Effects of Nicotine

We can no longer afford to regard cigarette smoking as a minor vice. It is neither minor nor a vice, but a physiological disorder of a particularly refractory nature, and all the evidence places it fairly and squarely in the category of a most pernicious, dependent disorder. The more one smokes, the greater is the hazard. This is called a dose-response relationship. The smoker's dose can be measured by the number of cigarettes smoked, the degree of inhalation, and the age smoking began. The person who has never smoked has the lowest death rate, and the one who has exposed him/herself to the greatest amount of cigarette smoke has the highest death rate (Figure 10.1). Many diseases and conditions are associated with smoking and although not all are causally related, they should not be overlooked (Figure 10.2). For instance, accident rates are higher for smokers than non-smokers. This includes fires in the home caused by the smoker who dozes off with a lighted cigarette in hand. The blood level of carbon monoxide is higher in smokers during the time they are smoking. Increasing attention is being given to the question of whether this carbon monoxide in the blood may be dulling the alertness of drivers to the point where this is a contributory factor in auto accidents.

Consider the anatomy of the cigarette. The modern flue-cured cigarette tobacco is acidic, about pH 5.5, is only mildly irritating, and the nicotine inhaled is 95% absorbed at about 0.2 mg of nicotine per puff. Pipe and cigar tobacco is air dried, has an alkaline pH of 8.5, and is quite irritating, but the nicotine is quite readily absorbed from the buccal (mouth) mucosa

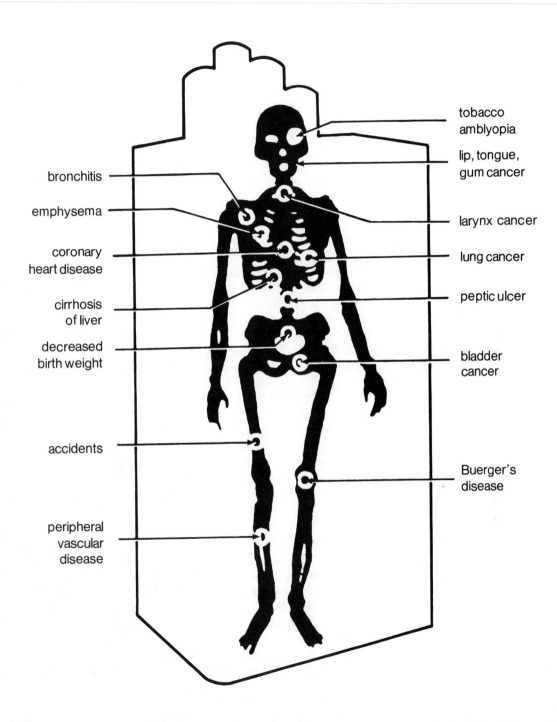

tobacco
amblyopia

lip, tongue,
gum cancer

bronchitis

emphysema

larynx cancer

coronary
heart disease

lung cancer

cirrhosis
of liver

peptic ulcer

decreased
birth weight

bladder
cancer

accidents

Buerger's
disease

peripheral
vascular
disease

Figure 10.2. Disease states associated with smoking. Reproduced with permission from **National Clearinghouse for Smoking and Health,** U.S. Public Health Service, 1973.

without inhaling. There is enough nicotine in one cigarette to kill a man if it were all injected intravenously, but only about 10% is absorbed. The killing effect, thus, is spread out over the remainder of one's life, shorter though it may be. Among the nearly 1,000 chemicals present in tobacco tar, many potent carcinogens can be found, but nicotine appears to be the chemical with the psychodynamic charm. Denicotinized cigarettes have generally not found much favor with the smoking public (Russell, 1971; **Smoking or Health**, 1977; Kozlowski, 1980).

Nicotine affects nearly every organ in the body, but its fat-solubility helps provide a quick entry into the brain. The brain cells have a high differential retention factor themselves, and quickly absorb nicotine, showing a 6-to-1 intracellular-to-extracellular concentration. Nicotine clears the brain in about 30 minutes which, coincidently, or understandably, in addicts, is the intervening period between relighting another cigarette. The modern cigarette is a highly efficient device for self-administration of the nicotine drug. It takes only 7 seconds for nicotine to be absorbed through the lung and reach the brain. In the heroin addict, it takes 14 seconds from injection in the arm for the drug to reach the brain. At 20 puffs per cigarette, and 1 pack per day, the average smoker gets nearly 150,000 nicotine shots to his brain per year (Russell, 1978).

Research on the neurological effects of nicotine shows that it has mixed stimulating and sedative effects. These mixed findings are exemplified by "Nesbitt's" paradox which states that, although nicotine is sympathomimetic (a brain-stem stimulator), when asked its effects the user invariably describes its sedating or calming action. Such mixed effects are seen in animal studies which show transient EEG and behavioral arousal due to stimulation of the brainstem activating system. The effects coincide with an apparent reduction of the impact of aversive events, either physical or psychological. The increase in blood pressure and heart rate (stroke volume remains unchanged) caused by nicotine may contribute to central nervous system (CNS) arousal. It has been observed that rats treated with

...long term smokers take little pleasure in smoking;
by this stage the controlling factor, in terms of intake,
has moved from overt pleasure to the chemical
dependency of nicotine in the primal brain region.
(Dunn, 1973; Kozlowski, 1980).

nicotine learn more quickly and remember better than controls. Even if the nicotine is given after training, enhanced peformance is still observed.

Once a rat has been trained it will perform a prescribed task better if given nicotine. Similar results are obtained in a variety of test situations, whether the animals are motivated by reward or punishment. Nicotine appears, therefore, to enhance performance and concentration directly, and this effect apparently cannot be attributed to reward or punishment, rather it is the nicotine itself (Dunn, 1973; Tachmes, 1978). Can this indicate that nicotine has positive value?

In the human animal nicotine enters the brain faster and more efficiently than most other psychoactive drugs. It has substantial behavioral effects on EEG habituation rates, arousal levels, and reflex activity of the skeletal muscles. It acts to suppress normal levels of these variables. An upper and lower boundary effect of nicotine consumption seems evident, the upper causing toxic aversive control, the lower causing withdrawal symptoms. Within this range smokers are free to fluctuate their intake according to the surrounding psychosocial influences. However either above or below the limits, smokers have either an aversive toxic symptom (feel uncomfortable) or a dependent urge (need to smoke) to fulfill. These boundaries are not seen in the novice or occasional smoker, but only in the person who has pushed intake to high tolerance limits. In the established smoker, it cannot be ascertained how much of the primary psychodynamic charm of nicotine has been eroded by the development of tolerance. For example, long term smokers take little pleasure in smoking; by this stage the controlling factor, in terms of intake, has moved from overt pleasure to the chemical dependency of nicotine in the primal brain region (Dunn, 1973; Kozlowski, 1980).

Plasma nicotine profiles of smokers show two types: "peak seekers," who smoke one cigarette per hour or less and enjoy the bolus effect produced; and "trough maintainers" who keep the nicotine level of the blood above a certain level by smoking a cigarette at least every 30 minutes. Either type of smoker is able to maintain his/her blood nicotine level within quite precise individual limits (Russell, 1978; Kozlowski, 1980).

*Until 1964 the well-documented fact that
cigarettes were definitely hazardous to one's health
had not been officially recognized.*

That unpleasant symptoms accompany withdrawal from nicotine addiction is quite evident from the testimonials of human suffering, but among lower animals, only rhesus monkeys have been rendered dependent on smoking and even have withdrawal symptoms when forced to stop. Rats, too, will demonstrate withdrawal, but since they can't inhale smoke their dependence comes from injectable nicotine. Nicotine-dependent animals when cut off, demonstrate a collapse of motivated behavior and are unable to perform learned tasks, foregoing rewards and accepting punishment for non-accomplishment. Interestingly, amphetamines seem to prevent this withdrawal syndrome (Lucchesi, 1967).

The withdrawal symptoms of human smokers include a generalized syndrome of depression, anxiety, irritability, poor concentration, sleep disturbance, sweating, intestinal upset, bradycardia (slow heart rate), hypotension, EEG changes, coordination difficulties, and faulty judgement. Nicotine injections will often correct such documented changes but only in the nicotine-dependent person (Russell, 1971).

A blind study of the recent advent of chewing gum containing nicotine demonstrated that smokers had a greater preference for nicotine gum than for non-nicotine placebo gum. The former gum reduces the recidivism rate of newly-won non-smokers significantly (Brantmark, 1973: Ferno, 1973).

Returning to Nesbitt's paradox, which ponders the issue of nicotine as the stimulator causing sedative feelings, it is probable that some of the calming effects of nicotine are associated with the reversal of the withdrawal symptoms in the dependent smoker. The sedating effects are observed only in long term smokers whose aversive tolerance (ability to tolerate toxic levels of nicotine) for cigarettes is high.

10.5.3 Dependency: Addiction vs Habituation

Until 1964 the well-documented fact that cigarettes were definitely hazardous to one's health had not been officially recognized. But in 1964 the Surgeon General of America published a very complete work on

Smoking and Health and pronounced, "the habitual use of tobacco is related to psychological and social drives reinforced and perpetrated by the pharmacological actions of nicotine on the CNS." However, he also stated that stopping smoking produced "no characteristic withdrawal syndrome other than symptoms which did not differ in any significant way from those observed in any emotional disturbance secondary to deprivation of a desired object or habitual experience." Thus, the terms "habituation" and "addiction" are in competition, and the argument about physical as opposed to psychological need persists in part even today (Smoking and Health, 1964).

In 1974 the World Health Organization added to the general confusion by using the term "dependence" in relation to drug addiction, suggesting that each drug produced its own type of dependence which either could be predominantly physical or psychological. In 1974, in its 20th report on Drug Dependency, the WHO stated that tobacco "is clearly a dependency-producing substance with a capacity to cause physical harm to the user, and its use is so widespread as to constitute a public health problem." In 1975, however, the WHO excluded tobacco from its list of dependency producing drugs (WHO, 1974).

The **mechanisms of psychological habituation or physical addiction** are the same. To label a drug **dependency producing** is enough; it need not be qualified with the terms "psychological" or "habit." The neuro-physiological mechanisms of the obvious "addictive drugs" are still confusingly complex, and the mechanisms of the less obvious "psychologically habituating drugs" are equally subtle, or more so. It would seem fair to say that all psychological mechanisms have a hitherto undiscovered physiological base. To argue "real" versus "imagined" is illogical.

10.5.4 Smoking-Cessation Programs

Doctors have been exhorted to counsel their patients to stop smoking, and the results of such pressure have been predicted to be 20% successful (Woods, 1978). The figures attributed to such a program may be optimistically high though, considering that an estimated 15% of smokers stop voluntarily during the peak 10 year period of their smoking, that is age 32 to 42. Men tend to stop spontaneously at a given rate, regardless of therapeutic ventures pressed upon them, while women tend to gain more from group support (Todd, 1969).

There is a myriad of choices with regard to the types of programs which are open to the public when they choose to stop smoking. Most models involve some sort of decision-making process, influenced both by internal and external variables. Once the decision is made, for instance, even "non-treatment" seems to be fairly successful. Subjects asked to stop on their own displayed consistent and significant success, especially if future aid was not expected (Bernstein, 1969; McFall, 1971). Various comparison studies have shown little relevance to success in the long term for differing modes of therapy. Some of the methods and conditions studied were sensory deprivation versus no-message therapy; satiation versus desensitization; anxious smokers versus the non-anxious; experienced therapist versus the non-experienced; smoking therapist versus the non-smoking therapist; and aversive therapy versus non-treatment. Proponents of each of these psychotherapeutic methods considered their own contribution as the "active ingredient" in promoting changes, but none actually rose to the top in terms of success. In fact, most of these studies averaged 30-40% short-term success, but only 13-16% of a success rate was achieved after 6 months (Thompson, 1966; Levenberg, 1976; Elliott, 1978; Pomerleau, 1978).

Hypnosis has been touted as a miraculous tool for aiding cessation in the smoker, but one famous study yielded only a 20% success rate at 6 months (Spiegel, 1978). However, the complexity of the treatment package, in which it is usually imbedded, would make it difficult to separate hypnosis per se from unsystematically applied social-learning techniques which often accompany it.

The latest methods in smoking therapy seem to emphasize every effective treatment successively, attempting complete cure.

Another recent study attempted to use both hypnosis and acupuncture to help patients stop smoking. When compared with treatment with acupuncture only, however, the combined treatment of acupuncture-hypnosis was no better than the single acupuncture treatment. The short term success of this experiment/treatment was 50% and its long term success 25%. This rather strong positive result may have been due to the fact that acupuncture elevates brain endorphins, which in turn have a calming effect upon the brain. Theoretically, this would alleviate the abstinence syndrome occasioned by the withdrawal of nicotine and make quitting cigarettes more comfortable. It was suggested that, although acupuncture is not unique in helping the smoker to quit, it may be a useful adjunct (Allen, unpublished data).

Thus far nobody has found a "best" answer, except perhaps that of beginning an exercise program. A survey of 141 runners showed that 35 were smokers prior to running, but only 3 of these were still smoking (Morgan, 1976). A ninety-one percent (91%) success rate is very encouraging, especially as these successes were not part of a designed anti-smoking campaign. That running appears to somehow affect smoking behavior is worthy of special note (Morgan, 1976). (Recall, running also elevates endorphins!)

The latest methods in smoking therapy appear to abandon any special analytic methodology or efforts to find a single trigger for change. Rather, the emphasis seems to be to use every effective treatment successively, attempting complete cure. Large multifocus centers, emphasizing careful follow-up and support with many personnel to ensure this, may achieve as much as a 38% long term success (Best, 1977). In the final analysis, there are many methods open to hopeful non-smokers; their motives should not be questioned, but their needs should be fulfilled instead. So, whether they ask for aversion therapy, group support, insight, guilt trips, sensory deprivation, hypnosis, satiation techniques, nicotine gum, or acupuncture, the helping profession should be ready for the chosen strategy of change for each individual. As long as it is the informed choice of the smoker, the means to the end of smoking is unimportant.

10.6 SUMMARY

Drugs in medicine and sport medicine occupy the same place as any other activity or habit in our lives: they may be used or abused; they demonstrate both benefits and hazards. In regular medicine, the use of chemical therapy is to bring the subnormal up to the normal. In sports medicine there is an emphasis on enhancing normal performance to the supernormal level. It is all a matter of perspective or degree. The list of ergogenic aids which purport to improve athletic performance range from the obvious abuse of stimulants, such as amphetamines and cocaine to the body building drugs, such as anabolic steroids. Some drugs, such as bronchodilators, are considered abusive but probably are not. They may merely bring subnormal conditions back to normal. Other more benign stimulants, such as caffeine, are used on such a worldwide basis that they are generally considered acceptable, though this does not mean that they necessarily are harmless.

Then there are the **curious hopefuls**, that miscellaneous collection of props and aids which probably work via the placebo mechanism. A few examples were given, but this list is constantly changing and those agents that you read about today will be different from what is offered tomorrow.

The use of iron was detailed for its benefits in enhancing the oxygen-carrying capacity of blood. Excessive iron does not lead to excessive hemoglobin. It will bring the oxygen-carrying capacity up to normal but will not surpass it. Blood doping, on the other hand, will actually elevate the blood heme levels well above normal and temporarily allow for an enhanced oxygen and nutrient-carrying capacity of blood.

Like all other people, athletes are exposed to the use and abuse of dangerous and addictive medications. Cannabis, benzodiazepines, alcohol and heroin have all been discusssed. It has been shown that not all chemicals are bad; some drugs, such as anti-inflammatories, possibly DMSO, and iron, are safe drugs which, in fact, can enhance the quality of life. Perhaps the safest of all is the placebo, whose effect may possibly be enhanced by the concomitant use of hypnosis. Smoking was discussed in detail as it is seen as the single most important preventable cause of ill health. Understanding and correcting this problem will have lasting benefit on the incidence of morbidity and mortality in society.

10.7 REFERENCES

Allen, M. Endorphins in Sports Medicine: A Review. **Canadian Journal Applied Sports Science,** 8(3): 115-133, 1983.

American College of Sports Medicine (ACSM). Position Paper on: Use and Abuse of Anabolic - Androgenic Steroids in Sports. **Medicine and Science in Sports,** 9: 11-13, 1977.

Anderson, K., Cate, B.W. and Jackson, D.S., et al. Crashing on Cocaine. **Time Magazine,** April 11: 18-27, 1983

Appenzeller, O., and Atkinson, R. **Sports Medicine and Fitness Training Injuries.** Baltimore: Urban and Schwarzenberg, 1981.

Berstein, D.A. Modification of Smoking Behavior: An Evaluative Review. **Psychology Bulletin,** 71(6): 418-440, 1969.

Berstein, D.A. and McAlister, A. The Modification of Smoking Behavior: Progress and Problems. **Addictive Behavior,** 1: 89-102.

Best, J.A., Bass, F. and Owen, L.E. Mode of Service Delivery in a Smoking Cessation Program for Public Health. **Canadian Journal of Public Health,** Nov.-Dec. 68: 469-473, 1977.

Brantmark, B., Ohlin, P. and Westling. Nicotine-Containing Chewing Gum as an Anti-Smoking Aid. **Psychopharmacologia (Berlin),** 31: 191-200, 1973.

Brecher, E.M. (ed). **Licit and Illicit Drugs.** Boston: Little Brown & Co., pp. 207-241, 1972.

Carrol, C. and Miller, D. **Health, the Science of Human Adaption,** 3rd edition. Dubuque, Iowa: Wm. C. Brown, 1982.

Clement, D.B. Anemia and Iron Deficiency in Athletes. **Sports Science Periodical.** Ottawa, Nov: 10-13, 1981.

Costill, D., Dalsky, G. and Fink, W. Effects of caffeine ingestion on metabolism and exercise performance. **Medical Science in Sports & Exercise,** 10(3): 155-158, 1978.

Dunn, W.L. **Smoking Behavior: Motives and Incentives.** Washington, D.C.: Winston & Sons, 1973.

Elliott, C.H. and Denny, D.R. A Multiple-Component Treatment Approach to Smoking Reduction. **Journal Consulting & Clinical Psychologists,** 46(6): 1330-1339, 1978.

el-Guebaly, N. Alcoholism and Drug Dependence. **Medicine North America,** 34: 3217-3223, 1983.

Ferno, O., Licktneckert S.J.A. and Lundgren, C.E.G. A Substitute for Tobacco Smoking. **Psychopharmacologia (Berlin),** 31: 201-204, 1973.

Gallagher, W., The looming menace of designer drugs. **Discover,** 7(8): 24-34, 1986.

Hamilton, C. and Banister, E.W. Variations in iron status with fatigue modelled from training in female distance runners. **European Journal of Applied Physiology,** 54: 16-23, 1985.

Haynes, R.C., Jr. and Murad, F. Adrenocorticotropic Hormone; Adrenocortical Steroids and Their Synthetic Analogs. In: Gilman, A.G., L.S. Goodman, eds. **The Pharmacological Basis of Therapeutics, 6th ed.** New York: Macmillan, 1466-1496, 1980.

Highbee, K.L. Fifteen Years of Fear Arousal: Research on Threat Appeals: 1953-1968. **Psychology Bulletin,** 72(6): 426-444, 1969.

Kozlowski, L.T. The Role of Nicotine in the Maintained Use of Cigarettes. **Drug Merchandizing,** Jan: 36-43, 1980.

Lamb, D.R. Anabolic Steroids. In **Erogenic Aids in Sports,** M.H. Williams, ed. Champaign, Ill.: Human Kinetic Publ., pp. 164-182, 1983.

Levenberg, S.B. and Wagner, M.K. Smoking Cessation: Long Term Irrelevance of Mode of Treatment. **Behaviour Therapy & Experimental Psychiatry,** 7: 93-95, 1976.

Lucchesi, B.R., Schuster, C.R. and Emley, G.S. The Role of Nicotine as a Determinant of Cigarette Smoking Frequency. **Clinical Pharmocology & Therapy,** 789-796, 1967.

McFall, R.M. and Hammer, C.L. Motivation, Structure and Self-monitoring: Role of Non-specific Factors in Smoking Reduction. **Journal of Consulting & Clinical Psychology,** 37(1): 80-86, 1971.

Morgan, P., Gildiner, M., and Wright, G. Smoking Reduction in Adults Who Take Up Exercises: A Survey of a Running Club for Adults. **Canadian Association of Health, Physical Education and Recreation Journal,** May-June: 39-43, 1976.

National Institute on Drug Abuse, Marijhuana and Health: Seventh Annual Report. Washington: Government Printing Office, p. 29. (Table on drug misuse, p. 234), 1979.

Olds, J., Travis, R.P. and Schwing, R.C. Topographic Organization of Hypothalamic Self-stimulation Functions. **Journal of Comparative Physiological Psychology,** 53(1): 23-32, 1960.

O'Reilly, J., Carpenter M. and Galvin, R.M. New Insights into Alcoholism. **Time Magazine,** April 25: 64-69, 1983.

Osler, Sir William. **A Way of Life.** An Address delivered to Yale Students, 1913, Thomas, Springfield, Ill., 1913.

Pate, R. Sports Anemia: A Review of the Current Research Literature. **Physician and Sportsmedicine,** 11(2): 15, 1983.

Percy, F.C. and Carson, J.D. The Use of DMSO in Tennis Elbow and Rotator Cuff Tendonitis: A Double Blind Study. **Medicine and Sciene in Sports and Exercise,** 13: 215-19, 1981.

Pomerleau, O., Adkins, D. and Perschuk, M. Predictors of Outcome and Recidivism in Smoking Cessation Treatment. **Addictive Behavior,** 3: 65-70, 1978.

Public Health Service, National Clearinghouse for Smoking and Health. **The Health Consequences of Smoking: A Report to the Surgeon General.** Washington: Government Print Office, p. 4-5, 1973.

Russell, H. Cigarette Smoking: Natural History of a Dependence Disorder. **British Journal of Medical Psychology,** March, 44(1): 1-16, 1971.

Russell, M.A.H., and Feyerband, C. Cigarette Smoking: A Dependence on High Nicotine Boli. **Drug Metabolim Reviews,** 8(1): 29-57, 1978.

Smoking, Marlboro Man, RIP? **The Economist,** 20, 1 August, 1986.

Smoking and Health. Report of the Advisory Committee to the Surgeon General of the Public Health Service. U.S. Dept. of Health, Education and Welfare, Public Health Service Publication, No. 1103, 1964.

Smoking or Health. The Third Report from the Royal College of Physicians of London. Pitman Medical, 1977.

Spiegel, H., and Spiegel, D. **Trance and Treatment, Clinical Uses of Hypnosis.** New York: Basic Books, pp. 210-219, 1978.

Tachmes, L., Fernandez, R.J., and Sackner, M.A. Hemodynamic Effects of Smoking Cigarettes of High and Low Nicotine Content. **Chest,** Sept. 74: 3, 1978.

Thompson, D.S., and Wilson, T.R. Discontinuance of Cigarette Smoking: "Natural" and with "Therapy." JAMA, June 20, 196(12), 1966.

Todd, G.F. (ed.) **Statistics of Smoking in the United Kingdom**, 5th ed. Tobacco Research Council, London, 1969.

Vaillant, G.E. **The Natural History of Alcoholism: Causes, Patterns and Paths to Recovery**. Cambridge, Mass. Harvard University Press, 1983.

Wilcox, A.R. The effects of caffeine and exercise on body weight, fat-pad weight, and fat-cell size. **Medicine and Science in Sports and Exericise, 14(4):** 317-321, 1982.

Williams, M.H. (ed.) **Erogenic Aids in Sports**. Champaign, Ill.: Human Kinetics Publishers, pp. 164-182, 1983.

Woods, D. Comments by Dr. Rosser. **CMAJ**, Aug 4, 121: 349, 1978.

World Health Organization. **Twentieth Report of Expert Committee on Drug Dependence**. Technical Report Series No. 551, W.H.O., Geneva, 1974.

10.8 STUDY QUESTIONS

1. The use and abuse of anabolic-erogenic steroids in sports has been strongly criticized by the American College of Sports Medicine. Why? Consider this question in view of the benefit risk features and the proof, or lack of proof, of benefits. List the common stimulants used by athletes and briefly outline for each the proported benefits and hazards.

2. How might an asthmatic use medications and approach a sporting event successfully? Describe the similarities and differences between blood doping and the use of iron.

3. What is the abstinence syndrome, and by what means will this syndrome be precipitated? List the common drugs associated with this problem.

4. Describe in general terms the similarities between hypnosis and the placebo response. In what way can anti-inflammatory drugs function in a curative or remedially beneficial manner for athletic problems?

5. Discuss smoking in terms of the risks, benefits, addiction, and methods to aid cessation.

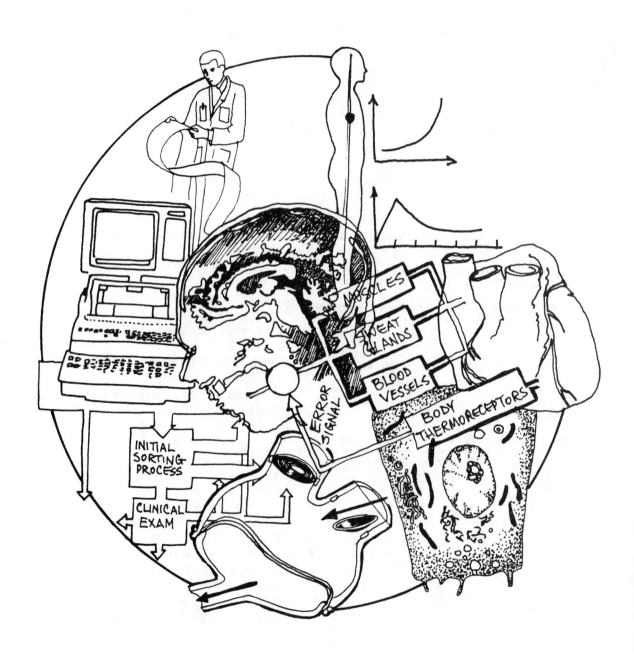

11

Bioengineering

Many of society's endeavours, paricularly medicine, will continue to be a blend—a synergy of science, engineering and technology.

OBJECTIVES

When you have completed this chapter, you should be able to:

- **Define** and **describe** the relationships among the disciplines of science, engineering, and technology.
- **Outline** some of the major contributions to health care delivery systems that bioengineering has made.
- **Explain** how systems theory helps in understanding the functions and structures operating within the human body.
- **Describe** several recent advances in bioinstrumentation that have made diagnosis and patient monitoring more effective and/or less "invasive."
- **Outline** the role of DNA in determining hereditary characteristics.
- **Explain** generally how the sex of a child is determined and how certain characteristics of the parents come to be expressed rather than others.
- **Discuss** the physical, social, political, and moral ramifications of genetic engineering.

KEY TERMS

BEAM	science
biomedicine	SQUID
construct (noun)	steady state
control systems model	systems theory
electrocardiography	systems modelling
engineering	technology
feedback loop	ultrasound

(Note: Key terms for **genetics** *sections of this chapter appear in the Glossary at the end of the chapter.)*

11.0 INTRODUCTION TO BIOMEDICAL ENGINEERING

Engineering in medicine emerged as a complex multidisciplinary endeavour during the late 1950s and early 1960s. Bioengineering, or Biomedical Engineering as it is now called, is already well advanced and accepted as a bonafide discipline in many countries throughout North America, Europe, and Asia. The interaction between a number of basic disciplines and medicine has spawned the interdisciplines of biochemistry, biophysics, biomechanics, and bioengineering. But it is the interaction between science, engineering, and technology that has had such impact on modern medical practice. In order to appreciate their potential for contribution to the health care field, we should understand the basic synergy of the disciplines of **science**, **engineering**, and **technology**.

Science has been described as the process of selecting a particular phenomenon (not necessarily a problem) to be studied, developing the methods to do it, executing the detailed procedures, collecting observations and assessing the results, and finally, proposing certain conclusions illuminating the phenomenon, together with some assessment of the relative certainty of these proposals (Harrison, 1984). A legacy of such activity is a base of knowledge, detailed methodologies of investigation that may have broad application, and a base of constructs underlying and explaining the knowledge gained. In a similar way, **engineering** investigates how to solve problems. Again here, the legacy of such endeavour is a gain in engineering knowledge, investigative methodologies, and the possession of principles and underlying concepts.

Technology principally devises methods for the production and delivery of goods and services of practical use, developed from a science or engineering knowledge base. Technological innovation results from four types of research and development. These are (1) the investigation of how to deliver goods or services more efficiently; (2) development of a more effective product or system; (3) creation of new goods or services; and (4) development of new applications of an existing product.

In modern society, separate roles for these three disciplines will become quite indistinct, with scientists becoming increasingly concerned with problem-oriented research, and engineers with the illumination of phenomena. Technology will continue to bridge the gap between temporary, developing, and well-defined substantiated practice. Many of society's endeavours, particularly medicine, will continue to be a blend—a synergy of science, engineering, and technology (Harrison, 1984).

Figure 11.1 shows the basic scientific activities studied in different engineering specialties, their medical correspondence, and the appropriate functional systems of the body that will benefit from contributions to knowledge in the field. The topics of interest (left-hand columns) are applicable to problems represented by the many different organ systems of the human body (right-hand columns). These new inter-disciplines of Bioengineering, Engineering, and the Life Sciences interact constructively across a broad interface, aiding in:

- an understanding of disease processes
- the ability to modify the consequences of illness
- an understanding of the life process and their control
- the capacity to make more precise diagnoses and improve treatment of illness
- the ability to manage complex administrative health care systems within hospitals or regional hospital groups more effectively
- the ability to develop a more rational system of patient care

Unfortunately, the benefits of modern scientific medicine have been accompanied and often obscured by sky-rocketing costs (x50 in the last 30 years) of sophisticated medical diagnostic and treatment facilities, which cost more than $20 billion in Canada in 1983 and $200 billion in the United States (see chapter 3). Currently the cost of health care in the USA (1987) is $365 billion.

There has been an explosion in medical technology in recent years, characterized by major developments in bioengineering. This stems from the latter's focusing upon basic knowledge discovered in the life sciences throughout the years and proposing practical applications for such knowledge in the construction of machines, materials, and processes that are useful in the practice of medicine.

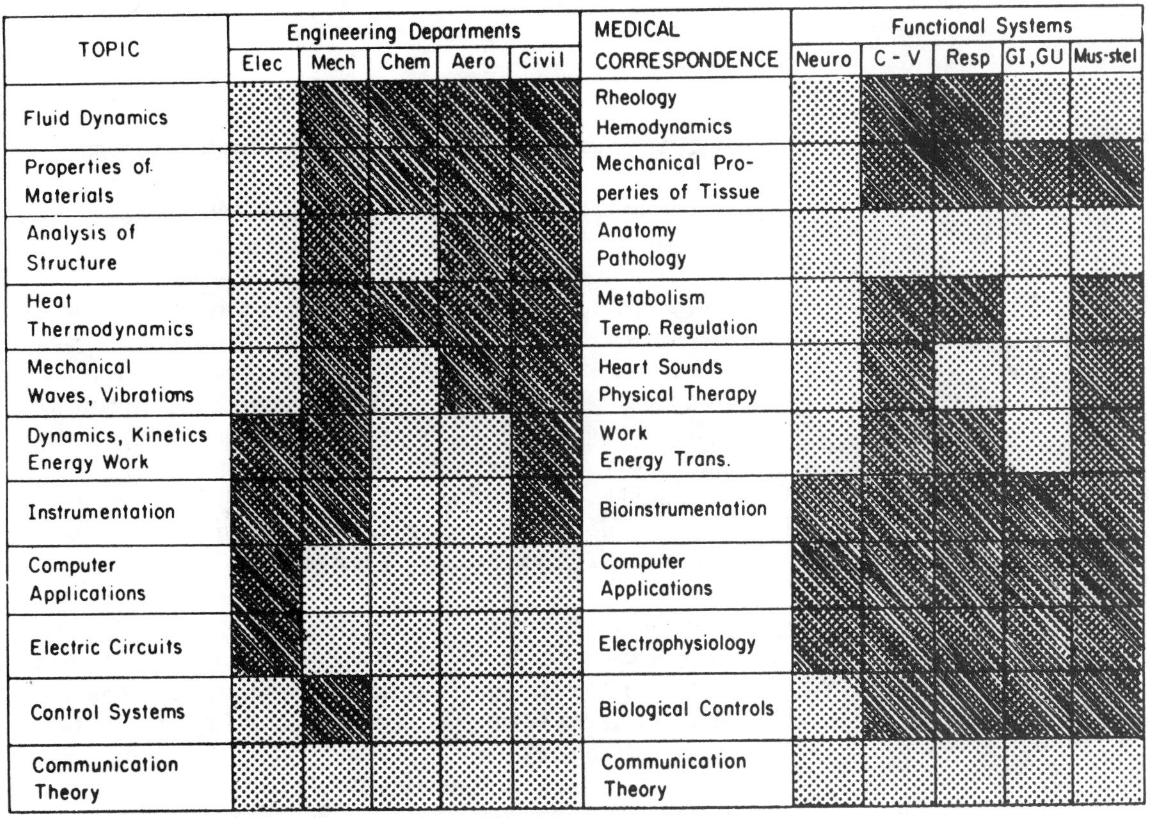

TOPIC	Engineering Departments					MEDICAL CORRESPONDENCE	Functional Systems				
	Elec	Mech	Chem	Aero	Civil		Neuro	C - V	Resp	GI,GU	Mus-skel
Fluid Dynamics						Rheology Hemodynamics					
Properties of Materials						Mechanical Properties of Tissue					
Analysis of Structure						Anatomy Pathology					
Heat Thermodynamics						Metabolism Temp. Regulation					
Mechanical Waves, Vibrations						Heart Sounds Physical Therapy					
Dynamics, Kinetics Energy Work						Work Energy Trans.					
Instrumentation						Bioinstrumentation					
Computer Applications						Computer Applications					
Electric Circuits						Electrophysiology					
Control Systems						Biological Controls					
Communication Theory						Communication Theory					

Figure 11.1. Basic scientific activities studied in different engineering specialties and their medical correspondence. Reproduced with permission from Rushmer, R.F., Medical Engineering: Projections for Health Care Delivery, Academic Press, page 11, 1972.

Increasingly, an objective science-engineering approach is being brought to the analysis of the complex interacting processes which are either producing disease, or operating within the health care delivery system designed to treat it. Recordkeeping, diagnosis, communications, instrumentation, cost analysis, and many other elements of health care practice are becoming increasingly reliant upon the systematic, quantitative, broad based, computer aided bioengineering approach rather than upon the subjective, qualitative practices used previously, which were limited both in terms of equipment and experience.

Table 11.1 shows the areas of basic and applied bioengineering to which the life sciences and engineering contribute. Some details of each of these individual areas are presented below.

11.0.1 Biomechanics and Biomaterials

Many structures of the body have analogs in common structures easily mirrored in everyday living. It takes little imagination to recognize such an analogy between a water pump and the heart, for instance, or between the material wrapping a package and the skin enveloping the body. The internal architecture of bone resembles the flying buttress shoring up the walls of old churches or buildings or the suspension cables supporting bridge structures. Water mains become arteries and veins, teeth become grinding pulverizing machines, the liver and kidneys become filtration-purification plants, and the muscles, become motors. It is little wonder that a fertile area of bioengineering has been the fabrication of synthetic materials to replace worn out body parts. Figure 11.2 shows the diversity of this particular aspect of bioengineering. Figure 11.3 shows various estimates of the cost of fabricating a bionic man or woman. The bionic industry is relatively young, most of its products being developed after 1950.

Spare parts sales and profit figures are closely guarded secrets. In 1983 alone, however, sales had an estimated value of $165 million US, with a potential to rise to the billions of dollars range. Large companies such as

Table 11.1. Basic and Applied Bioengineering Correlates in Medicine. Reproduced with permission from Rushmer, R.F. Medical Engineering: projections for Health Care Delivery, Academic Press, 1972.

BASIC BIOENGINEERING

Biomechanics

Properties of Tissues
Stress-strain relations
Visoelastic properties
Tensile strength
Compliance
Contraction-relaxation
Damping

Biomaterials
Support materials
Artificial joints
Bone substitutes
Artery-vein substitutes
Dialysis membranes
Nonthrombogenic surfaces
Artificial skin

Transport Mechanisms

Mass Transfer
Hydrodynamics
Diffusion
Active transport
Secretion
Excretion
Digestion
Absorption

Energy Transmission
Electromagnetic waves
X-ray
Ultraviolet
Visible light
Infrared
Microwaves
Radiowaves
Mechanical waves
Subsonic
Sonic
Ultrasonic

Simulation

Mathematical Modelling
Systems
Sequences
Interactions

Biological Models
Comparative Anatomy
and Physiology

Bionics
Sensors
Networks

Control System Analysis
Neural controls
Neuromuscular
Autonomic
Visceral organs
Glands
Temperature
Blood pressure
Hormonal Controls
Metabolic Controls
Psychological responses

APPLIED BIOENGINEERING

Instrument Development

Research Tools
Physical measures
Chemical composition
Microscopy
Isotope

Clinical Instruments
Neurology
Cardiology
Respiratory
Gastrointestinal
Genitourinal
Musculoskeletal

Diagnostic data
Automation
Chemistry
Microbiology
Pathology
Multiphasic screening

Computer Applications
Data processing
Analysis, Retrieval,
and Diagnosis

Therapeutic Techniques

Physical Therapy
Surgical instruments
Respiratory treatments
Radiation therapy
Radiation therapy

Monitoring
Intensive care
Surgical, postop
Coronary care
Ward supervision

Artificial Organs
Sensory aids
Heart-lung machine
Artificial kidneys
Artificial extremities
Arms
Legs

Health Care System

Organization
Medical economics
Longrange planning

Methods Improvement
Support function
Service functions
Nursing
Facilities design
Medical care

Operations research
Optimization of labs
Support functions
Personnel
Processing
Scheduling

Cost-benefit Analysis
Cost accounting
Evaluation of results
Beneficial economy

Environmental Engineering

Pollution
Air
Water
Noise
Solid waste

Human fertility

Population Control

Aerospace
Environment control
Closed ecologic systems
Physiological adaptation

Underwater
Compression effects
Heat conservation
Communication

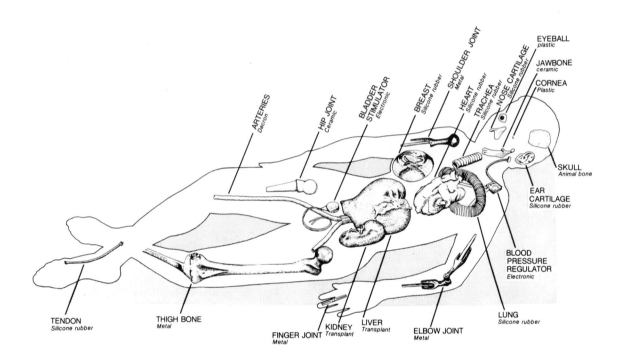

Figure 11.2. Showing the variety of replacement body parts which can now be fabricated from synthetic and/or organic materials.

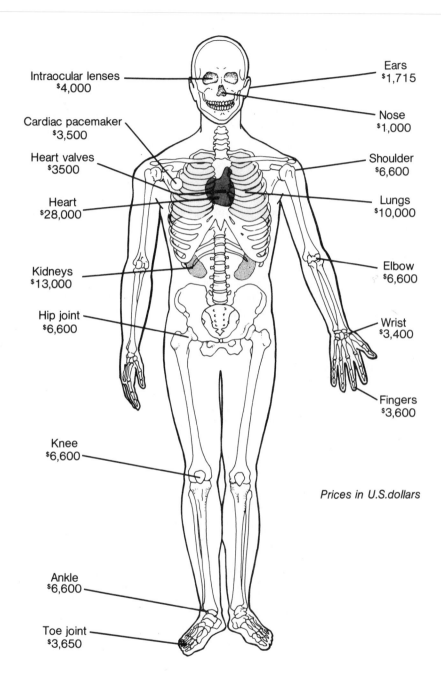

Figure 11.3. Estimated prices, in U.S. dollars, of various body replacement parts in 1984 (not including hospital costs, doctor and nursing costs or physcial therapy).

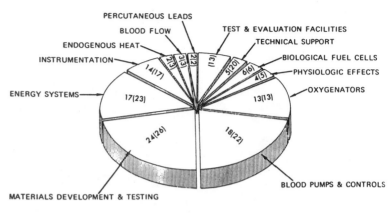

Figure 11.4. The number of research reports on subjects deemed necessary, in 1969, to solve the problem of developing a total heart replacement. Numbers in parentheses represent the total number of contracts. Reproduced with permission from Hastings, F.W. and Harmison, L.T. Medical Engineering: Projections for Health Care Delivery. Artificial Heart Program Conference National Heart Institute, Washington, D.C., June 9-13, 1969.

Pfizer, Bristol-Myers, Johnson and Johnson, and Dow-Corning dominate the American market. The largest commercial markets are for joints, intraocular lenses, heart valves, and blood vessels, with yearly sales of between $500-$700 million, U.S. An indication of the need for material in the United States each year is that 180,000 synthetic arteries are implanted and 170,000 coronary artery bypass procedures are done. Arteries for the extremities, such as the arms and legs, are replaced with umbilical cords. Once considered garbage by hospitals they are now assiduously harvested. Patient technology has also witnessed the growth of hard-to-synthesize materials in nutrient-baths. A major breakthrough of this type has been a technique to grow skin, cultured from an individual's own skin, in enough quantity to cover the worst burn case. In this way, life-saving skin grafts may be given without risk of rejection of the graft, as would be the case with donor skin or synthetic material.

The high cost of artificial replacements reflects to some degree, the large research and development operation needed to perfect a part. Figure 11.4 shows the number of research reports on subjects deemed necessary, in 1969, to solve the problem of developing a total heart replacement. The number of contracts awarded for such work, by the U.S. National Heart and Lung Institute are shown in brackets in the figure. Figure 11.5 (a, b, and c) shows a milestone accomplishment of this program in the diagram of the "Jarvik-7" heart, which was used in 1982 to keep the Seattle dentist Barney Clark alive for 112 days post surgery.

Drive-line tubes tunneled under skin and brought out in the left upper abdomen through specially designed skin buttons to minimize risk of infection. Buttons are introduced and tubes passed through via a separate, medial skin incision

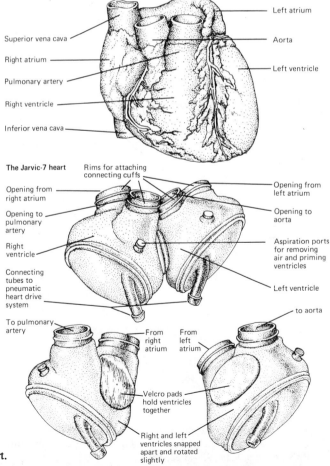

Drive lines emerging through skin buttons

Figure 11.5(a). The Jarvik-7 pneumatically driven artificial heart consists of two separate ventricles with air chambers. These ventricles are constructed of a smooth surface made of segmented polyurethane. The diaphragms consist of highly flexible four-layer sheets of polyurethane, and thus are infinitely pliable. This picture shows the placement of drive lines to the pneumatic heart driver.

Left atrium

Superior vena cava

Aorta

Right atrium

Left ventricle

Pulmonary artery

Right ventricle

Inferior vena cava

The Jarvic-7 heart

Rims for attaching connecting cuffs

Opening from right atrium

Opening from left atrium

Opening to pulmonary artery

Opening to aorta

Right ventricle

Aspiration ports for removing air and priming ventricles

Connecting tubes to pneumatic heart drive system

Left ventricle

To pulmonary artery

From right atrium

From left atrium

to aorta

Velcro pads hold ventricles together

Figure 11.5(b).
Comparison of human heart to Jarvik-7 artificial heart.

Right and left ventricles snapped apart and rotated slightly

FUNCTION OF ARTIFICIAL VENTRICLES

┌──── Diastole ────┐

Aortic or pulmonary artery valve closed

Mitral or tricuspid valve open; blood flows in from atria

┌──── Systole ────┐

Aortic or pulmonary artery valve open; blood flows out

Mitral or tricuspid valve closed

Biomer diaphragm, multilayered for flexibility and durability (Graphite between layers for lubrication)

Diaphragm depressed

Air

Diaphragm pushed up

Air

Air blows out to pneumatic heart driver

Air flows in from pneumatic heart driver

Response to increased circulatory needs (Frank-Starling law)

┌──── Diastole ────┐

┌──── Systole ────┐

Increased venous return in response to exercise further depresses the diaphragm in diastole

Stroke volume is increased during systole. Heart rate is unchanged

Valve function

┌──── Mitral or tricuspid valve ────┐

Diastole (valve open)   Systole (valve closed)

┌── Aortic or pulmonary artery valve ──┐

Diastole (valve closed)   Aystole (valve open)

Figure 11.5(c). How the artificial ventricles and valves function.
Figures 11.5 a, b, and c adapted and reproduced with permission from Devries, W.C. and Joyce, L.D., **Clinical Symposia** (CIBA), 36(2): pages 8, 9, and 22, 1984.

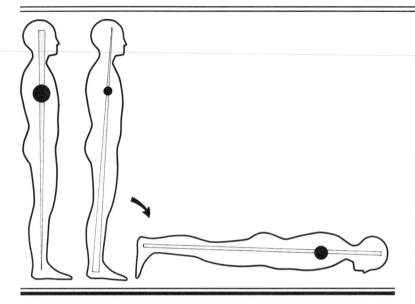

Figure 11.6. Showing differences in blood pressure, head-to-toe, as the heart and circulatory system work with and against gravity. The longer a person remains upright without moving, like a soldier on parade, the greater will be the pooling of blood in the feet due to the force of gravity acting on the blood columns in the blood vessels. Less blood flows back to the heart (smaller filled circle). Less blood gets to the brain (narrowed column) and the soldier faints.

11.0.2 Transport Mechanisms in the Body: Basic Physics

The body balances the transport of many substances within itself to maintain a co-ordinated, reactive, dynamic state. Fluids, gases, solutions, electrical (nervous) current, and heat are all in a state of constant flux (change) within the body as it adapts to internal and external stresses. The flow of much of this material obeys the laws of motion and energy transfer applicable to any other material in the universe, whether or not it is part of a living system.

Consider, for instance, the circulatory system, which consists of the blood, the blood vessels (veins as well as arteries), and, of course, the heart. Figure 11.6 shows a diagram of a man or woman standing upright and quite still. When this happens, although the heart is pumping, it has a more difficult job getting blood **uphill** to the brain than **downhill** to the feet. If the average blood pressure at the heart level is 100 millimeters of mercury (millimeters of mercury measure the force exerted by the heart on the blood), then blood flow to the brain is diminished relative to the feet. This is because the weight of the blood in the blood vessels obeys the laws of gravity and wants to flow earthwards, that is toward the feet. Thus, the strength of the contracting heart pumping blood headwards is opposed by the mass of the blood column above the heart and the force of gravity acting on the blood driving it footward. Similarly, the blood pressure is greater in the feet because the force of the heart on the blood footwards is aided by gravity, which also helps blood to fall to the feet.

Blood pressure at the head and feet may be calculated from the density of the blood, the lengths of the columns of blood above and below the heart respectively, and the force due to gravity. Many body functions may be calculated in a similar way from the laws of physics. Although they are not always absolutely precise, they allow good estimates to be made of the consequences of natural forces acting upon body systems.

One result of the pull of gravity on blood in the body is that, for example, a guardsman on duty, motionless in the erect (at attention position), for an hour or more will eventually faint. This is because blood will pool into his feet, and not enough blood will flow to his brain. Consequently he will lose consciousness and fall over. Luckily, when he does fall over, the blood flow to his brain is reestablished since the heart and brain are now on the same level, so he will slowly regain consciousness.

The movement of materials around the body, since they obey physical laws and have physical properties such as mass, density, electric charge, specific heat and so on, may be measured using physical (bioengineering) techniques. Electromagnetic flowmeters attached to the large vessels of the heart can be used to measure blood flow to and from the heart. These ideas will be developed further in the discussion of instrumentation used in the diagnosis of disease or organ dysfunction, another facet of bioengineering.

11.1 SIMULATION: MODELLING AND UNDERSTANDING PHYSIOLOGICAL FUNCTIONS

All body tissues need oxygen and substrates (food), and thus the distribution system for these substances is critical to survival. Disease or organ dysfunction compromises efficient function of interrelated systems. We would often like to know the effect that impairment of one process has upon another or upon the integrated activity of the whole bodily system. We would not only like to know the **qualitative** nature of the effect, that is, where it appears, what is its nature, and so on, but also we would like to know the **quantitative** nature (size) of the effect and how the size changes with single, double, or multiple deficiencies in various parts of linked systems. The linked systems of respiration and circulation can be described with the rather formidable equation above (Equation 1). It relates the volume of blood pumped by the heart each minute (represented by the symbol Q) in a steady state, that is, sitting quietly, to the volume of air breathed each minute (V_A) and to many other properties of the system.

$$\frac{P_{\bar{V}CO_2} - P_{ECO_2}}{\dot{V}_{CO_2}} = \frac{1}{f\dot{Q}} + \left[\frac{0.86}{\dot{V}_A} \times \frac{V_d}{V_t} \right]$$

Equation 1.

The actual operating system in the body, however, is dynamic not static. It operates at changing levels of ventilation because of the varying demands for metabolic energy made on it during different intensities of effort by the body. Thus, each part of the system varies and influences the others in a very complex way. Even Equation 1, complicated as it is, does not adequately describe transient changes in the components of the system as shifts occur from one level of activity to another. A branch of Engineering mathematics called **systems theory** has developed a particularly effective method for studying the contribution of each element or component of a system to its overall output and the interactive feedback that one component exerts on another. The method is particularly useful in the study of transient conditions before attainment of steady state conditions.

11.1.1 Systems Theory

Luckily, we do not always need to know the details of a system to understand how it reacts to stimuli. Systems theory allows simple understanding of even complex systems. Systems are made up of components, each of which is responsive to forces imposed upon it. Thus if a rocking horse is pushed, it will rock back and forth until it comes back to equilibrium again and is motionless once more. Almost all physical (inanimate) and living systems have similar responses to forces (stimuli) imposed upon them (if they are disturbed) and their reaction to the stimulus depends upon the intrinsic properties of their own system. Although we may not know the details of the biological mechanism of the structure producing an observed reaction, various characteristics of it may be measured such as the delay in the system between its stimulation and its response. This may be illustrated with several examples, as shown in Figure 11.7. As we shall see, systems theory also allows the interactions of different subsystems to be understood.

In all of the systems (K, A, B, C, D) of Figure 11.7, the output from the system is represented in the graphical plots to the right as some product of

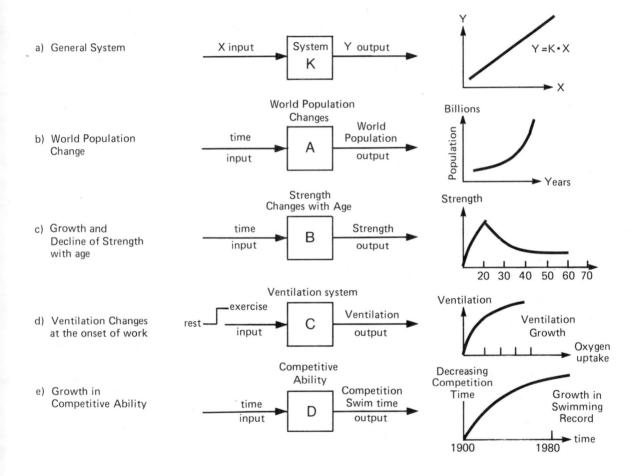

Figure 11.7. Showing several examples of how systems theory diagrams can help us conceptualize relationships among parts of a system. In these diagrams the input x is multiplied, added to, raises some number to the power of x etc., etc., in order to give a best estimate of y. When this can be done so that the estimated pattern of the input (x) and response (y), models (patterns) the real experimentally observed response then the equation relating y to x represents the system k, A, B, etc.

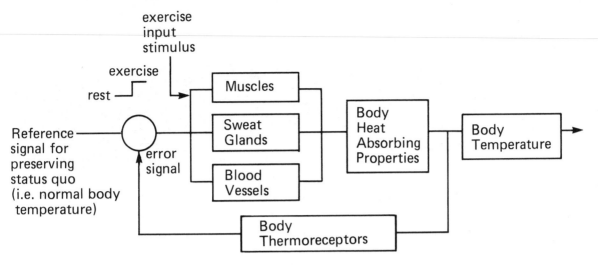

the input, and the characteristics of the system represented by K, A, and so forth in the "black box." Very often, in the first place, we are only interested in characterizing the properties of the system for given inputs (X) and outputs (Y). The power of systems modelling stems from the fact that the response of most human systems (Y), to input stimuli (X), may be represented by only a few basic mathematical manipulations of the input X (such as multiplying X by a constant K, so that $Y=X\cdot K$ or raising some number to the power of X, so that $Y=ae^{-bx}$).

We may now return to the idea of building a model of a larger system, whose subsystems themselves (K, A, B, etc.), have already been studied singly with regard to certain input stimuli, such as the passage of time, exercise, stress, and so on. Such separately measured characteristics combined together may then be used to explain the system overall.

The combination of several subsystems into a composite system to control body temperature is shown in Figure 11.8. A basic difference of this system, compared with the one-element subsystems (discussed previously), besides its complexity (i.e. several elemental subsystems grouped together), is the introduction of a connecting loop from the overall output (body temperature) back to the input signal. The latter is the body's own standard of what the body temperature should be for optimal comfort and operation. The model now becomes, in the terminology of the engineer, a **control systems model**, and the connecting loop is called a **feedback loop**. The feedback loop provides a real value of body temperature for comparison against the body's standard. If the steady state (resting) system is disturbed in a way that causes its temperature to rise (i.e., during exercise), an increasing temperature signal is fed back to the reference input temperature signal for comparison. The difference between the two is called the **signal error** (the difference between ideal and real temperatures). This, in turn, will influence various components of the system, such as the blood vessels or the sweat glands, to change in order to dissipate the excess heat and return the system to its original condition.

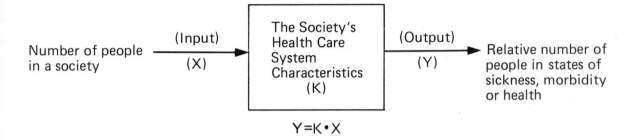

Figure 11.9. Systems model of a society and its health care system.

The usefulness of modelling physiological processes lies in the understanding it brings to our study of complex, interacting subsystems. Once the model system and its components are conceptualized and basic mathematical equations relating the input and output of each subsystem are developed, then the correspondence of the conceptual model output may be compared with reality for varying disturbing effects on the (human) system. The possible effects of different, currently uninvestigated, conditions may then be inferred without actually performing investigations to determine them experimentally.

In a similar way, models of hospital operations may be constructed from all the different sub-systems, contributing to an efficiently run total system. The flow of patients through different hospital services, their requirements for food, laundry, drugs, surgery, and so forth may all be modelled, and the most efficient grouping of services for optimal hospital operation may be arranged. Indeed, these ideas also apply to the provision and grouping (relevant to population use, cost, and other factors) of regional health care services, including not only hospitals, but also long term care, preventive care, check-up clinics, exercise clinics, rehabilitation centres, and physiotherapy clinics. By using models, the question of where to place the money available for health care most effectively may be evaluated better. The question, "If we changed the emphasis of care from 'here' to 'here,' what would be the feedback effect on other subsystems of the model (e.g. other parts of the health care system)," could be answered. We could also determine the effect of such action on the output of the model toward the ideal of providing for the greatest number of people needing services in the region served by the system (see for example Figure 11.9).

11.2 BIOINSTRUMENTATION
Over the years a wide variety of instrumentation has been developed in basic science for the purpose of investigating many scientific phenomena. The principles of operation of instruments such as those used in sonar,

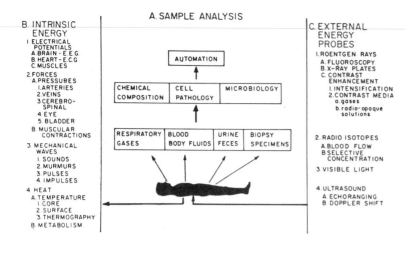

A. SAMPLE ANALYSIS

B. INTRINSIC
ENERGY
I. ELECTRICAL
POTENTIALS
A. BRAIN - E.E.G.
B. HEART - E.C.G.
C. MUSCLES
2. FORCES
A. PRESSURES
I. ARTERIES
2. VEINS
3. CEREBRO-
SPINAL
4. EYE
5. BLADDER
B. MUSCULAR
CONTRACTIONS
3. MECHANICAL
WAVES
I. SOUNDS
2. MURMURS
3. PULSES
4. IMPULSES
4. HEAT
A. TEMPERATURE
I. CORE
2. SURFACE
3. THERMOGRAPHY
B. METABOLISM

AUTOMATION

CHEMICAL
COMPOSITION | CELL
PATHOLOGY | MICROBIOLOGY

RESPIRATORY
GASES | BLOOD
BODY FLUIDS | URINE
FECES | BIOPSY
SPECIMENS

C. EXTERNAL
ENERGY
PROBES
I. ROENTGEN RAYS
A. FLUOROSCOPY
B. X-RAY PLATES
C. CONTRAST
ENHANCEMENT
I. INTENSIFICATION
2. CONTRAST MEDIA
a. gases
b. radio-opaque
solutions

2. RADIO ISOTOPES
A. BLOOD FLOW
B. SELECTIVE
CONCENTRATION

3. VISIBLE LIGHT

4. ULTRASOUND
A ECHORANGING
B DOPPLER SHIFT

Figure 11.10. Principle sources of information for diagnostic purposes include (A) analysis of samples from the body such as chemical composition, cellular structure or presence of bacteria; (B) analysis of intrinsic electrical, mechanical or thermal energy generated within the body; and (C) external energy sources which provide information regarding structure and function of internal organs. Reproduced with permission from Rushmer, R.F., Medical Engineering: Projections for Health Care Delivery, Academic Press, p. 22, 1972.

electro-magnetic measurements, and electrical measurements, with suitable modification, have also been applied to studying the fluids, gases, tissues, and energetic emissions of the human body by both invasive and non-invasive techniques. Figure 11.10 shows several properties of the human body, which may be sensed, sampled, and probed for diagnostic and therapeutic purposes in this way.

Major advances in data gathering procedures have been made using non-invasive techniques. Table 11.2 shows a list of the organ systems that may be explored quite sensitively with relatively little discomfort to the patient. These range from blood and urine analysis, to such techniques as ultrasound (Figure 11.11), multiple cardiovascular recording (Figure 11.12), or thermography. All these forms of data are used to supplement the physician's own diagnostic skill during physical examinations (Figure 11.13).

Ideally, the best diagnostic instrument would be one pointed at the body that would be able to present a complete visual or numerical picture of any abnormality. In fact, some modern procedures known as **medical imaging** are fast approaching this capability.

Earlier techniques of ultrasound and ultrasonic holography are being increasingly supplanted by newer, more sophisticated, imaging techniques (unfortunately all are more costly). Some of these newer techniques are computerized tomography (CT) and nuclear magnetic resonance (NMR), also called magnetic resonance imaging (MRI). The latter depends on the ability to manipulate the nuclei of elements, such as phosphorus, carbon, hydrogen, and oxygen found in the body, by magnetic fields and radio waves. NMR technique identifies the elements present in a body scan by their chemical form, concentration, and location, and it converts the signals from their magnetic excitation to shades of grey or colour that define the outline of the organs according to their elemental concentration profiles. Figure 11.14 shows the advances that have been made in the definition of internal organs, using such techniques, during the

Table 11.2. Chemical test groups considered useful in eliciting evidence of diseases in various organ systems. Reproduced with permission from Rushmer, R.F., Medical Engineering: Projections for Health Care Delivery, Academic Press, page 207, 1972.

Specific changes	Test Groups
Heart/vessels	Cholesterol, total lipids, ß-lipoproteins, BUN, creatinine, urinary protein, total protein, albumin, zinc sulfate test, sodium, potassium, chloride
Liver	Bilirubin, alkaline phosphatase, thymol turbidity, serum iron, TIBC, GOT, GPT, LDH (amylase and/or others), total protein, albumin, zinc sulfate test
Lungs	ESR, Protein-bound hexose, sialic acid, haptoglobin
Kidney	BUN, Creatinine, urinary protein (uric acid), hemoglobin, hematocrit, serum iron, TIBC, ESR, protein-bound hexose, sialic acid, haptoglobin
Blood	Hemoglobin, hematocrit, serum iron, TIBC, total protein, albumin, zinc sulfate test, ESR, protein-bound hexose, sialic acid, haptoglobin
Skeletal system	Calcium, phosphorus, alkaline phosphatase, total protein, albumin, zinc sulfate test, ESR, protein-bound hexose, sialic acid, haptoglobin
Endocrine Diabetes	Blood glucose (after glucose load), urinary glucose cholesterol, total lipids, ß-lipoproteins, ESR, protein-bound hexose, sialic acid, haptoglobin
Thyroid Parathyroid	PBI, T3, cholesterol, total lipids, ß-lipoproteins, Calcium, phosphorus, alkaline phosphatase
General Changes	
Inflammatory, neoplastic, etc.	ESR, protein-bound hexose, sialic acid, haptoglobin, hemoglobin, hematocrit, serum iron, TIBC, total protein, albumin, zinc sulfate test

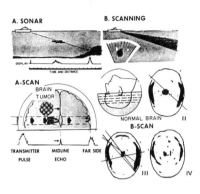

Figure 11.11. (A) Transmission time of sound waves indicate distances to reflecting targets in sonar just as ultrasonic pulses can be utilized to indicate the distance to midline structures of the brain to detect displacement in the presence of a brain tumor. (B) Scanning techniques provide two dimensional displays of reflecting surfaces which indicate the location of structures within the brain which cannot be detected by x-ray. Reproduced with permission from Makow, D.M. and McRae, D.L., Symmetrical scanning of the head with ultrasound using water coupling. **Journal of the Acoustic Society of America,** 44: 1345-1352, Pergamon Press, 1968.

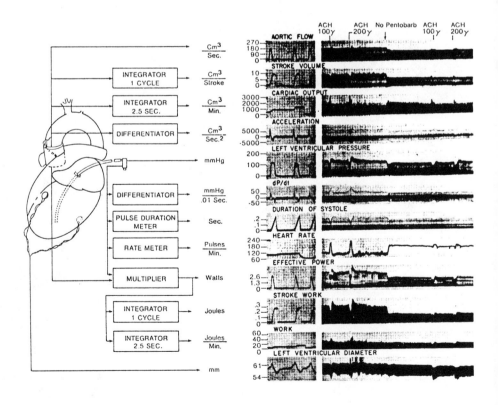

Figure 11.12. Multiple simultaneous variables, directly registered or derived, can be presented as deflections on paper moving at various speeds. Reproduced with permission from Rushmer, R.F., Cardiovascular Dynamics, 3rd ed., W.B. Saunders Co., page 169, 1972.

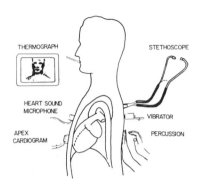

Figure 11.13. Physical examinations are the special province of physicians who depend largely on their subjective senses. Supplemental technology is available in the form of thermography for surface temperature distribution, phonocardiography, and apex cardiography for heart sounds and apical impulse and the prospect of vibrators to elicit information about resonance to supplement percussion. Reproduced with permission from Rushmer, R.F., Medical Engineering: Projections for Health Care Delivery, Academic Press, page 233, 1972.

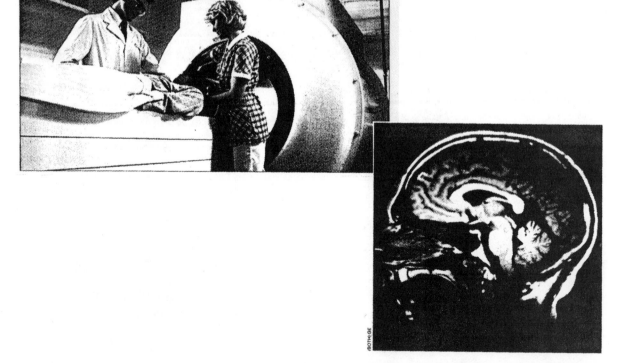

Figure 11.14. NMR scan and proton imaging of the brain's internal anatomy. Reproduced with permission from **High Technology Business Magazine** (August, 1984). Copyright © 1984 by Infotechnology Publishing Corporation, 214 Lewis Wharf, Boston, MA., 20110

relatively short period between1977 and the present. It is claimed that the NMR technique will one day allow chemical analyses (usually obtained from a blood sample and after considerable laboratory work) to be completed much faster and without even taking a sample, by the simple expedient of the patient placing one hand inside the magnetic bore of the apparatus.

Another device, producing electrical images of the brain, is the Superconducting Quantum Interference Device (SQUID). The SQUID measures the magnetic component rather than electrical component of the electroencephalogram (EEG) to visualize brain waves through a process known as Brain Electrical Activity Mapping (BEAM). In this way, several hypotheses have been developed linking highly variable small-scale magnetic fields in the brain to sensory brain activity. More stable, coherent, whole brain fields have been linked to the brain's innermost thoughts and reflections.

11.3 BIOENGINEERING HEALTH CARE SYSTEMS

Modelling an optimal regional health care system, using systems theory methods, was discussed earlier. Insight into the internal organization of service units within the hospital may similarly be sought, with a view to producing optimal efficiency and cost effectiveness. Perhaps the two areas of operation upon which engineering has had the most significant impact, however, are in monitoring patient care and data acquisition and reduction.

11.3.1 Medical Monitoring

Monitoring the condition of a patient is a prerequisite to providing care, whether under emergency, acute, or chronic conditions. The essence of this procedure is to allow the swift recognition of symptoms enabling appropriate lifesaving action to be taken. Bioengineering has contributed increasingly to the storage and presentation, in readily interpretable form, of information obtained from physical examinations or measuring devices.

PATIENT MONITORING—PACIFIC MEDICAL CENTER

PATIENT LOG. UNIT 3 DATE 818   TOWELL M

TIME	SYS	DIA	MAP	APID	LAP	CVP	HR	PRT	RRT	MV	TV
817***2254UXIMTER		AVD	7.0	HB	13.4	AO2 99 VO2 60					
1117	0	0	0	0.00	0	0.00	0	0	14	19.53	1354
1118	116	74	89	1.48	0	0.0	65	66	0	0.00	0
1121	0	0	0	0.00	0	0.0	0	0	10	15.65	1444
TIDAL VOLUMES UNBALANCED 1853.-1444.											
1121	117	78	92	1.33	0	0.0	72	71	0	0.00	0
1130	0	0	0	0.00	0	0.0	0	0	10	13.09	1299
TIDAL VOLUMES UNBALANCED 1616.-1299.											
1130	108	60	76	1.64	0	0.0	66	66	0	0.00	0
1132	0	0	0	0.00	0	0.0	0	0	11	17.48	1543
TIDAL VOLUMES UNBALANCED 1877.-1543.											
1132	105	61	75	1.37	0	0.0	70	71	0	0.00	0
1140	0	0	0	0.00	0	0.0	0	0	4	7.76	1707
TIDAL VOLUMES UNBALANCED 2005.-1707.											
1140	102	62	76	1.12	0	0.0	63	64	0	0.00	0
1210	112	59	76	1.65	0	0.0	71	71	11	15.12	1343
1220	0	0	0	0.00	0	0.0	68	0	8	12.53	1470
1223	0	0	0	0.00	0	0.0	0.0	0	10	16.73	1629
TIDAL VOLUMES UNBALANCED 2003.-1629.											
1223	0	0	0	0.00	0	0.0	62	0	0	0.00	
1230	102	66	81	0.79	0	0.0	66	53	13	19.81	1463
1240	104	57	71	1.35	0	0.0	60	57	10	19.82	1908
1241	108	64	77	1.17	0	0.0	62	64	10	17.73	1759
1250	139	75	95	2.20	0	0.0	93	93	12	20.74	1621
1251	128	69	87	2.18	0	0.0	84	85	7	12.36	1644
1300	112	64	79	1.47	0	0.0	65	63	7	14.16	1888
1310	122	70	88	1.49	0	0.0	84	84	4	10.76	2190
1312	110	69	84	1.21	0	0.0	78	78	9	17.35	1921
1315	0	0	0	0.00	0	0.0	0	0	14	26.44	1854
TIDAL VOLUMES UNBALANCED 1555.-1854.											
1315	117	74	91	1.21	0	0.0	104	84	0	0.00	0
1316	0	0	0	0.00	0	0.0	0	0	14	24.51	1693
TIDAL VOLUMES UNBALANCED 1341.-1693.											
1316	119	73	91	1.27	0	0.0	87	84	0	0.00	0
1321	0	0	0	0.00	0	0.0	0	0	7	11.20	1482
TIDAL VOLUMES UNBALANCED 1263.-1482.											
1321	119	74	92	1.09	0	0.0	75	75	0	0.00	0
1323	0	0	0	0.00	0	0.0	0	0	9	15.09	1606
TIDAL VOLUMES UNBALANCED 1412.-1606.											
1323	119	73	90	1.35	0	0.0	82	83	0	0.00	
1330	0	0	0	0.00	0	0.0	0	0	11	19.15	1675
TIDAL VOLUMES UNBALANCED 1463.-1675.											
1330	138	73	93	2.23	0	0.0	89	90	0	0.00	0
1340	121	68	85	1.62	0	0.0	75	75	9	15.61	1732
1350	0	0	0	0.00	0	0.0	0	0	5	10.62	2048
TIDAL VOLUMES UNBALANCED 1251.-2048.											
1350	108	66	79	0.95	0	0.0	69	70	0	0.00	0
1353	0	0	0	0.00	0	0.0	0	0	8	16.07	1886
TIDAL VOLUMES UNBALANCED 1558.-1886.											
1353	105	69	82	0.81	0	0.0	66	66	0	0.00	0
1400	127	65	85	2.19	0	0.0	69	68	9	14.97	1557
1410	0	0	0	0.00	0	0.0	0	0	7	15.32	1924

Figure 11.15. Intensive care units frequently present many different measured quantities as columns of figures which represent much information but are extremely difficult to interpret. Modified and reproduced with permission from Rushmer, R.F., Medical Engineering: Projections for Health Care Delivery, Academic Press, page 168, 1972.

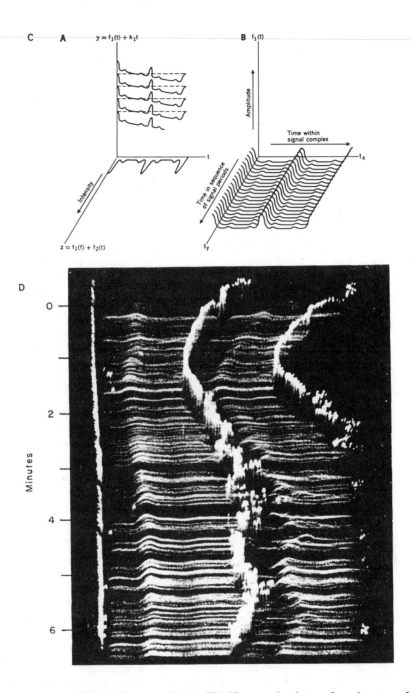

Figure 11.16. Continuous waveforms (A) can be packed into a small space (B) while preserving the waveforms by means of the contourgraph (D). Each complete electrocardiographic recording of a single heart beat is "cut and stacked" as it were in a box. Thus not only can the amplitude of the various parts of the "single beat" signal and the intervals between them be observed from left to right in the box (i.e., along the t_x axis) but the consistency of these intervals "beat to beat" may also be observed in the "back to front" direction of the box (along the t_y axis). Any developing abnormality of the signal may be instantly seen. Reproduced with permission from Webb, G.N. and Rodgers, R.E. The countourograph. **Institute of Electrical and Electronics Engineers Inc. U.S.A. Spectrum**, June 1966.

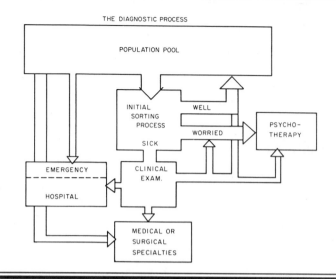

THE DIAGNOSTIC PROCESS

POPULATION POOL

INITIAL SORTING PROCESS

WELL

WORRIED

SICK

PSYCHO- THERAPY

EMERGENCY

HOSPITAL

CLINICAL EXAM.

MEDICAL OR SURGICAL SPECIALTIES

Figure 11.17. Systematic model of routes by which patients move through the health care system. Reproduced with permission from Rushmer, R.F., Medical Engineering: Projections for Health Care Delivery, Academic Press, page 184, 1972.

The efficiency and understanding of communicated information appreciates in direct proportion to the number of forms in which it is presented, such as in words, numbers, or pictures. A combination of the latter two forms supplements understanding gained from any one form alone. Thus, information contained in rows and columns of numbers is not considered to be as understandable as a graphical display of similar information (compare Figures 11.15 and 11.16). In Figure 11.16, the signal from one cycle of events (many events of human function are cyclical, with periods of seconds, hours, days, or weeks) is displayed along one graphical axis and the correspondence of each cycle with the previous one is displayed along the axis perpendicular to this. Gross variations in cyclic activity (which often are indicative of functional abnormality) are readily observed using this format. Notice the variation in time, within the cycle, where the peak wave form occurs. If the waves were corresponding perfectly, the peaks would all lie in a straight line under one another. Data transmission of this nature is often used in intensive care units, where rapid recognition of an abnormal pattern in a waveform is essential so that immediate corrective action may be taken.

11.3.2 Medical Records

A model of the diagnostic process for a patient entering a health care system is shown in Figure 11.17. The initial process of sorting patients into categories such as well, sick, worried well, or early sick is usually accomplished by interview, obtaining both general personal data and specific insights into the current complaint. However, extensive questionnaires (up to 1,200 questions long) can be expensive, time consuming, and variably recorded if personally taken (by physician or nurse). Extensive research is currently ongoing into methods of codifying such data in computer compatible form for storage, retrieval, and analysis. In fact, wholly computer-conducted interviews are regarded as more thorough in obtaining general medical histories than investigations by physicians. Computer question-

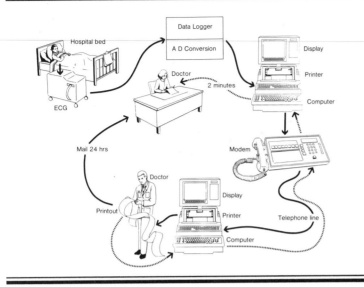

Figure 11.18. Electrocardiograms and other forms of diagnostic data may be sent instantly from the recorder in the patient's room to a city many miles away, via microcomputer/PBX networks.

naire analysis prior to patient examination may also be linked to preliminary computer sorting of symptoms. After review of symptoms by a primary physician, appropriate allocation of the patient to specialist services on an initial hospital visit is possible (Rushmer, 1972). A great deal of research is also presently being undertaken to develop new medical taxonomies (lists of medical sub-sections) designed for maximum information transfer in computer-compatible systems.

11.3.3 Communications

Modern engineering technology increasingly allows long range communication between computer data bases along conventional telephone links or private branch exchange (PBX) networks. By this means, Figure 11.18 diagrammatically indicates early transmission and analysis of electrocardiographic data between cities many miles apart. Development of more expensive, modern micro processing systems has encouraged the growth of both patient monitoring and interdepartmental communication systems for data transmission in written, graphical, numerical, and verbal modes. Thus, there is an increasing emphasis on building, accessing, and communicating well-structured data bases of patient problems, diagnoses, treatment progress, and overall evaluation to the exclusion of tedious, traditional, diagnostic, and record keeping procedures.

The direct role of the computer in the diagnosis of patient illness and prescription of treatment has been implemented most successfully in clarification of diagnoses in electrocardiography, but curiously as yet, little evaluation seems to have been done on the relative effectiveness and accuracy of computer use in diagnosis and prescription in medicine, compared with that of the physician.

11.3.4 Environmental Engineering

Engineering now pervades nearly every aspect of daily living. It is no less effective in health care activities outside the direct hospital setting than it is within it. Engineering plays an important role in the design of protective devices for limiting pollution of the natural environment by contaminants of every kind (radiation, chemicals, noise, heat, etc.) (see chapter 4). Safe working environments also owe much to good engineering, particularly in man's exploration of the alien environments of space, arctic regions, the deserts, and the oceans (see Figure 11.19). Bioengineering aspects of such activity certainly exerts an important 'preventive health care' effect on the environment of the workplace. The cooperative role of engineers, physiologists, and psychologists in solving the problems of an industrial society, and the so called man-machine system interface, has generated the science of ergonomics and professional ergometric, or human factor engineers (see chapter 5).

11.4 GENETIC ENGINEERING AND THE GENETIC ORDER

Although not strictly regarded as conventional engineering, the efforts of molecular biologists, geneticists, and engineers working together have pioneered, at one and the same time, the most exciting and forbidding aspect of medical engineering.

An on-going debate in science is concerned with the influence heredity and the environment have upon individual behavior. Genetics, the science that involves the transmissions of traits from one generation to the next, concerns the former. Practical applications of genetics are numerous. Engineering efforts in the field have been mostly for the benefit of mankind, such as in the synthesis of insulin, the manufacture of interferon, the formation of oil-eating bacteria, to name only a few. Genetics has provided explanations for phenomena such as twins, likeness or dissimilarity of children to their parents, and predictions of the occurrence of a certain hair color, eye color, or other characteristics. There are also "hot" topics in genetic engineering with moral, legal, and ethical considerations for society, such as: (1) cloning humans; (2) the possible escape of a deadly strain of manufactured bacteria from a laboratory that could threaten to decimate the human race; and (3) the effect of environmental pollution leading to

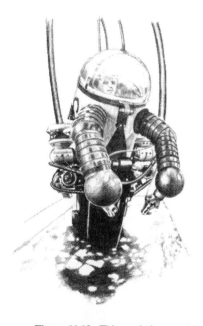

Figure 11.19. This revolutionary submersible, called the "WASP" because it resembles the insect, makes diving under arctic ice possible. Reproduced with permission from MacInnis, J.B., **National Geographic**, 164(1): 104A-104D, 1983.

possible detrimental human mutations. Many of the health issues arising from genetics will continue to have great impact on society. A knowledge of its underlying principles can help not only our basic understanding of these issues but also clarify our role in accepting or resisting this far-reaching human interference in basic natural processes.

11.4.1 The Cell: Unit of Life

In order to understand how heredity works, it is necessary to become familiar with the cell, how it divides, and the results of its division. The average human somatic (body) cell is surrounded by a cell membrane that contains **protoplasm** (Figure 11.20). Within the cell is a nucleus that contains a **nucleolus** and **chromosomes**; the cellular material between the nucleus and cell membrane is called the **cytoplasm. Ribosomes** are the tiny structures found in the cytoplasm that are the sites of protein synthesis. The cell also contains other organelles aside from the nucleus and ribosomes which, although important for the cell to maintain its life, are not essential in the discussion of heredity or genetics.

11.4.2 The Genetic Code

The carriers of genetic information in the cell are the chromosomes. Sections of chromosomes that have been known to carry hereditary traits (phenotypes), such as eye color, hair color, or other physical characteristics, are called **genes.** On a molecular level, the chromosome is comprised of the protein **deoxyribonucleic acid (DNA)**. Thus, genes may be considered as sections of the coiled double strand of DNA. The force or directive power, which fashions an integrated set of cells in a person, lies in the complex DNA molecule, or more specifically, in the chromosomes. Every cell in an individual (with the exception of the special case of mature red blood cells) has a nucleus containing an exact copy of the same genetic material. Even though the cells in our body differentiate in order to play different roles, that is, as skin, blood, liver, lung tissues, and so on, the same DNA

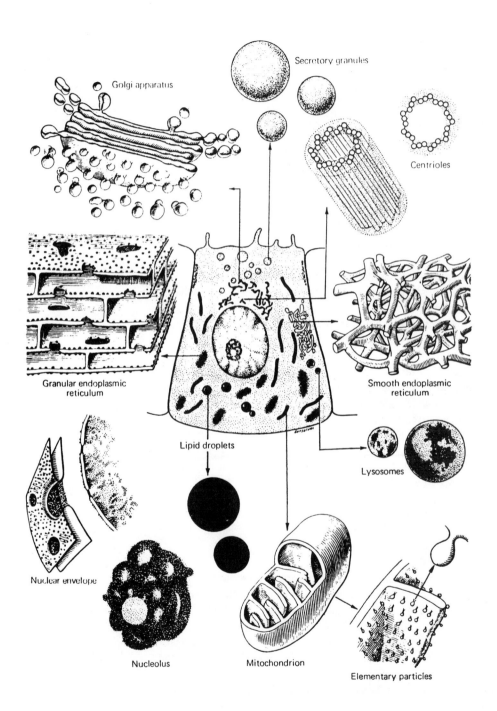

Figure 11.20. Diagram showing a hypothetical cell in the center as seen with the optical microscope. It is surrounded by its various structures as seen with the electron microscope. Reproduced with permission from Junqueira, L.C., Carneiro, J. and Contopoulos, A., Basic Histology, page 26, 1977.

directs the fashioning of specific tissue. A rather humorous parallel relates the DNA within a chromosome to a library containing information on how to construct an individual. Here, the specialized skin cell is one which goes into the **library of characteristics** and takes out books on sweating, sun tanning, effect of skin lotions, and so forth to determine what it needs to be an effective tissue.

What makes individuals biologically unique may be found in their DNA complement. Structurally, the DNA molecule looks like a long ladder which has twisted many times so that it takes the form of a spiral (it is called a **double helix**). On each rung there are two chemicals that bind the spiral together. These are called **nitrogenous bases**, of which there are four types: Adenine (A), Thymine (T), Guanine (G), and Cytosine (C). It has been determined through experiment that on the **rungs** of the DNA molecule, Guanine always bonds with Cytosine and Adenine always bonds with Thymine. Therefore, there can only be four permutations or combinations of these bases on the rung: A-T, T-A, G-C, and C-G. Although this may seem rather simplistic, the complexity and diversity of life is owed to the sequence in which millions of nitrogenous base pairs are arranged in the DNA molecule.

From the viewpoint of genetics, there are essentially two kinds of cells in the human body: (1) Germ cells (ova or spermatozoa), whose function is to reproduce the species, and (2) somatic cells, which are all of the other body cells. The structural difference between the two is that the latter contains **23 pairs** of chromosomes in the nucleus, while the former contains only **23 single chromosomes**—one from each pair. The reason why germ cells contain half the number of chromosomes is because if each parent contributed a somatic cell, the resulting children would carry around 46 pairs of chromosomes. The second generation would have 92 pairs of chromosomes, and so on, ad infinitum. Since our chromosome number has remained constant for millions of years, this concept is invalid. The person who developed the idea of germ cells and somatic cells was

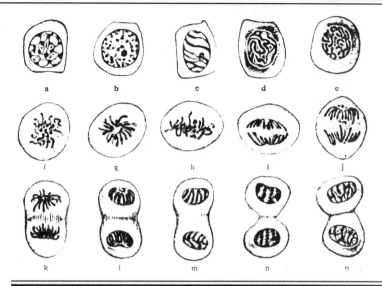

Figure 11.21. Mitosis. Epidermal cells of a mouse. These drawings are arranged in sequence from early prophase into telophase: a to f = Prophase; g and h = Metaphase; i and j = Anaphase; k to o = Telophase. Reproduced with permission of the publisher from Weiss, L. and Greep, R., Histology 4th ed., page 68, © 1977 by Elsevier Science Publishing Co., Inc.

F.L. Weismann, in 1882. His observation overthrew Lamarck's theory on the inheritance of acquired characteristics, to which some people still cling today. To take one example, Lamarck believed that the reason for the giraffe's long neck was attributable to generations of giraffes stretching their necks to eat the leaves on trees. To this day, there is no evidence that whatever natural changes an individual undergoes in a lifetime will be passed on to the offspring. Armed with this and the fact that, in animals and man, the **gamete-producing (sex)** cells are set aside early in embryonic life, we can put to rest such myths as a man lifting weights before fathering a child to ensure a strong son or a mother reading **Plato's Republic** during pregnancy to ensure a bright child.

11.4.3 Mitosis and Meiosis

When a mature sperm fertilizes a mature ovum, the resulting fusion of cells is called the **zygote**. Once the zygote has been formed, **mitosis** is one of the two types of cell divisions that follows in its life. It is through mitosis that the fertilized egg divides into the over 100 trillion cells that form the adult. The importance of mitosis, therefore, is mainly for growth and cell replacement. In this process the nuclear membrane of the relatively large cell breaks down and the chromosomes, which have now formed a duplicate set of genetic material, line up along an axis near the centre of the cell (see Figure 11.21). Next, one set of 46 chromosomes migrates to the top and the other to the bottom (i,j,k) of this equatorial plane so that cleavage to form two daughter cells may proceed (the daughter cells are identical to the mother cell).

The second type of cell division, called **meiosis**, occurs some time after the zygote has been conceived so that the gametes (sex cells) may be produced. This process occurs to a certain number of somatic cells that are labelled the **primordial sex cells**. Like body cells, germ cells undergo mitosis in the first division. The second division, also called the reduction division, results in a reduction in chromosome numbers from 23 pairs to

23 single chromosomes. There is **no doubling** of chromosomes before division as in mitosis.

It seems that what goes on in meiosis is opposite to that of mitosis. While somatic cell division maintains the stability of the organism, the purpose of sex cell formation in the organism is to generate as many combinations of gametes as possible so that humans, with the help of nature, advance biologically. It follows then that maintaining an infinite variety of gametes is a high priority. This is carried out mainly through random assortment of the chromosomes. When a man produces sperm, some of the chromosomes produced come from his mother and the remainder from his father. Since each chromosome of the 23 could be from either the mother or father, you can see that a great many combinations are possible.

11.4.4 Sex Chromosomes
In the end, the fertilized egg (ovum) contains 23 pairs of chromosomes, 22 of which are called **autosomes**. The last pair of chromosomes, on which the existence of any sexually reproducing species depends, are called the sex chromosomes. Each parent contributes one sex-determining chromosome to the zygote. The normal ovum always contains an X chromosome but the sperm can contain two types of sex chromosomes. If the sperm contains an X chromosome, the result of fertilization is XX (a female). If the sperm contains a Y chromosome instead, then the result of fertilization is XY (a male).

> X (Ovum) + X (Sperm) = XX (Female)
> X (Ovum) + Y (Sperm) = XY (Male)

It is the sperm that determines the sex of the child, not the female germ cell. (In some other cultures, it is thought that the mother determines the sex of the child). Although the exact gene has not been located, it has been suspected that a certain portion of the Y chromosome causes the development of the male gonads, while repressing those of the female.

Another difference between autosomes and sex chromosomes is that in most cases, autosome pairs are alike in shape, length, and position of genes. Each member of the pair is called a **homologue**, and each homologue comes from one of the parents. (As far as the sex chromosomes are concerned, only in the female (XX) are they homologous). The various genes on one homologue that have corresponding genes on the other are called **alleles**. An allele can be either one of two types, dominant or recessive. On a homologue, the way in which alleles behave and explain certain genetic phenomena hinges on whether the inheritance of certain characteristics or conditions are controlled by one factor or a combination of factors. In single factor inheritance, two general situations with respect to alleles on homologous chromosomes can exist. Both of the alleles may be identical or they may not. **Homozygous** (identical) alleles can be either both recessive or both dominant. A number of diseases that are due to **homozygous recessive alleles** are diabetes mellitus, congenital deafness, and albinism. On the other hand, **homozygous dominant alleles** have been associated with such abnormalities as Huntington's chorea, dwarfism, and polydactylism (six fingers on each hand).

If, alternatively, the alleles are **heterozygous**, then one of the alleles is dominant and the other is recessive. The **dominant** allele masks the ability of the **recessive** allele to express itself so that the phenotype, or observable characteristic, appears to be homozygous dominant. An example is that of eye colour. The allele for brown eyes is dominant while that for blue eyes is recessive. If a child receives an allele for blue eyes from one parent and an allele for brown eyes from the other, then the child will have brown eyes. In this case, dominance is **complete**. There are two other types of dominance that occur in the heterozygous condition. **Codominance** is the situation where both alleles of the hybrid (individual with heterozygous alleles) are expressed. An illustration of this concept is seen in blood types. Individuals with type A blood have a specific polysaccharide on the surface of their red blood cells, which could be called A. Individuals with type B blood have B on the surface of their blood cells. Individuals with AB blood contain both polysaccharides A and B in their blood. The existence of this shows no masking as found in **complete dominance**. The third type of dominance is called **incomplete dominance**. One's type of hair is a trait determined by this type of dominance. Curly hair is dominant over straight hair. Incomplete dominance results in wavy hair.

Many of the more interesting human traits such as intelligence, temperament, or body type are thought to depend on a combination of alleles. The realm of polygenic inheritance for such complex traits is not clear and beyond the scope of this chapter.

11.5 THE FUTURE OF MANKIND

In the past, humans lived with their endowed phenotypes (traits). When genetic mistakes occurred, they were usually discovered after the fact, and those unfit to survive died naturally. This was the survival of the fittest. Modern medical science allows people to transcend such natural genetic control, allowing survival of those who, in the past, would have died. It may be said that we have distorted the priorities of our genetic selections, and now there is an abundance of poor genetic material which, through the miracle of modern medicine, has the opportunity to create more of its own kind.

11.5.1 Gene Manipulation

Gene manipulation is a process whereby new combinations of genetic material are formed by inserting nucleic acid molecules, produced by whatever means outside the cell, into any virus, bacterial plasmite, or other bacterial system. These nucleic acid molecules are then allowed to be incorporated into a host organism in which they do not naturally occur but in which they are capable of continued propagation. Gene manipulation such as this implies genetic engineering. What this means is that genes from one organism can be isolated and then, by one of several steps, relocated into a new organism. The host organism continues to grow with the genetic material within it, and in many cases it has now **inherited** a new capability brought to it by the new genetic material.

In many instances, this work is done with primitive bacteria such as Escherichia coli (**E.coli**), which may take up the exogenous DNA of other plant and animal cells. Subsequently, the new **E.coli** will function, in part, as the previous plant or animal cell would have and produce whatever the DNA messenger requires.

In the world of biology and biochemistry this is an exciting event, for now it can be possible for a simple E.coli to become a chemical factory. For example, genetic materials (the DNA chain) responsible for the production of human insulin may be transposed into the E.coli, which then takes it up as its own genetic material. It continues to duplicate this new molecule during the replication of its own molecule in cell division (mitosis). E.coli may be cultured in vast amounts in bacterial cultures, and the production of human insulin thus becomes a cheap and reliable process.

One can only begin to imagine the consequences of such practise, for now it is theoretically possible to change bacteria, viruses, and maybe, in the future, human germ cells. The chances of re-engineering human genetic make-up to produce the person of the future may be a far fetched dream, and it might sound frightening, but it may be our link to the future.

11.5.2 Survival of the Fittest

Up to the present, human survival has been that of the fittest. The bigger, the stronger, the more aggressive, and the more hostile have had the edge, and their genetic material has passed on to the present generations, which also have these instincts. When backed into a corner, mankind is a most formidable beast. This aggressive type of response was necessary in our ancient primeval past (as was the case with the GAS response to stress; see chapter 6), but in the world of atomic warheads, such aggressive reflexes could be catastrophic. These reflexes **must** be tempered with intelligence.

In a subtle way we are already beginning to change man's genetic make-up. Those that would not be suitable for survival and adaptation to the modern world, such as those with Tay-Sachs disease, are often terminated before they are even born. People with chromosomal and genetic disorders are now counselled to seek the growth of their families through means other than procreation.

The next step is to identify many of the subtler diseases that predispose people to such handicaps as arthritis, cancer, arteriosclerosis, diabetes, Alzheimer's disease, and many other crippling diseases in our society. Already it is possible to spot in the present generation the prototype of some of the diseases in future generations. It is possible that, in a future of even greater world population stresses, to have a license to procreate one may have to prove the health and safety of their genetic make-up. This would be the modern version of the **survival of the fittest** for high technology survival.

The possibility of genetically engineering new traits into our genetic stock is close at hand. Such manipulations will undoubtedly have some grotesque mistakes, but the outcome could be a human race containing all those traits which are admired. Endowed with only **the best** characteristics of present day man, such future beings may appear and act quite differently from the present Homo Sapiens. Perhaps we will feel proud, in the same manner the Neanderthal man might have felt proud that he gave birth to modern humankind—to you and me.

11.5.3 Moral Aspects of the New Technology

Modern medical techniques have brought us to the threshold, and sometimes beyond, in preserving or denying our very existence, designing and nurturing life by artificial methods, or preserving life in limbo, awaiting a time when even more **modern** medicine and technology will resurrect and refurbish an existence.

Thus, the practice of medicine reflected in our Health Care Systems is a major force in our lives. Healthiness is considered critical for happiness. The legal and moral aspects devolving from our increasing power over preservation and manipulation of life, or over its very creation or abortion, as the existing techniques of medicine are refined and new ones are discovered, can only complicate our lives in the future. It will force reconsideration of many accepted tenets of the past and the development of wise and sympathetic laws for the future.

11.6 REFERENCES

Carroll, C. and Miller, D. **Health: The Science of Human Adaptation,** 3rd ed. Dubuque, Iowa: WCB Co. Publishers, 1982.

Curtis, H. **Biology,** 3rd ed. New York: Worth Publishers, Inc., 1979.

Devries, W.C. and Joyce, L.D. The artificial heart. **Clinical Symposia (CIBA),** 36(2): 1984.

Eisenberg, A. and Eisenberg, H. **Alive and Well: Decisions in Health.** New York: McGraw-Hill Co., 1979.

Grossman, J.H., Barnett, G.O., McGuire, M.T., and Swedlow, D.B. Evaluation of computer-acquired patient histories. **Journal of the American Medical Association,** 215: 1286-1291, 1971.

Medical Imaging High Technology, 69, August, 1984.

Harrison, A.J. Science, engineering and technology. **Science,** 223(4636): 1, 1984.

Jones, K.L., Shainberg, L.W. and Byer, C.D. **Health Science,** 2nd Ed. New York: Harper and Row, 1971.

Junqueira, L.C., Carneiro, J., and Contopoulos, A. **Basic Histology,** 2nd Ed. Los Altos, CA: Lange Medical Publications, 1977.

Kimball, J.W. **Biology,** 3rd ed. Menlo Park, California: Addison-Wesley Publishing Co., 1974.

Kogan, B.A. **Health,** 3rd ed. New York: Harcourt Brace Jovanovich, Inc., 1980.

MacInnis, J.B. Exploring a 140-year-old ship under arctic ice. **National Geographic,** 164(1): 104A-104D, 1983.

Pai, A.C. **Foundations of Genetics: A Science for Society.** New York: McGrace-Hill, Inc., 1974.

Rothwell, N. **Human Genetics.** Englewood Cliffs, New Jersey: Prentice-Hall, Inc., 1977.

Rushmer, R.F. **Medical Engineering: Projections for Health Care Delivery.** New York: Academic Press, 1972.

Rushmer, R.F. **Cardiovascular Dynamics,** 3rd ed. Philadelphia, W.B. Saunders Co., 1970.

Weiss, L. & Greep, R. **Histology,** 4th Ed. New York: McGraw-Hill, 1977.

11.7 GLOSSARY

Alleles: Paired genes located in corresponding chromosomes (homologues) that determine inherited characteristics.

Amino Acids: Nitrogenous compounds that are the building blocks of proteins and the end products of protein digestion.

Amniocentesis: Removal of some amniotic fluid from the amniotic sac for tests and analysis.

Amniotic Fluid: Clear fluid that surrounds and helps protect the growing fetus.

Autosomes: Paired chromosomes that are not sex chromosomes.

Capillary: Small blood vessel located between an arteriole and venule where oxygen is exchanged for carbon dioxide.

Cell: Small body of protoplasm containing a nucleus; the nucleus is the basic structure of all plants and animals.

Chromosome: A small rod-shaped body found in the nucleus of cells at the time of cell division. Chromosomes are composed of DNA, loosely bound with proteins, are constant in number within any species, and contain the genes, or hereditary material.

Codominance: In genetics, this is the situation where both alleles of the hybrid are expressed. An example is a person who has genes for blood types A and B—the A and B genes both are dominant, so the resulting blood group phenotype would be AB.

Deoxyribonucleic Acid (DNA): Double-strand coil of chemicals responsible for the production of body proteins containing all the biological directions for hereditary characteristics.

Down's Syndrome: Congenital, chromosomal abnormality that causes mental retardation.

Gamete: A mature germ cell.

Gastrointestinal: Pertaining to the stomach and intestine.

Genes: Tiny protein structures found in chromosomes that transmit all hereditary characteristics and genetic information.

Genetics: A science dealing with the study of genes and heredity.

Genotype: The combination of genes specific to every individual.

Germ cell: Ex-determining cell; ovum and sperm; gamete.

Gonad: Sex gland; testis in the male and ovary in the female.

Hemoglobin: Substance in red blood cells that carries oxygen from the lungs to the tissues and gives blood its red colour.

Heteroxygous: Possessing different alleles for a certain characteristric.

Homologue: One that corresponds to a part or organ in another structure.

Homozygous: Possessing identical alleles for a certain characteristic.

Incomplete Dominance: Also termed "variable expressivity," this is where a dominant gene produces a variable effect (as opposed to "all-or-none" expression).

Karyotype: Typical arrangement of chromosomes in a single cell.

Klinefelter's Syndrome: Male chromosomal abnormality associated with an XXY chromosome combination.

Meiosis: Cell division occurring only in sex cells whereby the number of chromosomes is reduced by half.

Mitosis: Cell division in which a somatic cell is duplicated and receives the exact number of chromosomes and characteristics of the parent cell.

Mutation: A basic change in an organism that makes it unlike its parents.

Nuclear Membrane: Membrane around the nucleus of a cell.

Organelles: Ministructures found within the cells that are responsible for specific functions.

Ovum: Mature female reproductve cell capable of being fertilized by a sperm cell.

Polysaccharide: A carbohydrate containing a large number of saccharide groups (e.g. starch).

Phenotype: Visible expression of a person's genes in physical characteristics.

Protein: Class of complex organic compounds containing amino acids that are found in plants and animals and are essential for the growth and development of all living cells.

Protoplasm: Intracellular material.

Red blood cell: Small cell that lacks a nucleus and contains hemoglobin, which carries oxygen to carbon dioxide from the tissues; erythrocyte.

Somatic cell: A cell other than a germ cell that forms all tissues and organs; a body cell.

Spermatozoon: Male sex or germ cell capable of fertilizing an ovum; sperm.

Syndrome: A group of signs or symptoms identifying a particular disease.

Teratogen: Agent that causes an abnormality or malformation of the fetus.

Turner's Syndrome: Chromosomal disorder in which the female has only one X.

Zygote: Fertilized egg cell.

11.8 STUDY QUESTIONS

1. Discuss "technology" in health care delivery. Include the following in your discussion:
   - Instrumentation
   - Communication
   - Diagnosis
   - Costs vs. advances
2. List and describe two or three types of body "replacement parts" that are common in medicinal practice today. What are the risks involved in such operations?
3. How can physics help us to understand the functions of the human body? How would you calculate the blood pressure at your head and feet?
4. Why is it useful to apply systems theory to the study of physiology? What are its limitations?
5. Draw a diagram illustrating the use of a systems model to show the operation of a health care delivery system with which you are familiar.
6. Describe the development of a fetus from the point of view of genetics.
7. Discuss the potential advantages and disadvantages of gene manipulation when it is controlled and used for therapeutic purposes.

Part IV

The Human Condition

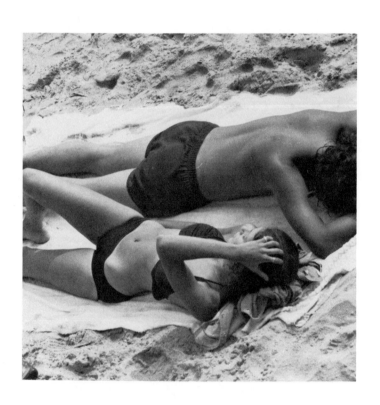

12

Human Sexuality

Over and above the rudiments of sexual behaviour, men and women
have continued to modify the basic sexual responses.

*Many of the urges that guide our current
sexual behavior were built into our species
over the millenia of our inheritance.*

OBJECTIVES

When you have completed this chapter, you should be able to:

- **Recognize** the similarities and differences in the sexual responses of men and women.
- **List** and **describe** the common disorders of sexual response.
- **Outline** the features and hazards of the sexually transmitted diseases.
- **Understand** AIDS.

KEY TERMS

AIDS	intromission
coitus	NSU
clitoris	orgasm
congestion	plateau
detumescence	resolution
erogenous	STD
gonorrhea	syphilis
herpes	trichomonas

KEY CONCEPTS/DEFINITIONS

- The sexual response in males and females is much the same and can be defined.
- Sexual satisfaction has numerous expressions.
- Sex can transmit contagious diseases.
- AIDS is not just a STD.

12.0 INTRODUCTION

Understanding human sexuality, figuratively speaking means to dissect the various components of sex, understand them, and reassemble them into a coherent explanation of the human sexual response. The basic tenet of sex is to procreate. Without sex mankind would cease to exist. As intelligent beings we may understand this concept, but what of our most primitive pre-primate ancestors, did they comprehend the greater purpose of sex? Likely not; but neither do the birds nor the bees, and yet they too successfully reproduce. Many of the urges that guide our current sexual behavior were built into our species over the millenia of our inheritance.

Over and above the rudiments of sexual behaviour, men and women have continued to modify the basic sexual responses. These are inherently complex, but our inquisitiveness has modified, extended, varied and, some would say, has debased so-called **standard sexual behavior**. Society is still struggling to understand the full dimensions of sexual behaviour.

We should also recognize that in the same way that humans evolved to fill a niche on earth, so too have many other organisms. Some of them are very pathologic to humans, and they have found a route into our bodies via sexual interaction of the species, to live and reproduce themselves. They cause sexually transmitted disease and imperil human health.

12.1 PHYSICAL PHASES OF SEXUAL RESPONSE
Our primitive ancestors probably had stereotyped sexual roles. Man was usually an aggressor and woman, too often, a target for such aggression. The intelligence of modern people, the law of modern society, and an emerging equality of the sexes has reduced, although not eliminated, this primitive stereotyping. However, when it comes to understanding sexual behavior, it is well to remember the primitive past; for that is where sexual relationships began and where atavistic responses sometime revert.

The clinical work of Masters and Johnson (1966) has now produced a reasonably clear understanding of how humans respond to sexual stimuli. The four phases of human sexual responses are:

1. an excitement phase
2. a plateau phase
3. an orgasm phase
4. a resolution phase

The art of lovemaking is not merely a biological act
but part of a shared mutual endeavor to fulfill the
psychological and physical needs of two people.

The art of lovemaking is not merely a biological act but part of a shared mutual endeavor to fulfill the psychological and physical needs of two people. Although it is unlikely, even among experienced partners, that all four phases of the sexual cycle will be experienced in perfect harmony, each partner may enjoy lovemaking both from their personal perspective and their partner's perspective and response. Psychologically and biologically, such a sharing requires a mutual awareness, consideration, and caring. Sexual responses vary enormously, even within the same person on different occasions. However, the nature and sequence of the sexual response cycle is quite predictable and follows certain physical changes which are similar in both sexes. The phases are normally identified in well-defined physical/physiological terms. The accompanying emotional changes are varied, complex, and still poorly understood.

THE EXCITEMENT PHASE

The first phase of a sexual encounter is sometimes termed **foreplay.** It is the time when participants gradually arouse each other sexually. The first phase of excitement is an anticipation of things to come. The individual response varies, but initially the blood pressure tends to rise and pulse rate and breathing rate increase. There are some early voluntary and involuntary muscle contractions, particularly in the lower abdominal region. These are part of a complex reflex spasm, the result of erotic involuntary activity in the central nervous system.

As the level of arousal intensifies, the male's penis begins to stiffen due to engorgement with blood. This is the vascular congestion (erection) phase with the trapping of blood within the corpus cavernosum (shaft) and spongiosum (bulbus and glans penis) which leads to its erect posture. Other sexually responsive tissues, such as the nipples, the end of the penis, and the scrotum become more sensitive to touch. There is a great build up of tension in the lower abdominal muscles during this phase.

The same response occurs in females. Although it is usually slower to start in females, it is perhaps more profound in the end than that of the male. The female's clitoris, which is the counterpart of the penis, becomes hardened through a similar vascular congestion or engorgement phase. This organ, although small, then begins to rise up from underneath its hood of skin called the prepuce.

In both the male and female at this level of engorgement, there is a secretion of clear, colorless, odorless, and tasteless fluid, which is secreted from the small glands within the urethral portion of the penis and in the inner two-thirds of the vaginal wall. The female secretes much more than the male, and this helps in lubrication. During this phase the nipples also become erect, particularly when stimulated directly but gently. A pink rash or flush often appears over the upper rib cage and breasts, but this pink flare is not usually seen (Zilbergeld, 1978).

Excitement is usually initiated by such behaviors as a deep seductive glance, holding of hands, and a phase called sensate focus. This is a process of touch and arousal of erogenous zones, which are areas of the body with extra sensitive nerve endings. One example of an erogenous zone is the edge of the lips where the skin meets the lip. When touched very softly and gently with the fingertips, this area is more ticklish and sensitive than the lip or the skin around the lip. It is an erogenous zone. The classic erogenous zones are the eyelashes, lips, deep ear canal, around the anus, around the vulva, clitoris, and glans of the penis. (Note that not all of these zones are commonly considered sexual areas.) As the excitement phase progresses, intromission, or entry of penis into vagina, may occur. If it does, it is usually near the end of the excitement phase rather than the beginning.

THE PLATEAU PHASE

During the **plateau phase** the engorgement of both the penis and the outer third of the vagina increase to a maximum. In the female, the clitoris may withdraw temporarily underneath the prepuce hood. The plateau phase is

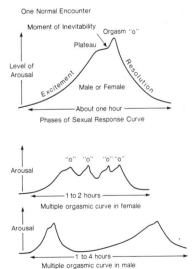

Figure 12.1 Male and female sexual arousal patterns.

*Although the sexual response in the pelvic region
has been much discussed, most experts in the
field concede that orgasm, in fact, is an
autonomic nervous system response controlled
from within the brain.*

so named because no further arousal occurs and the level of excitement
tends to level off. For the naive lover this may be a phase of disappointment
and concern that all is lost; however, this plateau phase is merely a lull in
excitement.

Since males often reach the plateau phase faster than females, the
considerate male partner will use mental restraint and other techniques to
delay the final resolution of sexual excitement so that his partner may
"catch up." It is interesting to note that the change in the average male
penis, from flaccidity to maximal erection, will increase from 50 to 100 per
cent in size. In the female, the congested vascular tissues of the outer third
of the vagina will actually swell from 100 to 300 per cent of the resting size.
Although this latter fact is not generally noticed (Lehrman, 1970), it attests
to a remarkable sexual response in the female.

THE ORGASMIC PHASE

There is a brief moment, experienced both in males and females, which
occurs just before orgasm: it is called the moment of inevitability, which
means that the climax has started and will not stop regardless of circumstances. A climax is the gradual increase of muscular tensions, followed
by a sudden explosive addition to the tension, followed by release. A
sneeze is a type of climax. A sexual climax is called an orgasm. The
intensity and duration of the orgasmic contractions vary considerably with
each individual, depending upon the psychosocial factors operating at that
time. Most of the fluids, making up the semen ejaculated during orgasm,
are forced by contractions from the seminal vesicles and the prostate gland
into the urethea. A small portion of that seminal fluid contains the sperm,
which is the active ingredient for procreation.

Although the sexual response in the pelvic region has been much discussed, most experts in the field concede that orgasm, in fact, is an autonomic nervous system response controlled from within the brain. The
autonomic nervous system consists of two portions: the sympathetic and

the parasympathetic branches. Normally, the nervous signals from each are in balance, but during the excitement phase the output from the sympathetic system becomes stronger and stronger until it reaches its maximum. At this point, muscular tensions within the body are very high and orgasm occurs, accompanied by a sudden decline of muscle tone within the body as the parasympathetic system rapidly takes over. All of this nervous system activity occurs within the brain stem, an area of the brain which has little analytical or co-ordinatory power but which initiates a comprehensive reflex response to incoming stimuli or afferent signals (Hite, 1980).

In the past there has been considerable debate about the true nature of the female orgasm and whether it is related to the frictional movement of the penis against the clitoris or vaginal wall. Of course, an orgasm which occurs in dreams with no pelvic contact present at all is still considered an orgasm. An important sociological survey of sexual responses in women by Hite (1976) found that 75% of normal, sexually responsive, and satisfied females had orgasm only after finger stimulation of the clitoris. This report more or less crushed the notion of **penis supremacy**, and recognized the true nature of an orgasm in the female.

THE RESOLUTION PHASE
All of the arousal of the excitement phase, that is, vascular congestion and engorgement, begins to reverse with the conclusion of the orgasmic phase. This loss of vasal congestion and swelling in both male and female is called detumescence. It represents the physical changes during the **resolution phase** as the body begins to return to the pre-excitement state. Mental relaxation occurs as well.

In the male the resolution phase also represents a **refractory phase**, in which he is unable to have another orgasm immediately. The young adult male, however, can become easily aroused again and go through the cycle perhaps once or twice more. The female usually is capable of having another orgasm soon after the first. In fact, she may experience several orgasms in a row. This may be enjoyable for the male, as he is able to be part of his partner's continued pleasure. Hopefully, though, this does not become the singular goal for either partner. It should be remembered that sex between two people is an even sharing of personal pleasure. For both sexes, the resolution phase offers a chance to reflect back on the previous phases of contact, the sense of communication, and the joy that the act has brought to one another. It is a time of quiet appreciation.

12.1.1 The Meanings of Sex

A discussion of the myriad sexual mores of men and women would fill several written volumes and, thus, the following discussion is not complete. Of the many patterns of activity which are called sexual, only a few will be discussed. The following descriptions apply to sexual responses in a generic way; that is, they are similar for self-stimulated sex, homosexual, or heterosexual behaviors.

SEXUAL EXPLORATIONS

During early infancy, in both males and females, there is a phase of self-discovery. We explore various parts, first discovering that we have hands and lips, and then we move on to other regions of the body. Inevitably, this leads to the erogenous zones and discovery of the unique pleasure afforded by their stimulation. With patience and persistence, we discover that continued stimulation produces an even greater pleasurable feeling. As adults we may sometimes observe young children wandering about innocently arousing themselves. At this point we must be cautious not to inflict a sense of guilt upon them for their simple act of self-discovery.

There is a latent phase in this behavior following the initial explorations during infancy. In young adulthood another exploratory phase begins, usually heterosexual. Having learned about one's self, the next phase is to learn about others. This may sometimes be a confusing and frightening phase of maturation, and, in fact, a great many individuals do not learn

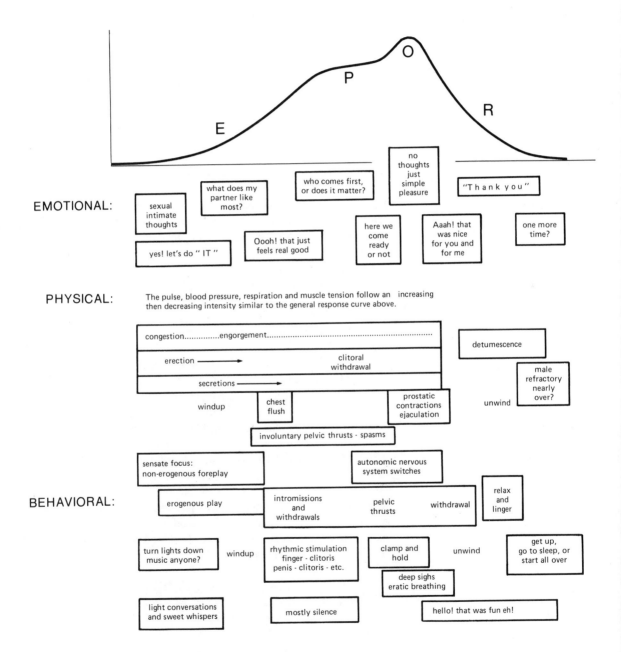

Figure 12.2. Response to normal sex profile.

from it. The present generation has a great advantage over past generations because, until recently, accurate knowledge of the opposite sex was not available. Most parents of today learned about their own sexuality through trial and error, repeated mistakes, locker room rhetoric, and the repetition of misinformation. And yet, despite the handicaps, many lead happy, sexually fulfilled lives.

RECREATIONAL SEX
In the juvenile, once the exploratory phase of self-discovery has been completed, the next phase is one of recreational self-stimulation. Most youngsters of both sexes engage in this activity. Ancient taboos about masturbation which have existed until fairly recently, make interesting jokes in light of today's knowledge. In fact, among most adults, masturbation is used on an occasional basis, even throughout a sexually normal and satisfactory marriage or other meaningful relationship.

In today's permissive society the recreational aspect of sex affects both heterosexuals and homosexuals. Short clandestine affairs and the so called **one night stands** are usually mutual masturbation arrangements, with no lasting relationship considered, and such contacts fall into the category of recreational sex. Unfortunately, such permissiveness may lead to numerous problems, both psychologically and physically. Physical problems are particularly troublesome, as will be discussed later under the topic of sexually transmitted diseases.

SEXUAL BEHAVIOR THAT SERVES TO PUNISH
Perverse as it may sound, some individuals consider sex to be the work of the devil, and any engagement in this activity is viewed as punishment, both of oneself and of others. Masochistic and sadistic attitudes toward sex are, as their names suggest, abusive. They should not be confused with normal forms of sexual behavior, which are characterized by mutual respect and caring. Sometimes teenagers use indulgence in sexual activity

*Eventually, most individuals hope to work through
their stages of exploratory and recreation sex and
discover a loving relationship which has lasting value.*

as a form of rebellion or punishment of others, particularly toward their parents. By means of this behavior they may feel that they are getting even with their parents. Often pregnancy results, and this will create even more strain on family relationships. Such dilemmas cause great psychological distress and require professional expertise in their treatment (Annon, 1976).

SEX AS A REFLECTION OF LOVE
Eventually, most individuals hope to work through their stages of exploratory and recreational sex and discover a loving relationship which has lasting value. Usually this is expressed in a marital relationship where sex becomes a part of the union. While sex certainly should not be the prime factor holding a relationship together, it remains a pleasure and joy that adds delightful uncertainty and excitement to a solid relationship. This does not mean that the love relationship settles down to singleminded and boring sex; it can have exploratory and recreational phases too. In fact, the trust and security of a solid relationship allows for numerous variations in sexual activity within the bonds of that union—straight or gay.

12.2 SEXUAL DISORDERS
There are a number of common disorders that are associated with unsatisfactory sex. Remember, although some experts may say that a certain sex pattern is abnormal, it may not necessarily be so. A common rule of thumb is, *if it doesn't bother you, and is not harmful to your partner or society, then it is not a problem.*

12.2.1 Anorgasmia
This term usually applies to lack of orgasm in the female. In the male this would be called impotence. Most females suffering this disorder do so innocently, and it is called **primary anorgasmia**. That is, they have never experienced an orgasm. The condition may arise from punishments

Table 12.1. Classification of physical causes of secondary impotence. Reproduced with permission from Masters and Johnson, *Human Sexual Response*, St. Louis, Little Brown Co., p. 184-185, 1980.

Anatomic	**Drug Ingestion**	**Neurologic**
Congenital deformities	Addictive opiates	Amyothrophic lateral sclerosis
Testicular fibrosis	Alcohol	Cord tumors or transection
Hydrocele	Alpha-methyl-dopa	Multiple sclerosis
	Amphetamines	Nutritional deficiencies
Cardiorespiratory	Atropine	Parkinsonism
Angina pectoris	Chlordiasepoxide	Peripheral neuropathies
Myocardial infarction	Chlorprothixene	Spina bifida
Emphysema	Guanethidine	Sympathectomy
Coronary insufficiency	Imipramine	Tabes dorsalis (syphilis)
Pulmonary insufficiency	Methantheiline bromide	Temporal lobe lesions
	Monoamine oxidase inhibitors	
	Phenothiazines	
	Reserpine	
	Thioridazine	
	Nicotine (rare)	
	Digitalis (rare)	

received for self-exploration as a child, engendering the feeling, *I will never touch this spot again, for it must be a very bad place since Mommy and Daddy become so upset.* Such a policy, while useful enough for avoiding further sanctions or punishment in the next several years of life, may affect her later attempts at developing a good sexual relationship. Having never been aroused, it is hard to know what is missed or how it is achieved.

Secondary anorgasmia is usually associated with a woman who has known and experienced normal sexual pleasures, but, in certain circumstances which could be construed as abnormal, she cannot be aroused to satisfaction. These circumstances are not necessarily of her making. Numerous psychological and physical disorders within the female or her partner could, and often do, lead to anorgasmia. The medical profession is becoming more adept at diagnosing and resolving these disorders.

12.2.2 Premature Ejaculation

To understand this very common disorder one need only consider our primitive pre-ancestor, the monkey. The sexual response in male monkeys is very fast indeed. From the first approach to intromission, to ejaculation, and to withdrawal may be as short as five seconds. Female monkeys must remain in a state of confusion, wondering what it was all about!

It has been proposed that in the youthful human male of Western society, a certain sense of urgency about self-stimulation (masturbation) was developed in order to get it over with before being caught. This, in the minds of some experts, is one of the factors leading to premature ejaculation in the adult male (Reuben, 1970). By definition, this term refers to the male reaching his orgasm before his female partner. If a male's partner is very slow in becoming aroused, and even if his orgasm came one hour after intromission and she had still not reached her equivalent phase, then it could still be called premature ejaculation. Of course, this is a slightly exaggerated example, but it does serve to point out the fact that the word **premature** really refers to male first and female second, especially if the female gets left out altogether.

Table 12.1. ... continued.

Endocrine	Genitourinary	Hematologic
Acromegaly	Perineal prostatectomy (frequently)	Hodgkin's disease
Addison's disease	Prostatitis	Leukemia, acute and chronic
Adrenal neoplasms (with or without Cushing's syndrome)	Phimosis	Pernicious anemia
Castration	Priapism	
Chromophobe adenoma	Suprapubic and transurethral prostatectomy (occasionally)	**Infections**
Craniopharyngioma	Urethritis	Genital tuberculosis
Diabetes mellitus		Gonorrhea
Eunuchoidism (including Klinefelter's syndrome)		Mumps
Feminizinge interstitial-cell testicualr tumors		**Vascular**
Infantilism		Aneurysm
Ingestion of female hormones (estrogen)		Arteritis
Myxedema		Sclerosis
Obesity		Thrombotic obstruction of aortic bifurcation
Thyrotoxicosis		

An occasional premature ejaculation is probably acceptable, providing the female partner is somehow assisted to a satisfactory conclusion to her sexual excitement. If a person feels cheated of the pleasure and satisfaction which he or she knows to be both possible and deserved (which is how our society regards sexual experience), problems are bound to occur. A sense of frustration, disillusionment, resentment, self-incrimination, and other negative or undesirable feelings may begin to affect the pair's relationship.

There is a rather common physical outcome associated with anorgasmia, which affects males and females similarly. In both cases where there is a lack of orgasm, there is no detumescence and, thus, the congestion lasts on and on. In the male this leads to a discomfort in the testicles and lower pelvic region, and in the female it is felt with a similar discomfort in the pelvic region. As one may imagine, there is one quick and easy method of relieving sexual tension (masturbation—for either partner) and thus reducing the vascular congestion. In some females, the gnawing morning after ache may be a very real physical discomfort which can create mental irritability as well.

There are a great many other disorders within the sexual response of humans, but the most common ones are those mentioned above. A brief review of the causes of secondary impotence (Table 12.1) will provide a focus for the overall complexity of sexual disorders.

12.2.3 Sexual Therapy

When couples or individuals seek advice for sexual problems their first recourse is to their family physician, who may indeed be well versed in the various therapeutic maneuvers and counselling skills necessary to help them. Alternatively, he or she may send them on to a sexologist, psychologist, psychiatrist, or sex gender clinic. The first prerequisite of therapy is the desire, by all those involved, to resolve the real or perceived problems satisfactorily. Often, sexual problems are really a reflection of underlying disorders within the marriage or union, and a lack of normal sexual activity is a sign that a couple needs to work on other aspects of their relationship also. In some cases it may be a needed excuse to terminate the relationship. In cases like this, sometimes sex therapy with unrealistic goals can do more harm than good.

Assuming that the relationship is sound except for the sexual responses, the first step is for the couple to learn what is normal. Quite often this educational process in itself will lead the couple to find their own solutions. Knowledge gives understanding and understanding goes a long way to providing a solution. There are many good books on the market dealing with sexual problems, most of which focus on teaching individuals to go back to the beginnings and rediscover such simple things as touch and the pleasure of arousing even the non-erogenous zones. People need to develop a sense of closeness and to go slowly without creating tensions or anxieties. A slow rediscovery of the erogenous zones and learning to bring sensual pleasures to one another without direct sexual contact is important. Such books also focus on the importance of the penis and emphasize the need for the male to develop self control and, when too aroused, to cool down in order to allow his partner to catch up. It is important to de-emphasize the importance of the penis, for it has been described as being inexpertly designed (Reuben, 1970; Araoz, 1982).

The resolution phase is crucial to improvement of the overall sexual relationship; it is the time of intimacy without the need to respond or perform. For one individual to reach an orgasm, roll over and fall asleep is not the path toward a closer, more caring sexual relationship. In truth, the lingering resolution phase is a way of both partners saying, *Thank you.*

12.3 SEX IN THE SILVER STAGES

A strange thing happens to people sexually as the years go by; the male sexual response becomes slower and lasts longer and longer, and the female is aroused faster and more easily. The smile and wink between a

*A strange thing happens to people sexually as the
years go by; the male sexual response becomes
slower and lasts longer and longer, and the
female is aroused faster and more easily.*

couple that says *you're not getting older, you're getting better* comes from
real experience. In their forties, fifties, and sixties, men experience occasions when they would like to be aroused but are not. Often there are good
reasons for this, for men at this stage in life often are very busy and stressed
in their careers, or they still may be in a resolution phase from previous sexual contact. Particularly in the over-sixties, the male resolution phase may
last for several days. This situation could cause alarm, but for an understanding couple, *there is always tomorrow* (Masters and Johnson, 1980).

Males may also be afflicted, in later life, by a condition irreverantly
termed **"brewer's droop."** Even mild social drinking over many years
can create changes within the liver which reduce the level of testosterone
in the male, and this in turn can lead to a slight lessening of the libido. In
particular, after several drinks or more, sexual arousal for the male may be
very difficult indeed. This can lead to frustration, for alcohol also reduces
sexual inhibitions. Unfortunately, the very drink which loosens inhibition
also develops a relative impotence (Edlin & Golanty, 1988).

In their late forties or fifties, women go through the menopause stage
of their lives. Although this is often accompanied by psychological problems, sexually there is very little change. Apart from some temporary adjustments in the lubrication phase (the secretion phase of sexual excitement), the normal sexual responses are usually retained. In fact, mature
couples have more time to be with each other, less stress from business and
the day to day pressure of life, and, thus, more opportunities to enjoy each
other sexually, as well as in other ways.

12.4 SEXUALLY TRANSMITTED DISEASES (STD)
A quite different aspect of sexual activity is the number of disease states
potentially associated with its practice. Sexually transmitted disorders are
just that; they are transmitted only by sexual intercourse. Some similar
disorders are contracted by means other than sexual contact, but these
disorders are not usually classified under the heading of sexually transmitted diseases.

12.4.1 Non-specific Urethritis
(NSU)/Non-gonoccocal Urethritis (NGU)

This miscellaneous collection of pelvic infections is perhaps the most common STD in all North America; approximately 5 million cases are known at present. There are several types of viruses, and/or bacteria or other agents, which are responsible for this group of disorders. All are characterized by a burning discharge from the urethea in both the male and female, and sometimes bladder infections as well. Tests for the usual common bacteria, including gonorrhea, are usually negative, and treatment consists of antibiotics. The usual positive response to antibiotic therapy is not consistently found, partly because there is more than one agent that causes the disorder. It sometimes resolves on its own. Long term serious problems are not common.

12.4.2 Trichomoniasis-Trichomonis vaginalis

The **trichomonis** is a small, flagellated microscopic organism that exists commonly within the vaginal mucosa and can be transmitted from female to male, and then back to female again (cross infection). It can exist in a dormant form in the female for many months or years, or it can occasionally cause a rampant infection. In the male it may be associated with a mild and transient **urethritis**, which is a burning in the male urethea upon urination, but the disorder is short lasting. Therapy is generally effective using appropriate medications. Both males and females should be treated at the same time to eliminate cross infection.

12.4.3 Gonorrhea (GC)-Neisseria gonorrhoeae

Gonorrhea is one of the most common of the venereal diseases. The term **venereal** is derived from Venus, the Roman goddess of love. Thus, venereal disease (VD) became associated with lovemaking. The increase in promiscuity in North America has led to an epidemic of gonorrhea, the results of which can be devastating for an individual. This infection can

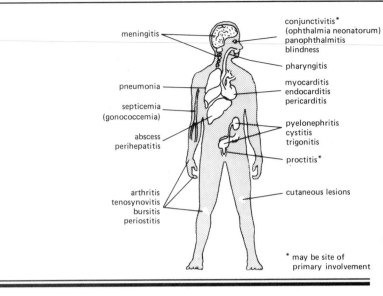

meningitis

conjunctivitis*
(ophthalmia neonatorum)
panophthalmitis
blindness

pharyngitis

pneumonia

myocarditis
endocarditis
pericarditis

septicemia
(gonococcemia)

pyelonephritis
cystitis
trigonitis

abscess
perihepatitis

proctitis*

arthritis
tenosynovitis
bursitis
periostitis

cutaneous lesions

* may be site of
primary involvement

Figure 12.3. Distant complications of gonorrhea. Adapted and reproduced permission from Carroll and Miller, p. 386, 1982.

come on within a few days of contact, and in the male it can lead to a stricture of the urethea, to infection of the testicles, and to infertility. Occasionally, GC infections can affect distant joints and other parts of the body, leading to a devastation of one's health (see Figure 12.3).

In the female, gonorrhea can exist quietly for weeks or even months before causing any symptoms. During this time it is very contagious to the male and must be considered a serious problem. When infection spreads in a female, it can infect the deep pelvic organs, the ovaries, and the peritoneal cavity leading to (occasional) fatality. Infertility in the female caused by gonorrhea is a prevalent problem. Unfortunately, this serious disorder can be contracted from only a single sexual encounter with an infected partner, and it may lead to chronic pelvic disorders and infertility in later life.

12.4.4 Syphilis (Treponema Pallidum)

Syphilis is a fascinating but serious venereal disease which has plagued the human race ever since its transmission to Europe from North America by members of Christopher Columbus' expedition force. Prior to that time, syphilis was present in the North American Indian tribes but was totally absent in Europe. It was a mild disease among the Indians. Within a year of Columbus' return syphilis had spread throughout most of Spain, much of France, and had a start in England. Within ten years this new and devastating mysterious disorder, which seemed to be "transmitted in the night air," was even found in Japan and China.

There are four phases of untreated syphilis:
1. primary chancre
2. secondary syphilis
3. latent phase
4. tertiary syphilis

Syphilis is caused by a fragile, sensitive bacteria, the **spirochete** identified as **treponema pallidum**. Like the gonorrhea micro-organism, spirochetes

---

You Can Help Control STD

1. Know the warning signals of sexually transmitted diseases.
2. Seek medical treatment upon recognition of early signs and symptoms of STD.
3. Refrain from sexual behavior likely to increase the risk of sexually transmitted desease, particularly promiscuous premarital and extramarital sexual activity.
4. As a male, use properly a condom or "rubber" as a prophylatic (disease-prevention) measure to reduce the chances of transmitting STD during sexual contact.
5. Wash your hands and external sex organs with soap and water before and after sexual contact.
6. Urinate as soon as possible after sexual activity to flush out any infectious agents from the urethra.
7. Warn your sexual partners of their exposure and possible infection if you develop warning signals of STD.
8. Encourage your sexual partner to seek medical care if you have become infected with STD.

Figure 12.4. Control of sexually transmitted diseases (STD). Reproduced with permission from Carroll and Miller, Dubuque, Iowa, Wm. C. Brown Co., p. 389, 1982.

are transmitted mostly through either heterosexual or homosexual practices, including intercourse, oral sex, and anal sex. Syphilis can be transmitted from an infected mother to the unborn fetus, causing a condition described as **congenital syphilis**. This latter disorder results in a very seriously disfigured and diseased child.

The **primary chancre** may be observed within ten to ninety days after contact when a small, painless ulcer (chancre) develops in the genital region. This looks as though it should hurt, but it doesn't. This chancre is highly contagious. Without treatment it disappears within four to six weeks and one may be left with the delusion that all is now well. By this stage the spirochete has spread throughout the body leading to secondary syphilis.

The **secondary syphilis** is seen with a rash on the palms of the hands and feet, some white blotches in the mouth, some loss of hair, and a low grade fever and mild sore throat. It can easily be passed off as some minor viral disorder and medical help often may not be sought. The rash and secondary phase disappear without treatment, just like measles.

The **latent phase** of syphilis is then entered and may last for several years without any indication that the disease is present. However, during this time the spirochete is invading internal body organs such as the heart, liver, brain, spinal cord, and joints. Sometimes the latent phase lasts only a few months before tertiary symptoms appear.

Tertiary syphilis is the result of the spread of the spirochete during the latent phase. After many years of latency (up to 20 to 40 years) serious problems arise. These include such problems as partial or complete paralysis, severe mental disturbances, blindness, bone destruction, liver disorders, heart disease, and weakening of the walls of the major blood vessels. Victims of tertiary syphilis are not always contagious. In fact, even during the latent phase contagion is not common.

Despite the advent of many syphilis tests, an occasional patient passes the medical screen and develops tertiary syphilis. Early in the disease the use of ordinary penicillin is very effective in eradicating the disease. However, the critical link in the process is the need for early identification. Public education is very important in spotting this and other venereal type diseases, for once they have progressed too far the damage done may be irreversible.

12.4.5 Herpes (Herpes Simplex Type II)

The exposure given to **herpes** today seems extravagant to those familiar with the truly serious venereal diseases. If one were to rely on the public press for knowledge about herpes, the impression would be given that it is of epidemic proportion and a very disabling disease indeed. Many individuals develop cold sores or fever blisters around the mouth or lips; these conditions are caused by a virus identified as Herpes Simplex Type I. A close relative, Herpes Simplex Type II, can infect the genital regions of both men and women, causing a slightly painful fluid-filled blister or lesion containing virus. Symptomatically they are similar to the cold sores in the mouth. Genital herpes is usually acquired by sexual intercourse, but it can also be transmitted by non-sexual intimate contact. Additional symptoms are those of painful urination, a general aching in the pelvic region, and a mild fever. Symptoms seldom last for more than a few weeks and then the sore gradually subsides. There are no medications which seem to eradicate herpes faster than its normal rate of spontaneous remission. For the victim of herpes, the chance of reactivation of their genital sores is possible under circumstances of stress, fatigue, or any other general illness which tends to debilitate them. When we are tired, overworked, or suffering from other problems, our general immunity is down a bit and our cold sores will rise to the surface; so it is with genital herpes. Only during the active phase of the cold sore or genital herpes sore are these viruses contagious. When the sore has subsided the condition can no longer spread. Some experts in the field of STDs suggest that the incidence of genital herpes has not changed in the last five thousand years. The only difference is that recently the public press has chosen to headline the disorder. Herpes does not lead to infertility, it does not cause pelvic inflammatory disease, nor does it cause other debilitating disorders. It is mostly a nuisance. However, herpes infection in the newborn infant can be a fatal disease. If a mother at term has genital herpes, it may be advisable to deliver the baby via Caesarian section in order to avoid herpes contact.

12.4.6 Warning Signals of Sexually Transmitted Diseases

- **Discharge - Female:** abnormal yellow or white vaginal discharge that causes irritation or itching. **Male:** a white, clear or often yellowish discharge from the penis or from the rectum.
- **Burning on urination** - painful and frequent urination and an urge to urinate, sometimes with only small volume.
- **Sores** - painful or painless sores or blisters in and around the vagina, on external sex organs, on the penis, or around the mouth or rectum.
- **Bumps and Lumps** - painless lumps, bumps, or warts in or around the vagina or penis or swelling of lymph nodes in the groin.
- **Itching** - an intense itching in the genital area that may result in an appearance of lumps, bumps, or pimple-like lesions in the genital area.
- **Lower Abdominal Pain** - with or without fever this condition may indicate serious pelvic inflammatory disease (PID) in females.
- **AIDS** - the warning signs for AIDS are not included above.

12.5 AIDS—(Acquired Immune Deficiency Syndrome)—1987

Since Gottlieb (in 1981) first identified a rare immunodeficiency disorder in four otherwise healthy young American homosexual men and French and American scientists identified the virus responsible, Acquired Immune Deficiency Syndrome (AIDS) has become recognized as a global health problem. It is reported in 74 countries. Cases in the United States number 29,435, of which 16,667 have already died. The U.S. Surgeon General estimates that unchecked spread of the disease could kill 100

Chancroid (soft chancre)—an acute bacterial infection spread by sexual contact with an open lesion. Characterized by painful genital ulcers and swelling of lymph nodes, chancroid usually is controlled by antibiotics.

Granuloma inguinale—a chronic and progressive ulcerative disease of the skin and the lymphatics of the genital and anal regions. This STD is relatively uncommon in the United States and is caused by bacteria-like Donovan bodies, intracellular microorganisms. Granuloma inguinale responds to treatment with tetracycline and streptomycin.

Lymphogranuloma venereum (LGV)—a few weeks after initial exposure to LGV, caused by certain forms of Chlamydia trachomatis bacteria, a small sore appears on the genitals or rectum. Sometimes, after the small lesion heals, the infection spreads to the lymph nodes and channels, which become swollen and filled with pus. Unlike most other sexually transmitted diseases, one attack of LGV appears to provide a measure of immunity against further infection.

Moniliasis—caused by a yeastlike fungal infection, this STD is often called candidiasis. Resulting in vaginitis (inflammation of the vagina), the infection is accompanied by a malodorous, cheesy white discharge of pus. Monilia organisms do infect the male reproductive tract, sometimes causing small sores on the penis, which are overlooked or considered negligible. The fungi of moniliasis, along with the trichomoniasis parasites and other infecting microorganisms, give rise to the "ping-pong" effect in sexual relations—the back and forth infection or reinfection between male and female if only one of the sexual partners receives medical treatment.

Pediculosis ("crabs")—an infestation of the pubic area, especially the pubic hair, by crawling, blood-sucking lice that look like crabs when magnified. This condition is marked by considerable itching and the appearance of pale blue spots on the skin. Crab lice are usually transmitted by intimate contact but may also be spread by bedding and clothing. Specific ointments and shampoos are available for effective treatment.

Scabies—an infectious skin disease caused by a small mite and characterized by intense itching and the appearance of small red bumps or lines on the body when the female mite burrows into the skin to lay her eggs. Formerly widespread only in areas of poverty or during wartime conditions, scabies is found frequently among the "clean." Sexual contact is becoming more important as a means of spreading this disease.

Venereal warts—papova virus-caused warts that often appear on the external sex organs and rectums of males and females. Genital warts usually occur one to three months after intercourse with an infected partner. Usually painless, the pink, cauliflowerlike bumps cause annoyance and discomfort. Although most of these warts regress in time, surgical removal is the preferred therapy.

Figure 12.5. Other sexually transmitted diseases. Reproduced with permission from Carroll and Miller, Dubuque, Iowa, Wm. C. Brown Co., p. 388, 1982.

Table 12.2. Adult AIDS cases diagnosed in 26 European countries through 31 March 1986, by risk group and geographic origin. Data from the WHO Collaborating Center on AIDS in Paris, France. Reproduced with permission from Quinn, T.C. et al., AIDS in Africa Science, 234: 956, Nov. 21, 1986.

Patient Risk Group	Europe	Caribbean	Africa	Other*	Total
Number	2,162	61	177	73	2,473
Male:Female ratio	16:1	1.4:1	1.7:1	16:1	10:1
Homosexual/bisexual male	73%	8%	5%	85%	67%
Intravenous drug user	11%	3%	0%	1%	10%
Homosexual male and					
intravenous drug user	2%	0%	1%	1%	2%
Hemophiliac	4%	0%	0%	1%	4%
Blood transfusion	2%	0%	4%	4%	2%
No known risk factor					
Male	4%	49%	50%	3%	9%
Female	2%	36%	30%	1%	4%
Unknown	2%	3%	10%	4%	2%

*Other includes patients whose major place of residence included countries of North and South America, Asia and the Middle East.

million people worldwide by the year 2000. Life expectancy for AIDS victims, from first diagnosis, is currently estimated to be 310 days, and a good proportion of that time is spent in a hospital at a cost of up to $1,000 per day. It is also reported that for every diagnosed victim there are 90 other people also infected and infectious who show no symptoms. Because the full impact of the disease, that is, destruction of the body's ability to fight viral diseases, takes some time to develop (even 5 to 10 years), it is estimated that of the 300,000 victims whose immune system will collapse in 1990, 57% are probably currently and unknowingly infected. Worldwide it is estimated that 7 million Africans, 1.5 to 3.5 million Americans, and 200,000 Europeans may already be infected. The patient risk groups, as a percentage of the total diagnosed cases through March 31 1986, are shown in Table 12.2.

The growth of diagnosed cases of AIDS in the United States resembles the current explosive proportions of World Population Growth. The latter has been reached only after 700 years, from an estimated initial population of 1 million, and a doubling factor of 50 years (Figure 12.6). These explosive proportions have been reached in only about eight years in the case of the AIDS virus. The problem has multiplied faster than the population growth because of the much shorter doubling time of incidence in this disease, estimated to be 6 months to 1 year.

In the face of this potentially catastrophic pandemic (worldwide) plague, the wisdom of the American Centers for Disease Control's (CDC) policy of keeping anonymous, even from "test positive," the results of random testing for AIDS in 60,000 blood samples, from 15 hospitals must be seriously questioned (Opinion, USA Today, Jan 21, 1987). Only recent testing of Army recruits in New York for AIDS has shown how far outside the original circle of victims (homosexuals, drug abusers, hemophiliacs, etc.) the disease has spread. Of this male and female, heterosexually active, population, 1 in 50 was infected.

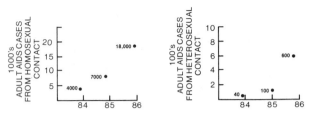

Yrs from 1st reported number of AIDS Victims.
Doubling period approximately ½ to 1 yr.

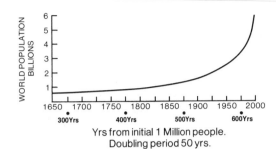

Yrs from initial 1 Million people.
Doubling period 50 yrs.

Figure 12.6. Showing the similarity in explosive growth between AIDS in the USA (mirrored world wide) and world population. Reproduced with permission from the **Economist**, July 5, 1986.

In the most affected areas of Central Africa it is estimated that 10% of the population is infected. Other places of high incidence are Haiti, New York, Florida, and California.

Currently another 300,000 Americans suffer from AIDS Related Complex (ARC), characterized by weight loss, fever, and lymphatic disorders. This complex is often a precursor to AIDS itself. Three million others carry some form of the virus that causes AIDS and may be classified as carriers.

The causative agent for AIDS is human T-lymphotropic virus Type III (HTLV-III)/lymphadenopathy virus (LAV). More recently it is called Human Immunodeficiency Virus (HIV). Presently there is a lack of either an effective therapy or preventive vaccine, and 10-30% of currently infected AIDS victims are expected to die in the next 5 to 10 years. Some suggest 100% will die.

AIDS has been traced from retrospective (looking back—tracing studies) epidemiological work to certain areas of Africa between the late 1970s and early 1980s. A marked increase in such diseases as meningitis, and Karposi's Sarcoma (now specific markers for AIDS), were noted in the population during that time.

The characteristic symptoms of AIDS described by the World Health Organization are shown in Table 12.3, and risk factors associated with the contraction of AIDS are shown in Table 12.4.

Since 1981 much has been learned about the AIDS virus, although ways to halt or slow its progress are still rudimentary. The AIDS virus is a retrovirus consisting of similar material to one of the genetic materials of the human cell, RNA (ribonucleic acid). When the virus invades a cell it uses an enzyme, reverse transcriptase, to change the viral RNA to DNA (deoxyribonucleic acid). DNA is the prime nuclear material of the cell, which directs replication during cell division. The invading DNA material of the virus is thus incorporated into the cell's replicating machinery. When the cell replicates itself the virus is also replicated and its numbers proliferate rapidly. The viruses finally overwhelm the normal function of the cell,

Table 12.3. Clinical manifestation of AIDS (MMWR, 1985).

AIDS in adults.
AIDS in adults is defined by the presence of 2 major and 1 minor sign listed, in the absence of other known immunosupressive diseases such as cancer or severe malnutrition.

Major Signs
1. Weight loss greater than 10% of body weight
2. Chronic diarrhea lasting longer than 1 month
3. Prolonged fever, intermittently or chronically

Minor Signs
1. Persistent cough for longer than 1 month.
2. Generalized puritical (constantly erupting) dermatitis—itch.
3. Recurrent herpes zoster (wet, blistery sores) for greater than 1 month.
4. Oropharengeal candidiasis (mouth yeast or thrush).
5. Chronic and progressive and widespread Herpes Simplex (cold sores).
6. Generalized lymphadenopathy (lymph node swelling).

The presence of generalized Kaposi's Sarcoma or cryptococcal meningitis are definitive in themselves for a diagnosis of AIDS.

which then dies and releases all the viruses to seek out new host cells to invade.

The HIV virus is so dangerous because it targets the helper T4 lymphocyte, an essential cell in the immunosuppressive action of the body against viral infection. Consequently it destroys the very cell that usually acts to form antibodies to combat this, or any other, invading viral antigen. During a period of time, therefore, the body's whole defensive system against infection is destroyed and viruses or bacteria of any type may now take hold and destroy the body. This is why such a variety of symptoms characterize the final state of the AIDS victim as he/she successively suffers from one opportunistic infection after another. Viruses and bacteria are always surrounding us in preparation to attack if immunosuppressive defense lets down. Like many viruses, the HIV may also produce defects in host cell DNA, leading to abnormal cancerous growth. AIDS victims show a high incidence of Kaposi's sarcoma (cancer of the skin and connective tissue). HIV also attacks macrophages, another type of defensive cell, and it may indeed use this cell to invade the central nervous system. AIDS sufferers often display signs of dementia.

It is easy to see why early diagnosis of AIDS infection is critical in any fight to preserve the immune system from total destruction. Clinical symptoms of the disease often take so long to appear that mass screening seems to offer the only hope for early detection of victims.

An inactive form of the HIV, is called a "provirus." Often undetectable, a provirus may infect a cell for years before some event, or combination of events, triggers its activity.

The immediate problems of AIDS research seem clear: first, diagnostic procedures for the condition must be improved; second, the HIV must be destroyed; and third, an effective vaccine against it must be provided. Continuing effective containment of this and other sexually transmitted diseases will only occur through effective educational programs at every level, which raise the consciousness of the public to the problem and enlist their cooperation in solutions.

Table 12.4. Behavioral risk factors associated with HIV infection in heterosexuals. Reproduced with permission from Fauci, 1985.

1. High numbers of sexual partners.
2. Increasing amounts of sex with prostitutes.
3. Being a sexual partner of an infected person.
4. Association with partners suffering from Sexually Transmitted Diseases such as Gonorrhea, Syphilis, and Genital Ulcers.
5. Participation in certain sexual practices such as anal intercourse.
6. Seropositivity of infants is significantly correlated with the seropositivity of mothers.
7. Use of unsterilized needles or skin piercing instruments used for medical purposes, drug abuse or rituals.

12.5.1 Diagnosis

Early diagnostic tests were based on identifying the presence of antibodies (proteins formed in the victim's blood to combat the virus) by means of their reaction with killed HIV preparations. These tests lack specificity because the killed virus preparation does not really represent an active virus. The virus preparation may bind wrong antibodies in the blood and produce a wrong color reaction. Victims may also test negatively for antibodies due to the long time lag before their production after infection. This is a central defect of all antibody testing for the disease. When antibody detection is confirmed, no distinction can be made between those really infected and those in whom the antibody presence merely reflects a passing encounter and successful defense against the disease. Thus, some tests have 50% or more false positive reactions. New approaches to diagnosis are being studied by the assay of other chemicals representative of the immune system's integrity, such as white blood cell adenosine deaminase activity and refinements of "killed" virus preparations where the virus is fragmented. AIDS antibodies in blood will bind to these fragments, and, subsequently, the addition of a second antibody which binds to the first will produce a colour reaction for a positive test.

12.5.2 Therapy

Two approaches are presently followed in therapy for AIDS: one approach is to attack the virus chemically (antivirals), and the second, is to stimulate the natural immune system (immunostimulants). Table 12.5 shows the present state of research and clinical trials with these types of drugs.

One drug of the above group, AZT, was authorized early for distribution to patients suffering from AIDS. The authorization followed the drug's success in clinical trials in prolonging the lives of patients within the first four months of suffering the first episode of pneumocystis carinii pneumonia (PCP), a lung infection. Patients with AIDS Related Complex (ARC) or significant AIDS progression, indicated by weight loss, thrush

Table 12.5. AIDS therapeutic drugs: manufacturer and status. Reprinted with permission, HIGH TECHNOLOGY BUSINESS magazine, (January, 1987). Copyright © 1987 by Infotechnology Publishing Corporation, 214 Lewis Wharf, Boston, MA 02110.

Drug	Action	Manufacturer	Status and Outlook
Ribavirin	Antiviral	Virateck/ICN (USA)	In clinical trials. Canada has approved for some AIDS patients.
AZT	Antiviral	Burroughs Wellcome (USA)	Toxic at higher doses. Approved for limited use in the U.S.
Foscarnet	Antiviral	Astra (Sweden)	Little data available. U.S. trials just beginning.
HPA-23	Antiviral	Rhone-Pouleric (France)	Little data available. U.S. trials still being planned.
Alph -interferon	Antiviral	Hoffmann-La Roche, (USA) Schering-Plough	Is effective on some cancers. Now being tested on AIDS.
AL-721	Antiviral	Praxis (USA)	Works by weakening virus membrane. U.S. trials just beginning.
Interleukin-2	Immune system stimulator	Celus, Amgen, Biogen, Immunex, Hoffmann-La Roche, Ajinomoto (Japan)	Boosts immune-system function. Could be used with antiviral.
Isoprinosine	Immune system stimulator, weak antiviral	Newport Pharmaceuticals (USA)	Is approved outside U.S. for other disorders. Clinical data in AIDS patients now being reviewed by FDA.
Dideoxycytidine	BDC antiviral	Hoffman-LaRoche under Federal license	As effective as AZT and less toxic in laboratory tests and early human trials.

fever, or herpes zoster, are also eligible for treatment. AZT crosses the blood brain barrier, a therapeutic property likely to be of increasing importance to any drug's usefulness, since up to 60% of AIDS patients have neurological symptoms. The drug is not without significant side effects such as the inhibition of normal production of blood cells by bone marrow, which then requires regular blood transfusions. Headaches are another unwanted symptom.

12.5.3 Prevention

Development of an anti-AIDS vaccine is a high priority goal. Vaccines arouse the immune system to produce antibodies (protective elements) against a foreign antigen (a virus or other organism or element alien to the body's normal function). Viral vaccines are produced in the body by injections of killed viruses or non-infective strains of the active virus. Tests of effective vaccines usually proceed in animal trials prior to human use. Unfortunately, no animal model responds to the HIV exactly as the human. Because the most effective and ongoing protection is from active vaccines (non-infective, living viral injections), it will be some time before this type of clinical trial is authorized.

For the moment, drug companies researching vaccines potentially effective against AIDS are using non-infective substitutes. Sometimes these are proteins, termed "viral antigens", whose amino acid sequences mimick those of the virus, and which may elicit the same body immune response as the virus itself. Regular vaccination with such a preparation would keep the body's antibodies continuously at an effective level, thus eliminating the long lag time before their usual production after infection.

It is clear from animal studies that AIDS antibodies can be raised by viral antigens (once a matter of some doubt and gloom). Whether they can be raised in humans against HIV remains to be investigated in human trials. A unique property of the antibody itself is being used in another approach to antibody stimulation against viral infection. Protective anti-

*Your next sexual partner could be that
very special person—the one that gives you AIDS.*

bodies (called the idiotype) generate their own antibodies called the anti-idiotypic antibody (the anti-id). Thus, synthetic, non-infectious anti-id molecules may be just as successful in raising protective antibodies against an antigen as the infectious antigen itself. In fact anti-id vaccines are already being developed against a variety of diseases including rabies, encephalitis, and hepatitis B.

A most important recent development is the discovery in Africa of an HTLV-virus strain HTLV-IV, which is non-infective and may be used potentially as an active vaccine for antibody stimulation.

12.5.4 Containment

Current suggestions on how to stop AIDS spread offer little immediate hope for success since one major component requires a fundamental change in the sexual mores of society. These include use of condoms during sexual activity, restriction of sexual activity to one partner, abstention from anal intercourse, and restriction from sexual activity with partners with herpes or syphilitic sores. The viral disease is spread mainly through intimate contact with a victim's body fluids such as blood, semen, or vaginal secretions. Thus, the avenues of infection are through breach and bleeding of the anal epithelial cells during homosexual intercourse; through bleeding incurred during intravenous drug administration using contaminated needles; through blood transfusions with contaminated blood or blood products (increasingly rare); or by direct infection from mother to fetus. There is increasing evidence that substantial transfer of infected blood is needed to produce infection, such as in transfusions or repeated use of heroin-type needles previously used by infected people. One study showed that accidental stabbings or cuts sustained by staff nursing AIDS victims resulted in only 2 infections in 543 incidents.

What seems to be of fundamental importance for any coherent management of the problem is to first obtain reliable estimates of both the pattern and degree of incidence of the disease by widespread population sampling.

AIDS is not prejudiced,
it can kill anyone.

Public screening procedures, of the kind previously used to detect tuberculosis from chest x-rays, which do not violate an individual's right to privacy, seems a rational procedure in the face of such an overwhelming threat to the general life and health of nations. An individual's knowledge of the results is a prerequisite of such procedures, so that early management of a person's problem may be instituted. Intermily it seems essential to protect the wider community of people by these methods while arousing greater awareness of the problem by public education schemes until a medical solution is found. Currently some $2,000 per annum is spent on each person's health care in the USA (some $400 billion). If care of terminally ill AIDS patients does indeed reach $1,000/day, the overall cost of health care is likely to rise precipitously and health care commitments to other areas will decline.

Despite the seemingly slow awakening to the long term consequences of the threat of AIDS, several encouraging moves aimed at raising the public level of awareness of the disease have been initiated. Britain has undertaken a massive public education program on AIDS, costing 40 million £, which describes in explicit terms its causes and consequences and the preventive measures to be taken against it. In the USA, the Institute of Medicine of the National Academy of Sciences issued a report (1986) calling for the allocation of $2 billion per year by 1990 to AIDS research and prevention—five times the present level of funding. Half of this amount would be earmarked for extensive and explicit public educational programs, and the remainder, would be used for research in prevention and cure.

The Surgeon General's own report (1986) recommended that sex education in school begin as early as the third grade and include information on the sexual practices that put children at risk from AIDS. At a conference of the nation's mayors in January 1987, it was reported that a survey of 73 of the largest school districts in the country showed that 40 were already providing AIDS instruction and 23 others planned to do so in the fall of 1987. Most mayors expressed support for extending AIDS education in schools. In another report, 51% of U.S. doctors (1500 surveyed in M.D. magazine) favored requiring an AIDS antibody test as a prerequisite for a marriage license. In addition, 78% supported tracing infected people to alert them of their risk, 79% supported high school education on AIDS and other Sexually Transmitted Diseases (STD), 28% favored some kind of quarantine for AIDS victims, 48% had treated AIDS victims, 43% favored testing of all Armed Service personnel for the AIDS antibody, 40% favored testing dentists, and 35% favored testing doctors and hospital employees.

Citizens of developed nations are once more in a privileged position to fight, contain, cure, and ultimately, maybe, prevent the spread of the HIV disease. However, in Central Africa the conditions surrounding the several million people infected with the HIV are conducive, not only to the contraction of further opportunistic viral infections, because of their already debilitated immunosupressive systems, but also to the increased expression of the HIV in the helper T4 lymphocytes mobilized to fight the new infection. It is currently impossible for these countries to control the spread of the disease, which may be occurring predominantly through transfusion and infection of children from serapositive mothers rather than through homosexual activity as is common in North America and Europe (see Table 12.2). The $60 million invested by the USA to screen its blood banks for HIV infection in 1985 is several times greater than the entire health care budget of many developing nations.

The estimated cost of caring for 10 AIDS patients in the USA ($450,000 per annum) is more than the entire yearly budget of a large hospital in Zaire. A little further reflection also shows that the cost of maintaining 8 million such victims in the United States at the above rate will consume the entire money appropriated to Health Care in 1986—some $400 billion. It is a small wonder that eradication of a disease with such potentially rampant proportions requires more than merely addressing the immediate medical problem. A nation's capacity to provide a solution may well be

Sex, drugs and rock 'n' roll
—at least rock 'n' roll can't give you AIDS.

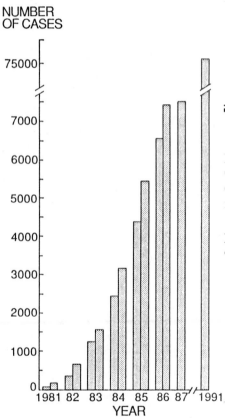

Figure 12.7. The number of AIDS cases is rising exponentially in the USA and may reach 76,000 by 1991. Data from U.S. Dept. of Health and Human Services, 1987 and the Coolfont Report, 1986, U.S. Public Health Service.

submerged in health care costs before a medical solution is found. Thus, public education programs on the enormity of the problem and the need for changes in human sexual habits are paramount. Additionally, without concern for containment of the disease in less affluent countries, containment in affluent societies may be impossible also.

Figure 12.7 shows we are faced with a pandemic disease of enormous proportions which will probably change the very fabric of our world— directly or indirectly it will touch us all.

12.6 REFERENCES

A plague on everyone. **The Economist,** Nov 22, p. 16, 1986.

AIDS Studies become part of Curricula. **USA Today,** Jan, 1987.

Annon, J.S. **Behavioral Treatment of Sexual Problems-Brief Therapy.** Harper and Row: San Francisco, 1976.

Araoz, D.L. **Hypnosis and Sex Therapy.** Brunner/Mazel: New York, 1982.

Barnes, D.M. Promising Results Halt Trial of Anti-AIDS drug. **Science,** 234(Oct): 15-16, 1986.

Carroll, C., & Miller, D. **Health, The Science of Human Adaption.** Wm. C. Brown Co.: Dubuque, Iowa, 1982.

Coolfont Report. Public Health Reports U.S. Public Health Service, 101(4): 341-348, 1986.

Editorial "Opinion." Don't keep AIDS Victims in the Dark. **USA Today,** Wed. Jan 21, 1987.

Edlin, G., & Golanty, E. **Health and Wellness: A Holistic Approach.** Jones and Bartlett Publishers, Boston, 1988.

Fauci, A.S., Masur, H., Gelmann, E.P. The Acquired Immunodeficiency Syndrome: an Update. NIH Conference. **Annals of Internal Medicine,** 102: 800-813: 1985.

Heil, M. and Hemley, R. Taking Aim at AIDS. **High Technology Journal,** p. 44-48, 1987.

Hite, S. **The Hite Report.** Dell: New York, 1976.

Institute for Medicine National Academy of Sciences Report. **Confronting AIDS, Directions for Public Health Care and Research,** National Academy Press, 2101 Constitution Ave., N.W. Washington, D.C. 20418, 1986.

Lehrman, N. **Masters and Johnson Explained.** Playboy Press: Chicago, 1970.

Masters, W.H., and Johnson, V.E. **Human Sexual Response.** Little, Brown and Co., Boston, 1966.

Masters, W.H., and Johnson, V.E. **Human Sexual Inadequacy.** , Little, Brown and Co., Boston, 1980.

M.D.'s for Premarital AIDS Tests. **USA Today,** Jan, 1987.

Morbidity and Mortality Weekly Reports (MMWR). Centers for Disease Control. 34:373-75, 1985.

Quinn, T.C., Mann, J.M., Curran, J.W., and Piot, P. AIDS in Africa: An Epidemiological Paradigm. **Science,** 234(Nov): 955-963, 1986.

Sex transmits AIDS. **The Economist,** July 5, p.14, 1986.

Surgeon General's Report on Acquired Immune Deficiency Syndrome, AIDS. Washington, D.C. PO Box 14252, Washington, D.C. 20044.

U.S. Dept. of Health and Human Services, Public Health Service, Health United States, Maryland, 1987.

Wiley, C., Lampert, P., Oldstone, M., Schrier, R., and Nelson, J. Brain Endothelial Cells Infected by AIDS Virus. Proceedings National Academy of Sciences, USA (in press) reported in **Science,** 233(July): 418, 1986.

Zilbergeld, B. Male Sexuality. Little, Brown and Co., Boston, January, 1978; and Bantam Books, New York, December, 1978.

12.7 STUDY QUESTIONS

1. Discuss briefly the stereotyped sex roles of males and females, and mention why these roles are not suitable in today's modern society.
2. Describe the instinctual nature of the sex drive.
3. There are four major physical stages of the sexual response. Discuss each briefly.
4. What is the moment of inevitability?
5. Discuss the role of the infantile sex exploration stage and the development of normal adult responses later in life.
6. What is the hallmark of the sexual responses of juveniles?
7. Discuss briefly the two major adult sexual disorders that can occur in physically and mentally normal males and females.
8. What is an erogenous zone?
9. Is sex beyond retirement age possible? Describe why or why not.
10. There are numerous sexually transmitted diseases (STD). Describe:
    The most common;
    The most serious;
    The most discussed;
    The newest.
11. List five warning signs of STD.
12. Write out in full the meaning of:
    AIDS
    ARC
    HTLV-III
    LAV
    HIV
13. When was AIDS first diagnosed?
14. When did HTLV-III first start incubating in the world?
15. What does opportunistic mean, and how does this apply to AIDS?
16. What body fluids carry HTLV-III, and how can they be a risk?
17. What is the most important step that society can take in the battle against AIDS.

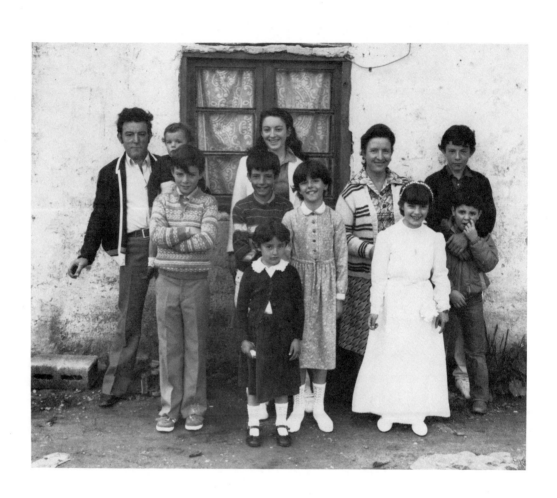

13

Reproduction

When one considers the multitude of hazards to life even
before it begins, it is amazing that any of us are alive today.

OBJECTIVES

When you have completed this chapter, you should be able to:
- **Understand** the role of conception in family planning and how contraception can be achieved with relative safety;
- **Understand** the hazards associated with conception, contraception, pregnancy, and childbirth;
- **Understand** the causes of infertility, methods of recognizing these causes, and some of the cures.

KEY TERMS

abortion	infertility
barrier techniques	insemination
blastocyst	IUD
conception	neonate
condom	oral contraceptives
contraception	parturition
diaphragm	seminal vesicles
endometrial cavity	spermacides
fallopian tubes	tubal ligation
fetus	vas deferens

KEY CONCEPTS/DEFINITIONS

- Conception can be planned. Medications and techniques are available to delay conception, to prevent it permanently, or to enhance it.
- Certain illnesses will hinder fertility.
- Abortions are not an ideal method of family planning.
- The events surrounding the birth process are critical; great care must be taken to avert complications.
- Most cases of infertility can be diagnosed by readily available means. Sometimes cures can be effected.
- Certain modern methods of family planning mean that nearly every infertile couple can acquire a child. Some of the techniques of achieving this end are unusual.

*Among the creatures of the world humans are the only
ones in whom sexual encounters show
an unpatterned character, often being pursued merely
for their pleasurable/social experience.*

13.0 INTRODUCTION

Among the creatures of the world humans are the only ones in whom sexual encounters show an unpatterned character, often being pursued merely to procreate (engage in sexual intercourse for purposes of acquiring offspring), but they do so in response to strong hormone urges during fertile periods. Only man and woman consider sex in terms of a social/recreational interchange. Moreover, we are the only creatures that temper procreative reflexes with forethought about possible progeny. In other words, we think ahead (in this case, 9 months or more ahead).

With so many factors complicating human life, such as age, economics, social pressure, job, politics, and health, it is nearly impossible to manage one's life without some plan, no matter how rudimentary. Family planning is now considered one logical means of creating and maintaining order in this aspect of one's life.

13.1 CONTRACEPTION

In the past, before the time of planned parenthood, when a doctor asked a young couple how many children they expected to have they might answer, "Oh! about five or six." Today, however, the average couple would probably suggest "a family of four," that is, two children. Today we have a choice, yesterday was more or less unplanned.

Most couples attempting to conceive a child do so with ease. About 30% will succeed in the first month, about 60% in the first six months, and about 75% within one year. About 30% of all potential parents experience some difficulty; however, more than half of these finally succeed with some medical assistance, and about only 10% of women in the childbearing age are irrevocably infertile. That means that 90% of all women have the potential to conceive and bring further life to the earth (Shane, 1977).

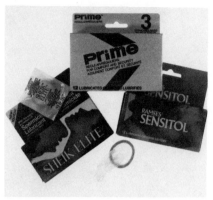
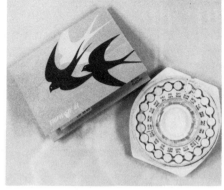
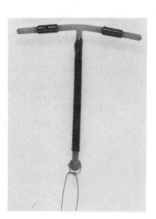

Figure 13.1. Condom, intrauterine device and pills. Regardless of which is used, fertility is usually restored with cessation of use of the device. Reproduced with permission from Carroll and Miller, page 309, 1982.

13.1.1 Temporary Reversible Methods

THE PILL

Approximately 40 million women have taken the Pill since its introduction about 20 years ago. This means that they have chosen one phase of their life in which to effect a temporary, but reversible infertility. The usual use of the oral contraceptive is to delay the first pregnancy. Often between pregnancies and after the last child is born, other contraceptive methods are elected.

In the early days of contraceptive pill use the side effects were more than a little disturbing. Engorged breasts, heavy pelvic bleeding, and emotional disturbances caused the pharmaceutical industry to look for a better, safer contraceptive.

Research has shown pill-users (particularly those of 35-40 years old and who smoke) to be at a greater risk of high blood pressure, heart attacks, and fetal blood clots than normal. For some time the pill was blamed for all sorts of ailments, but particularly for cervical and other cancers. However, recent studies have shown that, in fact, the Pill actually has a protective effect against the occurrence of endometrial cancers (of the womb) and ovarian cancers, and it has been shown not to be a factor in the cause of breast cancer. This is reassuring, considering the widespread use of the Pill and its advantages over some of the other methods of contraception. The content of the contraceptive pill has also been improved, and the present day low dose or "mini pill" has very few side effects, for most women at least. The latest improvements in the Pill represent fine-tuning of an established method.

The contraceptive pill is now also being advocated for the post-menopausal phase, when the normal hormonal functions of the ovaries have ceased and the body is without its normal supply of the hormones estrogen and progesterone. Here, the contraceptive pill, with its balanced estrogen and progesterone contents, serves a useful purpose in maintaining youth-

Technique	Pearl index Pregnancy per 100 woman-years
Birth Control Pills:	
• triphasics	0.06
• combination	0.03 - 1.20
• sequential	1.0 - 2.0
• mini	3.0 - 4.0
• progestin only	2.0 - 3.0
Intra-uterine devices	1 - 6
Barriers:	
• diaphragm + spermicide	2 - 20
• condoms + spermicide	3 - 36
Rhythm	1 - 47
No protection	60 - 80

Figure 13.2. Contraception effectiveness of common methods of birth control.

fulness in the body tissues, which would otherwise experience an accelerated aging. The bones, in particular, are prone to accelerated aging, and many women who do not undertake hormonal replacement past the age of menopause will develop osteoporosis (weak and softened bones).

One side effect of oral contraceptive use is a certain moodiness or depression. Recent studies have shown that the contraceptive pill causes a degradation of vitamin B6 within the liver, and this leads to a mild depression. Clinical trials have shown that the supplementary use of vitamin B6 while taking the contraceptive pill helps alleviate the moodiness associated with the medication. It is also a useful adjunct in the treatment of premenstrual tension (Adams, 1973).

OTHER FORMS OF TEMPORARY CONTRACEPTION

1. Intrauterine Devices (IUD)

The IUD is a plastic coil made in various shapes fitted in the uterus. The most common is the Lippes loop. The IUDs function in one of two ways:
• Through a friction effect, which prevents the fertilized ovum from implanting on the uterine wall, or
• Through speeding up the passage of the ovum through the fallopian tubes by some unknown mechanism, thus preventing its fertilization in the fallopian tubes.

The IUD is sometimes uncomfortable to insert, particularly in women who have never been pregnant. Other common problems with the IUD are involuntary expulsion, perforation of the uterus, persistent bleeding and cramps, increased menstrual flow, occasional pelvic infections and low back pain, and loss of the retrieval string, requiring occasional operations in hospital to remove the device. More than 25% of women who have IUDs inserted have them removed within three months because of such side effects.

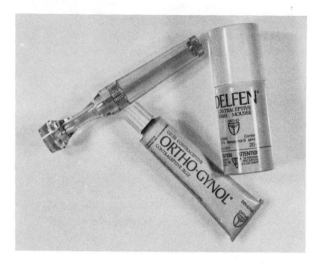
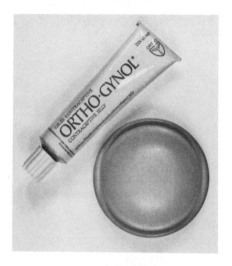

Figure 13.3. Several kinds of contraceptive foams with applicators are shown. Also shown are a diaphragm in container, vaginal jelly for lubrication, and indication of how to insert the diaphragm.

2. Condoms

Condoms are used for two purposes: to prevent pregnancy and to reduce the chance of transmission of sexual diseases. In fact, the "condom" was originally developed in the 16th century by an Italian anatomist, who suggested using a moistened linen sheet over the penis for prevention of venereal diseases (VD). Syphilis was rampant in Europe at that time. By the 18th century, parts of the sheep's intestine were used as condoms, and even today, animal membrane condoms are still available, but they cost about twice the price of the usual rubberized devices.

Problems with the condom as a contraceptive include the fact that it is easily dislodged during early foreplay, but it may be easily forgotten if not applied early enough. The lack of normal sexual sensation and stimulation with the presence of a condom leads some lovers to leave it off "just once" in order to enjoy sex more naturally. This one occasion may often lead to a pregnancy. <u>Synthetic condoms may prevent HIV transmission.</u>

3. Diaphragms

A diaphragm is a rubber shield which forms a barrier between the cervix and the vaginal canal. It is inserted intra-vaginally prior to each sexual encounter and removed again afterwards. It was initially designed as a barrier to prevent sperm from entering the cervical canal and passing upward to find an ovum. Because of great variation in the size and shape of the female internal genitalia, expert sizing and fitting of a woman's diaghragm is necessary. Besides being fitted and sized properly, the effectiveness of the diaphragm also depends on proper insertion each time and the auxiliary use of spermicidal jellies and creams, which are inserted in the diaphragm's cup to act as a spermicidal barrier between the diaphragm and the cervix. This is not a messy technique and does not detract from the enjoyment of sex (see Figure 13.3). In addition, the device should be inserted up to two hours prior to intercourse, and must remain in place for at least six hours after the last ejaculation into the vaginal canal. These

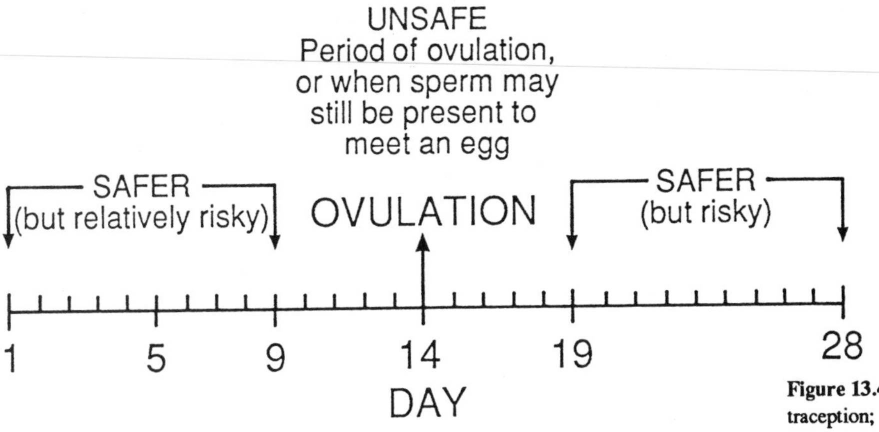

UNSAFE
Period of ovulation,
or when sperm may
still be present to
meet an egg

┌──── SAFER ────┐
(but relatively risky)   OVULATION   ┌──── SAFER ────┐
                                      (but risky)

```
├─┼─┼─┼─┼─┼─┼─┼─┼─┼─┼─┼─┼─┼─┼─┼─┼─┼─┼─┼─┼─┼─┼─┼─┼─┼─┤
1       5       9       14      19              28
                      DAY
```

Figure 13.4. The "rhythm" method of contraception; safer and unsafe days when intercourse may or may not lead to pregnancy. Note: this system is not reliable in women with irregular period times.

practical considerations make the diaphragm somewhat inconvenient, and from that standpoint, it is a less desirable contraceptive method than some other methods. Nevertheless, it is not painful or dangerous and is considered very effective if used properly. For many individuals, it is a very suitable contraceptive method. Many couples find this a nice addition to their lovemaking, it allows them to slow down and prolong the encounter.

4. Rhythm

As a means of contraception, the rhythm method often results in pregnancy. In fact, the older generation of today many times gave birth to their own sons and daughters as a result of mishap with this method. Natural forces, otherwise well controlled by human evolution, encourage women to be more receptive sexually at the time of ovulation at mid month (day 14). Given opportunity and a conducive social setting, women may still be "more than normally aroused" during the ovulation period. Such urges often interfere with the plans of a rhythm method. However, an older generation probably knew the limitations of the system and accepted families of six or more without undue resentment.

Basal body temperature (BBT) recordings are a useful index of fertile potential (see Fgiure 13-4). The subtle drop in first taken morning temperature may indicate that ovulation has taken place. This is quite valuable for the female who wishes to become pregnant, but it is less helpful as a guide to the rhythm method, especially if a well established pattern of BBT is not known, since fertilization of an ovum may occur over a 6-8 hour period after intercourse. However, a woman whose BBT is consistent over several months may be able to predict her fertile period quite accurately. She may then abstain, use condoms, diaphragms, jellies, or "coitus interruptus." This last practice is an adjunct to natural or rhythm method contraception; it means to interrupt intercourse just prior to male ejaculation, to "pull out," and if necessary, to accomplish orgasm by the manual technique of masturbation. Coitus interruptus is perhaps the oldest of all contraceptive methods known, but is the least trustworthy.

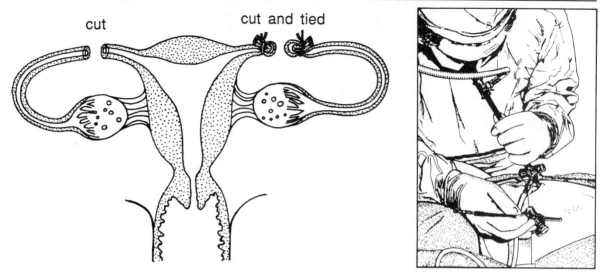

cut

cut and tied

Figure 13.5. a) The results of fallopian tube ligation by culdoscopy are shown in this diagram. **b)** Laparoscopy, one method of surgical sterilization for women, is used to sever the tubes and cauterize the ends. It can also be used for various other abdominal operations.

A unique form of coitus interruptus was practiced by some ancient peoples of Europe. They cut a small hole into the urethra at the base of the penis, which meant that all urine and semen would pass this way except if a finger should plug the artificial exit. When a woman wished to conceive, she merely plugged the hole with a finger as her mate ejaculated so that she could receive his sperm from the usual orifice. This literally placed the decision for conception in the hands of women—a concept that most modern contraceptive methods are trying to emulate.

13.1.2 Permanent Sterilization

TUBAL LIGATION

Permanent female sterilization is achieved by removing or disrupting a section of the fallopian tubes, thus preventing the ovum from reaching the uterus. Of course, it also prevents the sperm from passing up the fallopian tubes to find the ovum on the other side of the ligation. This common operation is performed using instruments which are able to visualize and grasp the fallopian tubes, cut out a section of the tube, and tie off the loose ends. These instruments are inserted either through a small incision in the abdomen, or through an intravaginal incision. The abdominal approach is called a laparoscopy, the pelvic (vaginal) approach is called a culdoscopy. There are numerous variations, but in all cases the end result is to disrupt the fallopian tube. The other functions of the uterus and ovaries are uninterrupted and they continue as before.

Failures of the operation do occur, however, and some fallopian tubes "recanalize" (reconnect themselves) to become patent again. This is doubly hazardous, since the pregnancy that develops is not only an unexpected surprise, but it may develop in the tube because the ovum becomes lodged in the tubal scars, fertilizes there, and stays to develop. This is a very dangerous situation and requires emergency medical attention. Fortunately, it is a rare event.

Other possible complications of this operation include pelvic infections, and although they are rare, they can be life-threatening. On occasion, a woman may enter the hospital for a tubal ligation and remain for several weeks or months to recover from an intra-abdominal infection. It is partly because of these complications of tubal ligation that another, easier technique has been developed for the male partner.

VASECTOMY

Most gynecologists, the doctors who perform tubal ligations, would prefer to have a vasectomy themselves rather than submit their wives to tubal ligation. Over many years and millions of vasectomies, this simple office operation has proven safe and effective. Through a small incision in the scrotum the two vas deferens are easily located and isolated, and after a small section is removed, the loose ends are tied off. This operation can be performed within minutes. The only side effects are a slight swelling and bruising of the scrotum, an occasional infection, and a short period of temporary abstinence from physical and/or sexual activities until the bruising subsides. Infections are easily handled with antibiotics, they are almost never serious, and because they may be observed in the early stages, medications may be started in time.

Vasectomy is considered irreversible. However, some doctors with special skills can reverse the operation. Such doctors are called "microsurgeons." The success rates of reversal operations have not been high so far, and for this reason the original operation should not be considered with the intent to reverse it later.

One minor side effect of both vasectomy and tubal ligation is the psychological fear that something sexual has been disrupted and that you are not quite a man or woman afterwards. This worry results from lack of information or understanding of the process. The notion is a fallacy.

Another minor problem with vasectomy is that the man is still fertile for a few months after the vasectomy as the seminal vesicles, which are on the caudal (headward) side of the vasectomy, still store many sperm. Some studies have shown as many as 30 ejaculations' worth of sperm are stored in the seminal vesicles. This may sound like a lot, but most of the fluid from the ejaculate comes from the prostate gland, with only a small addition of the active sperm from the seminal vesicles. Doctors performing vasectomies will usually ask for a semen sample at the second and third months to verify the absence of sperm. Only then should all other contraceptive methods be stopped.

13.2 ABORTIONS

13.2.1 Spontaneous Abortion

There are three different kinds of abortion. The most common type occurs during early pregnancy and is an unintentional expulsion of the fetus from the uterus. This is a spontaneous abortion (sometimes referred to as a miscarriage).

A spontaneous abortion occurs in at least 30% of all conceptions. This figure applies worldwide and equally to both upper socio-economic classes of Western societies and the poorest areas of third world countries. Most of these miscarriages occur within the first trimester, which is the first three months of pregnancy. Miscarriages normally are not caused by automobile trips, strenuous activity, falls, or emotional shocks. When a woman is threatening to miscarry within the first trimester most doctors today will reassure her that nature is taking its course. In the past, great effort was spent to preserve such pregnancies and such patients were hospitalized, given medications, and rest in an attempt to stop the process. The problem was that these extra efforts were hazardous to the woman, and in some cases it caused harm to a fetus which was not going to abort anyway. In most cases, if a pregnancy is to terminate spontaneously, such measures will not stop its predestined course.

Parents need to be relieved from possible guilt feelings and encouraged to take such a loss in their stride and try again, keeping in mind that two-thirds of conceptions result in full-term pregnancies.

13.2.2 Therapeutic Abortion

Legal intentional removal of the fetus by qualified medical personnel is often referred to as a therapeutic abortion. Historically, most therapeutic abortions were performed to protect the health of the mother. In the past, her health had to be in definite and absolute danger before a legal abortion would be performed, and even then the abortion was often performed too late. In recent years, due to legal and social changes, women have, more or less, a personal right to decide whether they will bear a child until term. Political and special interest group pressures, however, do not allow this choice to be made easily. The right of women to obtain **abortion on demand** is currently a highly debated issue in many countries. Both sides of the issue are supported by rational and emotional arguments, and the moral aspects of the case are far from simple.

The structure of the present medical care system in industrialized nations requires that abortions be performed in a hospital and that a committee of physicians within the hospital, a **therapeutic abortion committee**, judge each application. In general, these committees serve the legal requirement which demands such a committee, but in fact they also bow to public pressure. The law states that, for reasons of "health," an abortion can be legally performed. The word "health" is purposely not often clearly defined and so the range of disorders which may fall in this category is very broad.

In addition, most conscientious hospital abortion committees attempt to educate both doctors and the public about more effective contraceptives, and they urge both the public and their fellow physicians to consider seriously the dilemmas created by the need for an abortion. Without doubt, there is a movement towards providing effective family planning coun-

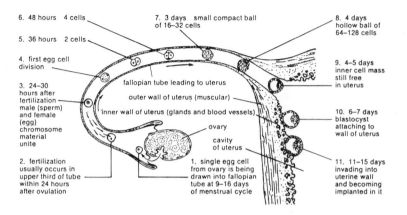

6. 48 hours   4 cells

5. 36 hours   2 cells

4. first egg cell division

3. 24–30 hours after fertilization male (sperm) and female (egg) chromosome material unite

2. fertilization usually occurs in upper third of tube within 24 hours after ovulation

7. 3 days   small compact ball of 16–32 cells

fallopian tube leading to uterus

outer wall of uterus (muscular)

inner wall of uterus (glands and blood vessels)

ovary

cavity of uterus

1. single egg cell from ovary is being drawn into fallopian tube at 9–16 days of menstrual cycle

8. 4 days hollow ball of 64–128 cells

9. 4–5 days inner cell mass still free in uterus

10. 6–7 days blastocyst attaching to wall of uterus

11. 11–15 days invading into uterine wall and becoming implanted in it

Figure 13.6. Fertilization and implantation. Reproduced with permission from Carroll and Miller, p. 28, 1982.

selling so that therapeutic abortions should not be necessary. Change comes slowly, however.

Most doctors performing therapeutic abortions find themselves caught between one section of the public, demanding their services, and another group who call the practice murder. Physicians recognize the growing problem of a burgeoning world population and also recognize the acute stress of an unplanned or unwanted child, both for the family and for the child, should it be born. Such doctors find themselves bound by a code which protects the interest of their patients, yet which respects the sanctity of life as well. This dilemma is complicated even further when they find themselves sitting on therapeutic abortion committees.

13.2.3 Criminal Abortion

A third kind of abortion is called criminal abortion. These abortions usually have been performed by unqualified individuals with improper training and poor technique. The results often were infection and death to the mother. In part, it was due to the outcry from such disastrous events that society urged the medical profession to provide safety with therapeutic abortions. Some elements of our society (such as pro-life groups) still consider all abortions, including those legally performed by doctors, to be criminal. Also, in many other parts of the world, therapeutic abortion still does not exist. In some countries any form of abortion is considered immoral and criminal.

13.3 CONCEPTION

Despite what we hear about cloning, artificial insemination, mechanical wombs, and test tube babies, the vast majority of the world population is conceived through sexual intercourse. The events and physical features of sexual intercourse are understood, but our knowledge of the process of conception and the formation of life is only superficial. The whole process of life is a mystery and a miracle in its complexity. Even that life as we know it exists at all must continue to amaze us, but to actually bring it forth from the midst of our own lives by means of a single pleasurable act is almost incomprehensible.

13.3.1 The Process

Conception occurs when one of the body's largest cells, the ovum, and one of its smallest, the sperm, are joined to produce a zygote. The male has an abundance of sperm available to be ejaculated, and, in fact, in the case of a normally fertile man, should have close to 100 million per cc of semen. The female releases but one ovum per month into the fallopian tubes to which the millions of sperm contained in an ejaculation converge. Despite all that are willing, only one sperm can enter the ovum and together they join to form a new life. (See Figure 13.6).

The process of fertilization usually takes place in the upper regions of the fallopian tube, and the **fertilized ovum** or **zygote** continues down from the fallopian tubes while dividing into numerous cells to form a **blastocyst.** It takes about one week to reach the wall of the uterus, where it implants into the uterine wall and grows. At this point it is called the **embryo,** and with continued cellular division and differentiation it is considered to be a **fetus** by 12 weeks. After the 40th week, approximately, the fetus leaves the uterus and becomes an individual human life on its own. (See Figure 13.7 for an overview of fetal development.)

13.3.2 The Diagnosis of Pregnancy

For the female who menstruates regularly the best sign of pregnancy is a missed menstrual period. Unfortunately, few women are regular, and the menstrual cycle varies somewhat with the state of health, tension, and so forth. In addition, not all women are familiar with their fertile moments and, thus, may not suspect the pregnancy until they have symptoms of morning sickness.

As noted above, the most common time to diagnose pregnancy is shortly after it is realized that a menstrual period has been missed. This is about two weeks past the time of conception and around this time the level of human corionic gonadotropic hormone (HCG) is quite elevated. This forms the basis for many pregnancy tests performed in doctors' offices. If the initial test is uncertain, then most doctors suggest a return visit in another week or so; if the woman is pregnant it is bound to show up then. In addition, the chemical diagnosis is usually accompanied by a physical examination which, normally, will show a slight softening of the cervix in the case of pregnancy. This is an early sign that the uterus is beginning to prepare to sustain the embryo.

13.3.3 The Protection of the Fetus

Since most planned pregnancies are cherished events, parents will make those changes in their living pattern which will give their baby the optimum chance, not only of surviving, but of thriving. Initially, this means a thorough physical examination to check on the present status of the mother's health and a series of blood tests to check for possible illnesses which could contribute to fetal risk. A well-balanced diet is stressed, containing a variety of foods from most of the major food groups. Some vitamins and minerals as extra supplements also are basic insurance. Iron, which is an extra requirement during pregnancy, is sometimes deficient in our diets. Most doctors suggest that women take supplementary iron throughout their pregnancy, and for several months after, to secure adequate tissue iron for both mother and fetus.

One of the routine blood tests is for the Rh Factor. The once common Rh incompatibility disorder contributed to more than 10,000 fetal or newborn deaths in 1969 in North America. It was called erythroblastosis or hemolytic disease of the newborn. This disorder is now almost totally controlled with a combination of maternal and newborn blood sampling, and subsequent injections of special medications are given to prevent

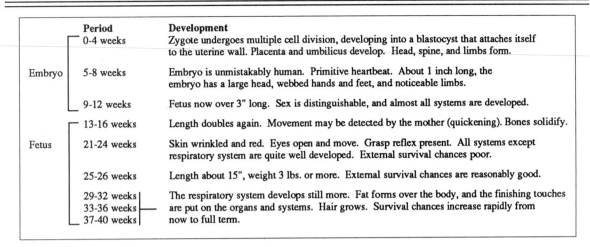

	Period	Development
Embryo	0-4 weeks	Zygote undergoes multiple cell division, developing into a blastocyst that attaches itself to the uterine wall. Placenta and umbilicus develop. Head, spine, and limbs form.
	5-8 weeks	Embryo is unmistakably human. Primitive heartbeat. About 1 inch long, the embryo has a large head, webbed hands and feet, and noticeable limbs.
	9-12 weeks	Fetus now over 3" long. Sex is distinguishable, and almost all systems are developed.
Fetus	13-16 weeks	Length doubles again. Movement may be detected by the mother (quickening). Bones solidify.
	21-24 weeks	Skin wrinkled and red. Eyes open and move. Grasp reflex present. All systems except respiratory system are quite well developed. External survival chances poor.
	25-26 weeks	Length about 15", weight 3 lbs. or more. External survival chances are reasonably good.
	29-32 weeks 33-36 weeks 37-40 weeks	The respiratory system develops still more. Fat forms over the body, and the finishing touches are put on the organs and systems. Hair grows. Survival chances increase rapidly from now to full term.

Figure 13.7. The first nine months. Reproduced with permission from Carroll and Miller, page 29, 1982.

formation of Rh antibodies within the maternal circulation. The effectiveness of these programs in modern hospitals is nearly 100%. Women no longer need worry about this previously devastating disease of the newborn (Carroll, 1982).

Rubella (German measles) is a serious complication in the first three months of pregnancy. More than 25% of women who develop rubella in the first trimester will give birth to a defective child. The problem affects the heart, ears, lungs, and often leads to profound mental retardation. Vaccines are available for rubella, but they should not be given during the early stages of pregnancy. Women anticipating pregnancy should have the rubella vaccine far in advance of possible conception if they are certain they never have had rubella. There are some accurate tests of rubella antibodies, which will confirm whether or not rubella infection has existed in the past and whether rubella resistance exists in the present. Women without resistance to rubella, and who are pregnant, should avoid contact with young children who may have the disease, especially during the danger period in the first 3 months of the pregnancy.

Radiation exposure of the mother during early pregnancy should, theoretically, be a concern, but today most doctors and dentists recognize the hazards of radiation to an unborn fetus and will shield the appropriate area of the body from potential radiation. In fact, the amount of radiation from the modern high technology radiograph machines is very low and does not pose a serious risk. Of course, other sources of radiation exposure such as may occur in the workplace for certain occupations, pose a risk (see Chapter 5).

The number of potent chemicals in our atmosphere and food chain is a source of growing concern to scientists today. The potentially hazardous chemicals which are ingested into our systems through food or inhalation are so great in numbers and complexity that it seems a hopeless task to find the dangerous ones among the not-so-dangerous. Many of these chemicals have very serious carcinogenic and mutagenic effects on human tissues, and the most sensitive time for these tissues is before birth.

*When one considers the multitude of hazards to life
even before it begins, it is amazing that
any of us are alive today.*

Similar in effect to chemical pollutants are the numerous non-prescription drugs available for use by the unwary today, many of which may have damaging effects on the fetus, particularly during the first 12 to 16 weeks of gestation. During this time most doctors warn their patients to avoid all drugs, unknown compounds, and herbs, just in case. At this phase of pregnancy a little paranoia is preferred over a lack of concern.

Among the drugs to avoid is alcohol. It has clearly been associated with birth defects. The babies of alcoholic mothers develop what is known as fetal alcohol syndrome, which involves mental retardation, disorder of the heart, and other physical abnormalities (see Chapter 10). Most doctors caution their patients to become abstainers during pregnancy.

Smoking is at least as hazardous as alcohol consumption. Although nicotine is the active addictive ingredient within tobacco, carbon monoxide also is present in great quantities and is a serious threat to the fetus. There are over a thousand other chemicals present within the smoke of the average cigarette, any one of which could be dangerous. Even smoking for the few months before pregnancy may cause an undernourished newborn nine months later. When planning a pregnancy it is wise to cease smoking at least six months prior to expected conception.

When one considers the multitude of hazards to life even before it begins, it is amazing that any of us are alive today. In ancient times, families planned for many children in the hopes that some would make it to adulthood. Today, in developed nations, we rely on quality of care and sustinence rather than on quantity to provide continuence of our race.

13.4 PARTURITION - THE PROCESS OF CHILD BIRTH

13.4.1 Delivery
Some time near the 40th week of gestation complex biochemical changes (possibly initiated by the fetus itself) occur within the female body to begin a process called "labour." The first sign of labour often is the breaking of the mucus plug, causing slight bleeding, and it is then followed some time

later with a loss of fluid from the amniotic sac. This is the sac in which the fetus "floats." This latter event may not occur until well into labour, but on occasion it occurs unexpectedly, before labour has begun. Uninitiated, prelabour or "Braxton-Hicks" contractions, which are a form of false labour, may precede the real event by up to two weeks.

As labour proceeds the cervix dilates to make room for the expulsion of the baby. By this time most women will be in a hospital and under the care of their physician or obstetrician who, with the assistance of nurses and midwives, will guide the mother through the various stages of labour and delivery.

In 80% of all deliveries labour proceeds uneventfully, with the need for only light analgesics or medications, if any, and with only some encouragement. In the other 20% there are some difficulties. Half of these difficulties are somewhat expected, since during the pre-natal period certain problems may be recognized which are known to lead to potential complications of labour and delivery. The other half are surprises, some of which can be life-threatening to both mother and child. It is because of this last 10% that doctors encourage mothers to bear their children in hospitals. Thus, in the event that quick decisions must be made and actions taken immediately in order to save lives, all facilities are on hand. Hospital delivery rooms, although usually somewhat sterile and aesthetically uninviting, do have all the supplies and equipment necessary to handle any obstetrical emergencies. Doctors and nurses today also are learning to fulfill some of the aesthetic expectations of delivery, and they have developed methods of delivering children which are non-violent, calm, and pleasant and which help to ease the child into the world with gentle dignity (Allen, 1977).

Another current trend is that Cesarean sections are becoming more and more common. Many first borns have mothers in their early to mid-thirties. Primips, that is women having their first child at this age, are more prone to problems of labour and delivery, and so Cesarean sections often are necessary to handle such emergencies and problems of delivery.

13.4.2 Complications of Delivery

The use of special x-rays and, more recently, ultrasound diagnosis, have led to better prediction of fetal abnormalities, twins, abnormal fetal positions such as breech, or oversized babies. Ultrasound also allows an accurate diagnosis of the stage of gestation.

Numerous blood tests can spot potential infections and also help determine the best time to initiate labour when it appears to be delayed. Monitoring devices available in hospitals can monitor the progress of the labour and the health and viability of the neonate. However, such fetal and maternal monitoring may be unnecessary, for 80% of births proceed uneventfully. The purpose of testing and monitoring is to diagnose the potential problem cases where special measures can be instituted to bring about a healthy mother and child.

Despite the best possible labour management, birth problems do occur and such disasters are a sad event for all concerned. The worst hazard is that of brain damage and, later, cerebral palsy and/or mental defection. It should be noted, however, that some of these conditions are not caused by birth trauma, but by other pre-existing disorders of the neonate. The complex problem of disorders in the newborn has been and continues to be an intensive area of investigation by neonatalogists.

13.5 UNWANTED INFERTILITY

Fertility is a marvel, infertility a mystery. The pathology underlying infertility may reside in the management of one's life or life style or it may be pure chance.

13.5.1 The Search for Causes

The first line of defence against infertility is the checkup. However, it is important that a couple not be subjected to the rigors of infertility investigations if the frequency and timing of intercourse or the nature of sexual contact is inadequate. Couples should have had at least one year of

Fertility is a marvel, infertility is a mystery.

unprotected intercourse before considering an intensive infertility investigation.

The fertility of a couple depends on the normal interaction of a number of factors. The male must be able to produce large numbers of healthy sperm; they must traverse the male reproduction system and be discharged at ejaculation into the (anatomically normal) reproductive system of the female. The sperm must then penetrate the cervical mucus and ascend through the uterus to the fallopian tubes where fertilization will occur. Simultaneously, the female must have developed and released the ovum at the correct time. The expelled ovum must have unrestricted entry to and passage through the fallopian tube and must have been transported to an area in the tube where fertilization will occur. Following fertilization the blastocyst must travel toward the endometrial cavity where nidation (implantation) in the uterine wall must take place in an endometrium uterine wall tissue which has been appropriately prepared by hormone action. The slightest defect in these basic events in either partner leads to infertility.

The age of maximum fertility in the male and female is approximately 25. After that, fertility begins to decrease, especially in the female, in whom it declines rapidly after the age of 30. The average length of time needed to achieve conception in a normal couple at age 25 is 5.3 months. Eighty percent of actively endeavouring couples will achieve a conception by the end of 12 months (Austin, 1972).

EXAMINATION OF THE MALE

This is by far the easier examination for fertility of the two sexes. A simple sperm examination may be performed by most medical laboratories and will quickly determine the potency of the semen sample. If this is normal, physical examination and inquiry into the sexual techniques and personal habits or current medications taken should determine if the male partner is or is not the prime factor in a particular infertility situation.

Some causes of low sperm count (under 10,000/ml) are those associated with past sexually transmitted diseases, past damage to testicles, childhood illnesses such as mumps during adolescence, congenital absence of a testicle, diabetes, or excess heat in the scrotal region, which decreases sperm production. Anatomical problems with the penis and testicles sometimes lead to an inability of the sperm to reach the required depot in the female. If the above factors are normal and, in particular, if the man has fathered other children with a previous sexual partner, then the need for a more extensive examination for the female is indicated.

EXAMINATION OF THE FEMALE
The history of the woman's menstrual pattern, including age at menarche (onset of menstruation), and the interval and duration of her current menstrual cycle is the first step taken. If there have been previous pregnancies, then one would look for intervening problems which may have occurred since the last pregnancy. A check for sexually transmitted disease, either current or past, and for pelvic inflammatory disease (PID) or intra-abdominal operations is also important. In addition, the reproductive history of a woman's family is informative, as certain congenital malformations of the pelvic organs are inherited.

The usual questions are again asked concerning sexual technique. In particular, the use of massage oils or lubricants is normally discouraged since they may kill the sperm. Postcoital douches also are discouraged at this time. The position during intercourse probably has no effect on reproduction, but some authorities suggest that the woman remain on her back with her legs up following the male orgasm to allow the pooling of the seminal fluid at the upper portion of the vagina in a position of close proximity to the cervix (entry to the uterus).

Certain drugs can impair fertility, particularly some of the major tranquillizers, analgesic medications and, of course, the Pill. Women involved in extensive sports and other physical activity may have temporary alter-

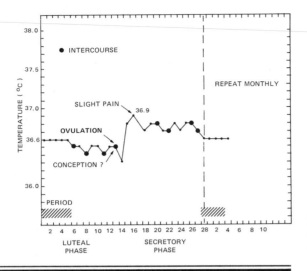

Figure 13.8. Recording basal body temperatures provides an acurate estimate of when ovulation occurs.

ation of their menstrual cycles and may be temporarily infertile. Ceasing intensive physical activity will usually remedy such temporary infertility. Cessation of the Pill will sometimes cause a rebound **hyperfertility**, and it is a method sometimes used by women to augment fertility.

During normal physical examination of a woman, a pelvic examination is performed to ascertain the position of the uterus; the presence or absence of fibroid tumors of the uterus; and the nature, size, and location of the ovaries. A general examination of both sexes will include a check on the relevant secondary sexual characteristics, such as facial hairs, breasts, male pattern baldness, and other signs or symptoms of hormonal or pituitary disease. In other words, does she look female and he male!

THE FIVE BASIC TESTS
Following the initial examination and check ups, the following five tests are designed to evaluate the anatomy, physiology, and fertility of the couple.

1. Basal Body Temperature Recordings
If a record of a woman's basal temperature is taken first thing in the morning by a very sensitive thermometer it is possible to determine whether ovulation is occurring regularly (see Figure 13.8). Sometimes two to three months of daily recording is necessary to compose an accurate pattern of this event.

As ovulation approaches, production of estrogen by the ovary increases, causing a drop in the basal body temperature. When ovulation occurs, the **corpus luteum** within the ovary produces progesterone, which directly or indirectly acts on the **hypothalamus**, causing a slight rise of the basal body temperature. The rise is usually no more than 0.5 degrees Celsius. The temperature should remain slightly elevated for the remainder of the menstrual cycle. If implantation does not occur, production of progesterone and estrogen by the corpus luteum decreases, and the temperature begins to fall as menses begins. If pregnancy occurs, the level of progesterone does not drop; the temperature remains elevated and menses does not occur. Thus, basal body temperature charts are also helpful in the early diagnosis of pregnancy.

2. The D and C

Further evaluation of the menstrual cycle is often necessary to check for progesterone effect upon the uterus. Progesterone, one of the major female hormones produced by the ovary after ovulation, produces a **secretory pattern** of the endometrium (the lining of the uterus). A biopsy (a small extracted portion of tissue examined under the microscope) showing a secretory endometrium is further evidence of ovulation. To be effective, this procedure, called a **dilation and curettage (D and C)**, is performed during the latter half of the menstrual cycle. This timing is necessary to determine the presence of this secretory phase of the endometrium. The D and C is a minor procedure, which is conducted either in the doctor's office or in the hospital. Unfortunately, the procedure also sometimes obliterates a newly implanted blastocyst. Such an inadvertent therapeutic abortion is especially disappointing, for it has destroyed the very thing that the test was designed to help evaluate and help produce.

If appropriate laboratory facilities are available, measurement of plasma progesterone concentrations may be performed. However, these levels fluctuate significantly from woman to woman and within any one woman from time to time, and, therefore, a series of tests must be done. Even then their diagnostic reliability is debatable.

3. Tubal Patency Test

Hysterosalpingography is a tubal patency test which is performed by injecting a special **radiopaque dye** through the slightly dilated cervix into the uterus and then forcing it up the fallopian tubes, at which point x-rays are taken. This outlines the course of the fallopian tubes and can determine the presence or absence of any abnormalities in the uterus, the fallopian tubes, and sometimes problems around the ovaries themselves.

Hysterosalpingography should be performed in the follicular phase (first half) of the menstrual cycle for two reasons: First, to avoid interrupting or eradicating an early pregnancy; and second, to avoid the secretory pattern of the endometrium, which occurs after ovulation and may prevent normal passage of the dye. The secretory endometrium after ovulation is thicker than the uterine lining before. A third reason is that the test itself may remove some obstruction in the fallopian tubes, which will subsequently allow the normal passage of the ovum and sperm through them. Thus, the test may act in a therapeutic manner.

4. Postcoital Examination
In this situation a couple is requested to have intercourse two to four hours prior to the examination and then a small amount of cervical mucus is examined for the presence of motile sperm. The presence of motile sperm is reassuring, but if the sperms present are all inactive there is the suggestion that the cervical mucus is either inadequate to support the sperm or that it may contain antibodies which destroy the sperm. Since this test is performed very close to ovulation, a peculiar ferning capacity of the cervical mucus, which may be observed at this time, helps to confirm that ovulation has indeed taken place.

5. Semen Analysis
This test is usually done first of all, before more complicated tests are done on the female. Semen analysis checks for sperm motility and morphology (anatomical integrity—perfectness of the sperm) as well as a determination of the absolute number of sperms present. A sperm count of 20 million sperms per cc of semen is considered a case of borderline infertility. Samples with more than 100 million sperms per cc of semen are considered normal. The semen sample must be collected either by masturbating into

a clean sterile jar or from ejaculations immediately after intercourse. The male should be sexually inactive for at least two days prior to the collection of the sample, and the laboratory examining the sample must use careful and exacting techniques to provide reliable results. The semen sample should be examined immediately after ejaculation, otherwise a false recording of the number of motile sperm may result.

By use of the five procedures outlined above causes for infertility can be determined in about 90% of couples. In most of these cases, corrective measures and therapy may often be successfully instituted, raising the chance of fertility to a near normal state.

13.5.2 The Diseases

During the above check ups a number of diseases may be found which themselves lead to infertility. A list of the sexually transmitted diseases has already given an indication of a number of disorders which cause infertility. These are described in the previous chapter on "Human Sexuality."

Certain genetic abnormalities of the male or female, such as deformed pelvic organs or penis, are obvious causes of infertility. Recent recognition of a sperm antibody development within the female has led to a unique type of therapy. In this condition the female has developed antibodies specific to her husband's sperm (thus destroying them) so that although he could not father her child another man might. However, if the female is not exposed to her husband's sperm for a prolonged period, then the antibodies specific to his sperm decrease and, thus, his sperm becomes able to survive long enough to reach the ovum and fertilize it. Thus, a solution to this cause of infertility is simple, Either abstain from intercourse or use a condom for five or six months. Then, at a time judged best for fertilization to occur, that is, when the female's basal body temperature is elevated, normal unprotected intercourse should occur. This must be one of the few times when condoms are worn to enhance fertility.

When examination of the female finds evidence of previous pelvic inflammatory disease, surgery is often necessary to release the scars and adhesions in the pelvic tissue and to restablish the lumen of the fallopian tubes. This requires very delicate surgery and only a few gynecologists specialize in these techniques. The removal of fibroid tumors from the uterus is fairly routine, but any subsequent pregnancy which may develop must be monitored carefully for the possibility of a uterine rupture, and consideration must be given to deliver the infant by elective (not emergent) Caesarian section.

Certain hormonal aberrations which have a bearing on fertility are sometimes found in people with anorexia nervosa, bulimia, high stress levels, and thyroid or pitutiary disorders. The therapy for these illnesses is beyond the scope of this chapter.

The recently recognized condition of amenorrhea (cessation of menstrual cycle and infertility in female long distance runners) poses some interesting questions. Perhaps women's bodies were designed to recognize that when they were very physically active, fertility would be a hazard. Research has not yet uncovered the answer to the phenomenon. However, what is known is that when such runners stop for a period of time they usually are able to become pregnant. A review of Chapter 9, on exercise and endorphins, illuminates this effect somewhat.

Despite all the tests and checks, about 10% of cases of infertility have no known recognizable cause. For such infertile couples the solution lies elsewhere, either in adoption or surrogate parenthood, until more answers are made available.

13.5.3 Enhancing the Family

ARTIFICIAL INSEMINATION

For many years the cattle industry has been using artificial insemination to bring the semen of the best bulls to their favorite cows. Nowadays, most major medical centres are finally providing the advantages of artificial insemination to solve human problems. This technique has its best application when the male partner of a couple is infertile but the female has normal potential fertility. Historically, this problem often was solved quietly and expeditiously by the woman merely finding a temporary lover. Henry VIII, of England, may have suspected this behavior of Anne Boleyn. As a result she lost her head.

As one mark of our changing times, today's women have a choice of anonymous donors, pooled donor samples, or, in some cases, the selection of sperms from Nobel laureates.

FERTILITY PILLS

For women with ovulation problems, new medications have been developed which stimulate ovulation. In general, they work by modifying the hypothalamic response to estrogens, causing the hypothalamus to respond with an outpouring of FSH and LH. FSH and LH are hormones from the pituitary gland which stimuate the ovary to produce a follicle (ovum container) and ovum.

The most common medication for this purpose is clomiphene citrate (clomid), which is taken from days five through nine of the menstrual cycle. Since the advent of this type of ovulation stimulation, there has been an abundance of multiple pregnancies. At one time triplets, quadruplets, and quintuplets were extremely rare, but with the use of clomid these events are no longer remarkable. A recent case of sextuplets in the Philippines followed the use of clomid.

SURROGATE PARENTS

Several years ago a Philadelphia journalist on a dare placed an advertisement in the newspaper requesting to rent a uterus for nine months. The ad specified that a couple with a barren wife wished to have the husband's child with another woman. The progeny of this temporary union would be adopted by the couple and cared for with the highest of standards. A moderate stipend would be paid to the owner of the uterus, and all medical fees and bills would be paid. This ad produced over 600 serious applicants, mostly from unmarried career women over 30 who wished to produce progeny but not be burdened by parenthood. The shock produced some serious thought. Several instances of such surrogate parenthood have now taken place.

ADOPTIONS

Infertile couples have the opportunity to apply to adopt children given up by their natural parent(s) through the services of adoption agencies. These agencies are governed by legislation, and they are usually staffed by conscientious social workers who carefully screen the prospective parents to find the best homes for their babies. At one time, there was an abundance of babies and a dearth of potential parents. Today the reverse is true. For every baby an agency must place there are 15 serious applicants. Unfortunately, not all of these applicants are suitable, and many of them are struck from the list early. Many couples are not only infertile but also are suffering illnesses which prevent pregnancy. Moreover, many may have social, financial, or other problems as well, which render them less than ideal or secure parents. They wish to adopt but may fail to realize that these same illnesses and problems may also be a handicap to normal parenthood.

The agency involved is fortunate, for it can choose the best and most suitable parents for the available child, acting as the child's advocate. Efforts are made to match the background of the genetic parents of the child to that of the adopting parents. In most cases everyone is a winner. The mother who gives up her child for adoption is virtually guaranteed that her child will be well cared for. The adopting parents have their child and can trust that efforts have been made to match that child to them. Most important of all, though, the child has a family who wants him or her.

A mysterious event often happens following adoptions. A couple, whose infertility was carefully examined and no cause found, finally adopts a child and shortly after this the woman becomes pregnant. It seems that the harder she tries the less fertile she becomes, and once she relaxes with the presence of the newly adopted child something seems to click. Some important and fascinating mind-hormonal change has taken place.

13.6 SUMMARY

Reproduction is one of the most fascinating events of the human species. Without it we would not be here. If left to nature our families would be somewhat lopsided. Some families would be large, some childless. Today, however, there is a value for and a technology capable of evening the load. The average family in North America consists of 1.7 children (Allen, 1977), and this is brought about through various methods of contraception, fertility enhancement, and in some cases, abortions. When the appropriate phase of life has concluded, and the 1.7 children are neatly tucked to bed, then the father may have a vasectomy or the mother a tubal ligation. They have had enough of the temporary contraceptive methods and the time has come to cut off the chance of further procreation. However, it is wise to wait until the family size has been established and the children's health secure before choosing sterilization, for problems do occur during conception and pregnancy, and the problems of the neonate can be serious and fatal.

When the desired number of children cannot be achieved, infertility is considered the cause. Numerous illnesses can create this state and, in most cases, may be diagnosed through a series of tests and examinations. A solution to the infertility is often found during the progress of such investigations, and remedies do exist. Fertility pills, artificial insemination, and, sometimes, adoptions are possible solutions.

13.7 REFERENCES

Adams, P.W., Ross, D.P., Folkard, J. et al. Effect of pyridoxine hydrochloride (vitamin B6) upon depression associated with oral contraception. **Lancet,** April 28: 7809-7811, 1973.

Allen, M.E. Obstetricians not needed in routine maternity cases. **B.C. Medical Journal,** 19:251, 1977.

Austin, C.R., and Short, R.V. (eds.). **Reproduction in Mammals,** Vol. 5. Cambridge University Press, 1972.

Carroll, C. and Miller, D. **Health, the Science of Human Adaption, 3rd ed.,** Dubuque, Iowa: Wm. C. Brown Co., 1982.

Dickey, R., Yuzpe, A.A. (ed). **Managing contraceptive pill patients,** 4th ed. Creative Informatics (Canada) Inc., London, Ontario, 1984.

Edlin, G. and Golanty, E. **Health and Wellness: A Holistic Approach.** Boston: Jones and Bartlett Publishers, 1988.

Family Living. **Sex Education Transparancy Series.** Hubbard Scientific Co., Northbrook, Ill., 1968.

Health and Welfare Canada. **Oral Contraceptives, Report 1985.** Minister of Supply and Services Canada 1985, Ottawa.

Shane, J.M., Schiff, I.S., Wilson, E.A. and Craig, J.A. The infertile couple, evaluation and treatment. **Ciba Clinical Symposia,** 29(2). Ciba Pharmaceutical Co., Dorval, Que., 1977.

13.8 STUDY QUESTIONS

1. Among the numerous methods of contraception, name two common effective temporary contraceptives, two less effective methods, and two permanent methods of contraception.
2. Discuss the best times and circumstances in family planning to use each of the above mentioned contraceptive methods.
3. Discuss the stages of conception.
4. Mention five influences on the growth of the fetus.
5. List three causes of infertility in the male.
6. List five causes of infertility in the female.
7. What are the five tests for infertility?
8. What legal methods are there of obtaining a child other than intercourse and pregnancy?

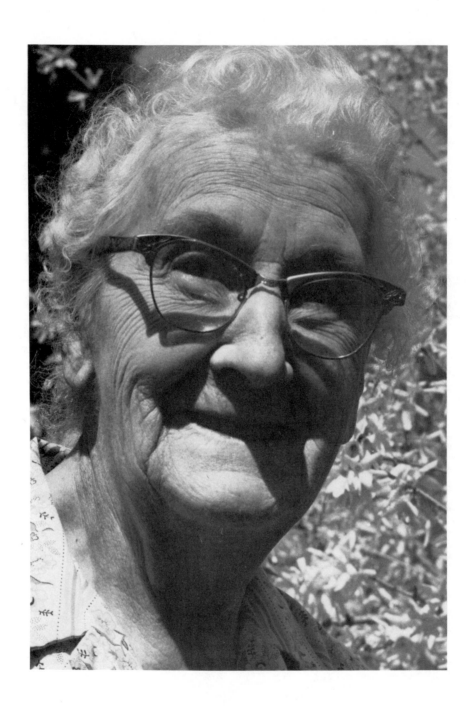

14

Aging, Death, and Dying

Aging is still a mystery, and we still have no firm medical
or scientific evidence favouring one theory over another.

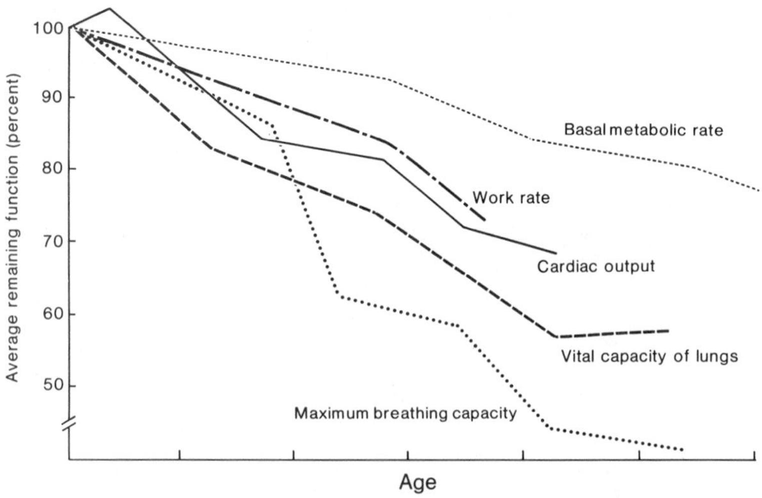

Figure 14.1. Shows the relatively steady decrease in body functioning which occurs throughout life. Reproduced with permission from Insel, P.M. and Roth, W.T., p. 98, 1976.

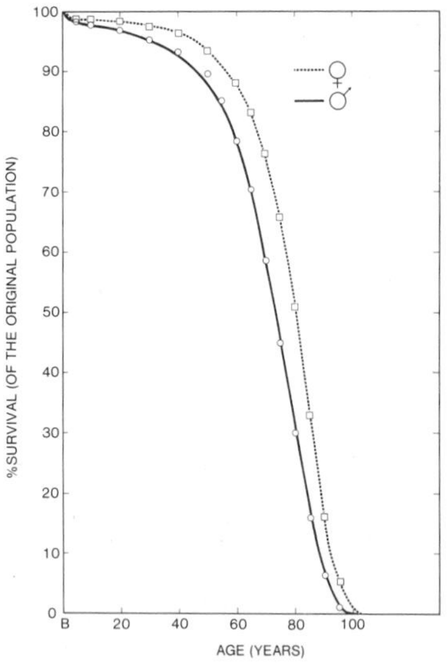

Figure 14.2. Survivorship curves for Canadian males and females in 1971. This graph shows the percentage of people who survived over a given period of time, in the sample studied. Reproduced with permission from Canada Year Book, 1980-81.

OBJECTIVES

When you have completed this chapter, you should be able to:
- **Outline** the principal theories of aging.
- **List** the common social problems associated with aging.
- **Distinguish** mean longevity from maximum longevity and geriatrics from gerontology.
- **Outline** how a diagnosis of death can be determined.
- **Summarize** various attitudes toward death.
- **List** the stages involved in facing personal death.
- **Discuss** the stages of grief and mourning.
- **Describe** the hospice movement and related organizations for the dying.

KEY TERMS

cross-linkage	hospice
DNA	juvenescent
enzymes	life expectancy
eschatology	mean longevity
euthanasia	maximum longevity
free radicals	senescent
gametes	senescence
geriatrics	senility
gerontology	thanatology

14.0 INTRODUCTION

Aging may be defined as the sequential or progressive change in an organism that leads to increased risk of debility, disease, and death. It is a process that proceeds inexorably from conception to death (see Figure 14.1). The words used in reference to one's age depend on the observer's stage of development. In other words, what is perceived as young or old depends on one's age. Thus, children refer to their grandparents as old (and often their parents also), and grandparents consider the children young. For

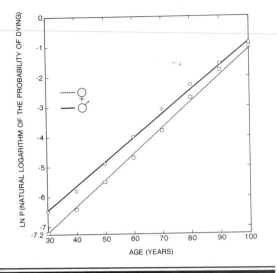

Figure 14.3. Probability of dying before one's next birthday versus age in Canadian men and women, 1971. The probability of not reaching the next birthday more than doubles every ten years after the age of 30, and is greater for men than women. Reproduced with permission from Canada Year Book, 1980-81.

statistical purposes, in this chapter "elderly" will be defined as persons 65 and over.

It is important to realize that not all individuals or groups of people age at the same rate. Any given point in the aging process occurs with a defined decline of basic physiological function. This point is unique in the developmental stage of the individual, and it can be reached faster or slower, depending on the person's rate of aging. Aging occurs throughout life, not only when the bodily functions slow down, the hair becomes grey, or the skin wrinkles.

The graphs shown in Figures 14.2 and 14.3 compare the rates of survival between men and women. Regardless of whether two individuals or the populations of two countries are compared, the basic shape of the plots remains the same. Figure 14.2 shows that, in general, women tend to outlive men. The difference seems greatest between 75 and 80 years and narrows gradually toward 100 years. In fact, for any age over ten years, in a large sample of men and women of equal number, a greater proportion of women will survive than men. The probability of dying for males and females before one's next birthday (Figure 14.3) is greater for men than women after age 30. This is primarily due to the higher probability that is already established by the age of 30. Throughout the remaining years this differential is maintained, although it gradually narrows to become almost coincident at 100 years of age. While this general trend may be observed, the difference is slight in comparison with the variation in rate of aging among individuals. People age at different rates because each individual is unique in constitution, and each is exposed to a different and changing environment throughout life.

Gerontology (the study of age) is a field that originated from our awareness of the finality of life. Note here that gerontology is different from geriatrics. **Gerontology** is a branch of science or knowledge that deals with the problems of the aged, whereas **geriatrics** is a branch of medicine. Gerontology is a realm of research that is gaining importance within

many other disciplines such as politics, economics, and medicine, not only because the percentage of people over 65 years of age is increasing, but also because the application of any knowledge gained in these fields can enhance both the quality and the length of people's lives. The subject of aging is multifaceted but may be examined from three different perspectives, dealing with
- biological/physiological processes,
- psychological/behavioral changes, and
- social/economic developments.

14.0.1 Longevity

Longevity (the length of life) depends on **intrinsic** factors, or an organism's genetic composition, and **extrinsic** factors of the environment. Longevity generally is measured in one of two ways: either in terms of **mean longevity** or **maximum longevity**. Mean longevity is a calculation of the average life span in a sample. Thus, mean longevity would be different for each town, city, region, and country. Maximum longevity, on the other hand, does not involve statistical calculation. It is the maximum length of life that has been attained by human beings, so far as it is known. This is estimated to be between 110 and 135 years of age.

Mean longevity is calculated as follows. Suppose there are five kittens in a litter. Further, suppose that one dies in the first year, two die at age five, one more survives until age seven, and the final one dies after 10 years. The average life span of the litter would then be equal to the sum of the ages at death, divided by the population size. Thus:

Mean longevity in years

$$= \frac{1x1 + 2x5 + 1x7 + 1x10}{5}$$

$$= 28/5 \text{ years} \quad = 5.6 \text{ years}$$

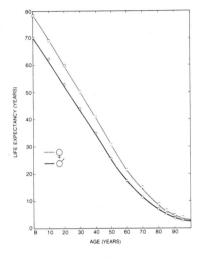

Figure 14.4. Expectation of life (in years) for Canadian men and women born in 1976. Reproduced with permission from Canada Year Book, 1980-81.

Also mean longevity = life expectancy (at birth)

$$= \frac{\text{sum of ages at death}}{\text{population size}}$$

For people, a similar calculation for the life expectancy (at birth) involves all the deaths in a given area during the census period (usually 10 years).

14.0.2 Life Expectancy

A term related to the mean longevity is **life expectancy**. This term applies to the statistical prediction of how long an organism will live beyond a given age. Generally speaking, one's life expectancy at birth is equal to the mean longevity of his/her social group or community. Life expectancy is a term that has a little broader meaning than mean longevity because the extra number of years a person can live decreases as one gets older. Thus, there may be different life expectancies at birth, at 1 year of age, or at 80. For example, a male born in 1976 (see Figure 14.4) could expect to live 70 more years. By the time he turns 70 (2046 A.D.), he would be expected to live for only about 11 more years. This prediction could not apply to a person born in 1970, 1980, or any other year.

If, on the other hand, one wished to compare life expectancy throughout history, a graph similar to the one in Figure 14.5 could be used. Since 1931, the life expectancy of men and women has increased by at least 10 years. This has been due mainly to the decrease in the mortality rate for infants from such diseases as smallpox, diphtheria, and polio through advances in immunology and antibiotic treatments. However, the gap between men and women during the same period also has widened from two years to seven years. A female born in 1976 could expect to live for 77 years, compared with 70 years for a male. The trend, on the whole, seems to be one in which the mean longevity actually is approaching maximum longevity. This means that more and more people are living to a certain

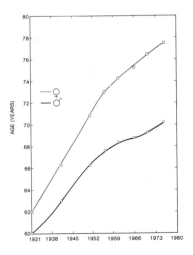

Figure 14.5. Life expectancy (at birth) for Canadian men and women (1931-1976). Reproduced with permission from Statistics Canada, 1979.

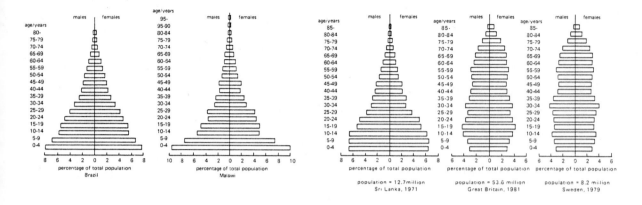

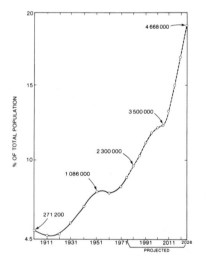

Figure 14.7. Population pyramids based on census data. Developing nations shown on this page whiled Developed Industrial Nations are shown on the top of page 447. Reproduced with permission from the **Health of Nations**, Open University, Health and Disease U205, Book 3, p. 15, Open University Press, 1985.

Figure 14.6. Canadian population aged 65 and over, as a percentage of the total population, from 1901 to 1976, with predictions to 2026. Reproduced with permission from Statistics Canada, 1979.

age (70 for males, 77 for females) so that the average life expectancy is higher, but longevity is not increasing.

With the mean longevity constantly rising, it would seem as though the population of Canada were steadily "getting older." A population may be described as "aging" if its median age is increasing as time passes or if the ratio of elderly people to the total population is increasing (see Figure 14.6). (The median is the age at which the greatest number of people are grouped, when an observation is made.) In 1981, there were over 2 million people at or over the age of 65, forming between 9 and 10% of the population. In the census year 2001 A.D., according to projections, there will be about 3 million "senior citizens" in Canada. By 2026 A.D., it is predicted, nearly one in five Canadians will rank among the aged. These statistics are similar in many developed countries. The transition toward an aging populace depends on the interplay between births, the number of deaths at different ages, and migration. The factors that have been responsible for modern trends in North America are

- a decrease in the death rate in older people as medical technology improves the treatment of heart disorders and other killer diseases,
- a decrease in the death rate due to infant mortality,
- an increase in the number of births since the turn of the century, and
- immigration from Europe and Asia.

The branch of knowledge that deals with the distributions of changes and trends in births, marriages, and deaths in a given population is known as **demography**. Figure 14.7 shows the age pyramids of several countries. The broad based pyramids of developing countries (Brazil, Malawi and Sri Lanka) reflect their high birth rate and child mortality rate. The square pyramids of such developed countries as Great Britain and Sweden reflect the aging populations of these countries as life expectancy has increased. The transition from broad based to square in just 70 years in the U.S.A. (1900-1970) is shown in Figure 14.8.

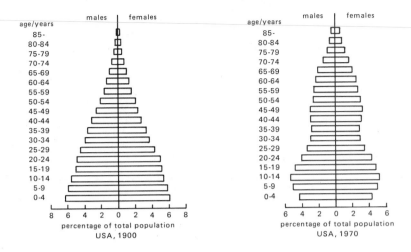

Figure 14.8. Population pyramids for U.S.A., 1900 and 1970. Reproduced with permission from the **Health of Nations**, Open University, Health and Disease, U205 Book 3, p. 16, Open University Press, 1985.

14.1 THEORIES OF AGING

Why is it that the Abkhaisians in Russia, the Vilcabamba in Ecuador, or the Hunzas in Kashmir can live over 100 years? At present, there are many theories, none of which include all of the answers. The state of gerontology is analogous to that of a crossword puzzle: There are many indirect clues, bits and pieces of information, but as yet, no solution that unveils the mystery. However, the persistent goals of this field of study are to determine the characteristics of aging processes and to determine the mechanism(s) by which aging occurs.

There are two major schools of thought through which attempts are made to explain aging. The genetic theories suggest that it is a programmed process. The nongenetic theories, on the other hand, try to explain how aging occurs, rather than why. All of these theories explain the phenomenon of aging biologically at molecular, tissue, and organismic levels. Scientific theories on aging are generally expected to meet the following criteria,

• the aging phenomenon must occur in all species,
• the process must progress with time, and
• the process must be deleterious in nature, leading ultimately to the death of the organism.

14.1.1 Genetic Theories

THE GENE THEORY
The gene theory is a rather fatalistic one in that it proposes that aging is a programmed process over which we have no control. It has two variations, but the theme is that destructive genes are "turned on" as one advances into old age. The first variation suggests that people and animals are born with one set of genes that change throughout their lives. The second version hypothesizes two sets of genes and labels one type **juvenescent,** and the other **senescent.** According to this theory, when the period of growth has

stopped, there is said to be a period of homeostasis during which reproduction occurs. The "aging" genes then supposedly gain ascendancy, leading to an increased probability of disease, debility, and death. (You will read more about how genes work in Chapter 11.)

THE RUNNING-OUT PROGRAM THEORY

According to this theory, human cells are programmed to reproduce only a certain number of times and then die. The theory has had a certain amount of empirical support. For example, Hayflick and his colleagues (1974) performed an experiment in which they placed some lung cells in a culture along with nutrient material that was free of bacteria. These cells doubled every 24 hours. All of the cells died after six months (or 50 cell divisions). Similar research also was done **in vitro**, as well as on other animal tissue.

The **paramecium** is a special example that supports the hypothesis of the genetic "program" of cells eventually running out. The paramecium (a one-celled organism resembling all body cells except the gametes) duplicates its genetic material by asexual reproduction and stops after a certain number of divisions. Further evidence in support of the theory is shown in the disease **progeria**, in which the body of a child assumes the appearance of an 80-year-old, with wrinkled skin and brittle bones. The number of times that each cell reproduces in a rare condition like this is far fewer than normal.

SOMATIC MUTATION THEORY

A series of experiments conducted by the biochemist H.J. Curtis and his colleagues (1971) provides evidence for the somatic mutation theory. The first involved irradiating (e.g. exposing to radiation) a portion of the liver in guinea pigs. Some cells were destroyed but were eventually replaced by the liver. However, when the chromosomes of the new liver cells were examined, it was found that they were abnormal. Curtis et al. then investigated another set of non-irradiated guinea pigs and noticed that, out of the group, the older animals had a greater number of **chromosomal abnormalities** than the younger ones. In a third experiment, the chromosomes of a strain of "short-lived" guinea pigs were compared with another strain of "long-lived" guinea pigs. The longer-lived ones had fewer genetic defects of their chromosomes. These experiments led Curtis to believe that aging is a time-dependent process resulting in increased chromosomal mutation.

14.1.2 Non-Genetic Theories

THE CROSS-LINKAGE THEORY
This theory was formulated over 40 years ago by Johan Bjorksten (1941). He knew that proteins could be irreparably damaged or denatured by certain agents. At that time the definition of cross-linkage referred to the denatured proteins in connective tissue (collagen). Connective tissue is what holds the cardiovascular and muscular systems together. When this tissue is altered, it results in a general loss of flexibility, as well as a loss in elasticity within the blood vessels.) On a cellular level, cross-linkage is the binding of large intracellular and extracellular molecules together, leading to the loss of flexibility in the cells of connective tissue (fibroblasts). The effect of cross-linkage is to bind essential intracellular molecules in such a way as to render them ineffective and to block the flow of other molecules, needed by the tissue, to them. Bjorksten and his supporters expanded this idea from connective tissue to DNA (the genetic material of the cell controlling its replication) within the cell nucleus, suggesting that if the genetic material was cross-linked within itself or with some external substance, then the "reading" of instructions (for cell maintenance and reproduction) would be hindered. Numerous cross-linked compounds have been detected in the experiments of Bjorksten.

THE FREE RADICAL THEORY
Harman (1956) proposed the free radical theory almost 30 years ago. **Free radicals** are one type of chemical agent that can bind with the cell. In

animals, free radicals are very reactive substances which are generated from oxygen-driven metabolism. This means that they are created by the body as oxygen is metabolized, through a process called "auto-oxidation." Although they exist for less than one second, free radicals have been known to damage unsaturated fats found in cell and nuclear membranes. If the attack is sufficiently strong, the membranes of the cells will be punctured, spilling out their contents. These transient substances also are capable of altering the cell's DNA, and this has very severe consequences for the continued survival of the cell or its death from abnormal (cancerous) cells formed by the alteration.

Once a free radical is formed it reacts quickly, producing more free radicals in a self-perpetuating cycle. If this were allowed to occur unhindered, damage to cells, and to the organism itself, would be very fast. However, the body also produces substances called **antioxidants**, which neutralize free radicals. Examples of these substances are superoxide dismutase and catalase; they are often referred to as "free radical scavengers." (Vitamin C and Vitamin E also act as free radical scavengers, but they are taken in by the body through diet, rather than being endogenously produced, that is, produced within the system through normal metabolic action.

The main idea of the free radical theory of aging is that, with age, the body is said to become less effective in producing the enzymes (antioxidants) needed to neutralize free radicals (Tappel, 1968).

THE ACCUMULATION THEORY

The accumulation theory is related to the three previously mentioned theories. It suggests that, as years pass, more and more substances build up in the cytoplasm, resulting in the cell's virtual suffocation and death. Examples of such substances are lipofuscin granules, aldehydes, histones, quinones, and free radicals. As these compounds accumulate they can have two effects. Lipofuscins, for example, are brown-colored pigments which are chemically inert. They do not react with chemicals in the

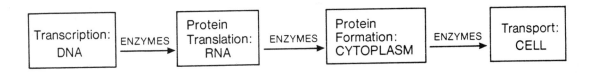

Figure 14.9. The process of coding by nuclear DNA for a protein's synthesis in the cell's cytoplasm.

cytoplasm, but float around and take up space that could be used by other chemicals for cell growth, maintenance, or repair. Such action may be compared to household "garbage" that piles up if it is not disposed of. The second potential effect of accumulated chemicals in the cell's cytoplasm is their possible reaction with whatever else is there. Free radicals and histones are examples of this effect.

THE ERROR THEORY

Another theory used to explain aging is the possibility of random error in genetic instructions for the construction of a protein.

When a protein is required to perform a particular function for the cell (hence for the organism), the DNA located in the cell nucleus codes messages (transcription) to another form of genetic material called RNA, which carries the instructions out into the cytoplasm and decodes them. The process of decoding (translation) leads to the assembly of a large number of building blocks of the protein (its amino acids) until the particular protein codon is made. All of these chemical reactions require **enzymes** (which themselves are particular types of proteins) to make them work. Figure 14.9 shows how enzymes act as catalysts. Depending on the size of the protein, its formation may require a few or many enzymes. The important point is that errors may occur at any stage in the process: in transcription, in translation, or in the very enzymes that catalyze the reactions. If the wrong protein is coded, the cell either will have to live with what it has erroneously produced or it will die.

Observations of cell processes for long periods of time have shown, however, that enzymes do not qualitatively change much due to random error, even though their activity does decrease somewhat. This would suggest that the error theory is not a likely explanation for how aging occurs.

THE AUTOIMMUNE THEORY

The autoimmune theory was proposed by Walford (1969) and supported by Adler (1974). The immunological system's function is mainly to destroy foreign substances within the body (see Chapter 7). Therefore, it must be able to recognize its own cells (i.e., all of the body's proteins) or it might very well destroy them as it does foreign invading proteins such as viruses (antigens). According to this theory, when a person is young and healthy the immunological system is able to distinguish self from non-self. But as time passes, this distinction becomes less and less clear, eventually leading to an attack by the body's defence mechanisms on its own cells during senescence. This theory explains *what* happens, but not exactly *how* it happens. It is unclear whether the action takes place because of some somatic mutation, genetic miscoding, cross-linkage, or other means.

THE WEAR-AND-TEAR THEORY

This theory simply assumes that the body is like a machine which, after long use, wears out. The theory is used to explain why the cells of the heart and nervous system, since they are incapable of replacing themselves, eventually die.

14.2 PROBLEMS OF THE ELDERLY

14.2.1 Retirement and Loss of Income

Among all of the social implications of aging, retirement at an arbitrarily determined age of 65 carries with it the greatest number of life changes for the ever-increasing number of people aged 65 and over. A primary factor affecting people as they retire is the drop in income that they experience. In North America, mandatory retirement is practised by government, educational institutions, and business in general. In the United States, public pressure against the retirement age of 65 has caused it to be raised to age 70. A similar pressure may emerge in Canada where retirement age is still 65 years, as the proportion of elderly increases, although unemployment problems may create counter-pressure, where people are urged to retire early in order to make more room for young people in the workplace.

*A primary factor affecting people as they retire
is the drop in income that they experience.*

Upon retiring from work, the retiree's income drops to a minimum of 60% of the average income for all ages in the categories of family and unattached individuals. In 1975, the average income for a Canadian family was about $16,000, while the average income for a family with a retired "head" was a little over $10,000. Similarly, an unattached person, on the average making about $6,600 (in 1975), would have this amount reduced to a little over $4,000, if he or she were age 65 or over.

The money that supports the elderly comes from three main sources: employment, pensions and investments, and transfer payments. Employment income paid to families with a head of household (main wage earner) aged 65 or over accounts for nearly one-third (32%, 1975) of the average family income because so many of these people work, either out of necessity or choice. Another 29% (1975) of their income comes from investments and private pensions. One problem that develops with the passage of time is that if the funds from this category are fixed, then inflation erodes the purchasing power of the recipients. Transfer payments for the age 65+ group have accounted for 39% (1975) of the total income going to such families. Examples of these types of payments are old age security payment, guaranteed income supplement (GIS), and spouse's allowance.

As with other sources of income, the patterns of spending for the elderly differ from the average younger person. In general, unattached individuals aged 65+ or families with an aged 65+ head spend a higher proportion of their income on food and shelter than do younger people. A 1974 survey of unattached individuals in 14 major cities across Canada noted that people in the age 65+ category spent a little more than half of their income on food and shelter, while about one-third was the average. Other noteworthy patterns were that the elderly spent a smaller proportion of their income on travel and, naturally, less on contributions to unemployment insurance and pension. Both groups spent an equal portion of their budget on recreation.

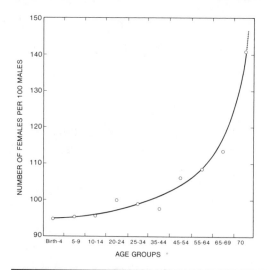

Figure 14.10. The number of Canadian females per 100 males, according to age groups, in 1977. Reproduced with permission from **Canada Year Book**, 1980-81.

14.2.2 Living Conditions

Contrary to society's belief, two-thirds of the nation's elderly are heads of families or are family members (a family is defined here as a group of individuals sharing a dwelling and related by blood, marriage, or adoption). The other third are unattached, mostly maintaining their own households. About 70% of those living alone are women. Since women often tend to marry men older than themselves, and have a greater life expectancy, they are three times more likely to become widowed. These women are unlikely to remarry because there are relatively few men left at that age (Figure 14.10 illustrates sex ratio as a function of age).

In Canada, only 10% of the elderly live in collective dwellings such as nursing homes, facilities for the handicapped, veterans' hospitals, and psychiatric institutions.

14.2.3 Housing

The fact that 6 out of 10 of the elderly own their own homes has been attributed to payments for the house accumulating from a lifetime of work. These houses are often humble dwellings, a considerable number having been built many years ago. Many of them are in need of maintenance and have become unsafe because of the rising costs of property taxes, repairs, and utilities. Three out of 10 old people live in apartments but they are no better off, since they must pay a large portion of their income in rent. This forces many to move into apartments in inner city neighborhoods, where the crime rate usually is high. There are many problems associated with this situation.

14.2.4 Crime

CRIMES COMMITTED ON THE ELDERLY

For those older people who are forced to live in a neighborhood with a high crime rate, life can be very dangerous. The violent crimes of burglary, robbery, and purse-snatching are well-publicized, but fraud is an even more prevalent problem. Days on which older people receive their retirement benefits are the most dangerous to them. Because of their physical inability to resist, they are the targets of thieves, primarily from the 15-24 year age group. Elderly people in large cities often lose so much sleep at night for fear of being robbed that they sleep during the day. Some don't even bother to go out and are virtually prisoners in their own homes. Examples of the fraudulent ways in which the elderly are exploited are the workings of con-men or medical quacks who promise ways of getting rich with a small investment, physical attractiveness, or renewed health. Cosmetic, pharmaceutical, real estate firms and even funeral directors have not escaped suspicion of taking advantage of the aged.

CRIMES COMMITTED BY THE ELDERLY

The crimes committed by the aged usually are less violent than is the norm in other parts of the population: drunkenness, liquor law violations, vandalism, gambling, and shoplifting food items are the most common. On the whole, the crime rate declines from adolescence onwards, and crime is much less common among the elderly compared with other age groups.

14.2.5 Patterns of Illness

CHRONIC CONDITIONS

Chronic conditions of illness are the usual type of medical problem found in the elderly. Compared to the national average of 11.3 days, the stay of the elderly in hospital averages 25.2 days. The three major causes of death are coronary disease, which claims about one third of each sex; stroke, which is more common in women; and cancer.

The treatment of older patients has illuminated some areas of health care that need improvement. The most conspicuous of these is the fact that, for most diseases of the elderly, there is, as yet, no cure. While conventional medicine, on the one hand, is geared toward curing diseases, the elderly, suffering chronic diseases, cannot wait for cures. They need alleviation of their current problems and a support that is lacking in today's health care organization. Often in medicine, an illness is diagnosed as having a single cause. In an elderly patient, however, the problem is more likely to be multi-faceted. The chance of making an inaccurate diagnosis in this case increases as a result because even if one disorder is treated, other, more fundamental problems may remain undetected. Furthermore, age may change symptoms of the problem, dulling the sharpness of a diagnosis, as in **angina pectoris**, for example (angina pectoris is a type of heart disease, usually associated with lack of oxygen delivery to the heart muscle). With increasing age, a person may not feel pain in the chest, which is the usual physical response to this condition.

MENTAL ILLNESS

The mental problems of senility and confusion that are often cited as problems of aging may, on further appraisal, be judged as due to physical problems. Poorly supplied arteries in the brain can cause disorientation, memory loss, and shifts in mood. The side effects of drugs also may produce dizziness and confusion. Other psychological or emotional problems that may be rooted in physical causes are mental depression due to ill health, emotional traumas of surgery, and psychological disorders caused by nutritional imbalances. About half of the mental disorders in old age are due to cerebral arteriosclerosis, which results in irreversible brain damage (see Alzheimer's disease discussed in Chapter 16).

14.3 INTRODUCTION TO DEATH AND DYING

14.3.1 What is Death?

"Death, like life, is change,...and change depends on the passage of time." According to Einstein, time is relative, and according to experience, time's arrow points forward. Thus, change occurs in only one direction through

*The mental problems of senility and confusion
that are often cited as problems of aging
may, on further appraisal, be judged
as due to physical problems.*

time—it does not backtrack. If change is moving forward through time, then an event at time (T1) must be different from one at T2, later on. We know that time is elapsing from the types of changes that occur in our environment. For example, spontaneous events seem to be inferred whenever there is movement from a state of order to one of disorder. A bottle on a high ledge will shatter if it hits the ground; the reverse is not likely to occur—shattered glass will not magically become a bottle. Similarly, if a bottle of Chanel No. 5 is opened in one side of the room, eventually the smell of perfume will reach the other side. In this case, the molecules change from being in a relatively ordered state (in a bottle) to a more random, disordered state (throughout the room). Likewise, a living body, which is a highly ordered state of hundreds of molecules, in time suffers a decrease in its order, or structure (it ages), and it finally comes to a state of maximum disorder (minimum entropy), known as death.

The above is a rather dispassionate account on a molecular level of what death is and why we die. However, on a more organismic or biological plane, a different explanation is offered. In the novel *Roots*, by Alex Haley, a grandfather tells his grandson that there are three types of people in this world: Those waiting to be born, those walking the earth, and those who have been here and died. This is connected to the idea of a gene pool. The people who are walking on the earth constitute the pool. The people who are either being born or dying, enter or leave this pool, respectively. Each individual in the pool is a unique combination of genes (i.e., genetic material) in nature's cauldron. From another perspective altogether, one sees that, in Darwinian terms, older people generally cannot adapt to the changing environment as well as they used to, so they die sooner. The genes—changing and competing for survival—allow the species as a whole to evolve; this evolution is the biological driving force that tends to create greater order in nature to combat the forces that cause death. This is said to be true not only for humans, but for any sexually reproducing species. In a sense, although the individuals in a species die, they live on through their offspring.

*Death is strange, irreversible, can only be experienced
alone, and cannot be anticipated by an individual.*

14.3.2 The Physical Meaning of Death

The subject of death may be discussed from many other points of view besides the scientific one, including the social, religious, cultural, and philosophical. All of these overlap to some extent. Various attitudes toward this final human experience will be discussed briefly later on, but first it is useful to clarify the physical meaning of death.

How do we determine if a person is dead? What is the definition of death? Before answering these questions, it should be pointed out that in recent years, medicine and the law have been forced to face this question in more detail as a result of cases where a person may be kept alive by means of a life support system, while the brain may be completely nonfunctional. To clarify this issue somewhat so that medical care could proceed, a Harvard ad hoc committee in 1968 set up criteria for defining death. They were

- unreceptivity and unresponsivity to external stimuli,
- lack of reflex movements such as pupil response to bright light, indicating a lack of central nervous system activity,
- flat electroencephalogram (EEG) readings, indicating a lack of brain activity, and
- at least one hour of observation by physicians during which there is lack of movement and breathing.

If these four conditions are constant over a period of 24 hours, then the person may be considered dead. It is apparent that several criteria have been taken into account here, besides the cessation of a heart beat. Earlier definitions from which the committee borrowed its criteria are

- **somatic death**—instant death of the body as in a car accident;
- **cardiac death**—the stoppage of heart beat;
- **brain death**—absence of electrical activity from the brain;
- **biological death**—when all parts of the brain have died; this does not include the other organs which could be used for transplants;
- **clinical death** stoppage of heart beat and respiration;

- **cellular death** the death of all of the cells of the body; the rate of cellular death varies among the regions of the body;
- **legal death** the definition of death that is determined by the physician or institution.

14.4 ATTITUDES AND UNDERSTANDINGS ABOUT DEATH

Thanatology is the study of death. It includes such areas as grief, social and psychological aspects of death, the awareness of death, and coping with this awareness. Thanatology is now taught in some high schools and universities; and some medical and nursing schools also are giving instruction in this area. In addition, more and more research is being undertaken in this field by physicians, psychologists, and scientists, as is shown by such well-known publications as: *On Death and Dying; Death: The Final Stage of Growth*, both by Dr. Elizabeth Kubler-Ross, and *Life After Life*, by Dr. Raymond Moody. Some reasons for studying this inevitable and irreversible event are

- to help people to cope with the prospect of their own death and the death of loved ones,
- to understand how a dying person should be treated,
- to consider the legal, moral, and ethical aspects of death,
- to comprehend the cultural and historical views of death and how they differ in other countries and other times,
- to develop a healthy outlook on death so that one can enjoy life better.

14.4.1 Emotional Stages of Dying People

From a personal point of view (the psychological aspect), one's "fear of death" may be partly attributed to the fear of the unknown and the fear of being alone; most people are "social animals" and thus need human relationships. Death is strange, irreversible, can only be experienced alone, and cannot be anticipated by an individual. To a varying extent, the fear of death affects everyone. In a study by Diggory and Rothman (1961) a list of attributes which were said to be lost through dying was developed. The list included

• loss of the ability to have experiences,
• loss of the ability to predict subsequent events,
• loss of body,
• loss of the ability to care for dependents, and
• loss suffered by friends and family.

After studying a large number of terminally-ill patients, Dr.Elizabeth Kubler-Ross, the Swiss psychiatrist, conceptualized the awareness of death in terms of five stages. Her observations need to be qualified somewhat: These stages are not absolutely distinct in all people—they may overlap, and the order in which they occur may vary among individuals. Moreover, a dying person may go back and forth from one stage to another. With these qualifications in mind, Dr. Kubler-Ross' five stages are described as follows:

STAGE ONE: When a person is informed that he or she is suffering from a terminal illness, their first reaction is shock or denial, or both. "No, it can't be me," is a typical response, (it is interesting that, in a well-known study by Oken in 1961, 88% of the physicians responding to a questionnaire did not inform their cancer patients of their condition, almost in accord with the idea that the condition would be denied.) This stage may be partly replaced with acceptance, if the patient has to take care of unfinished business matters or arrangements for surviving children.

STAGE TWO: This is a stage of emotionally experiencing impending death. It involves a shift from denial to an attitude of, "Why me?" This occurs once the person has accepted that the whole thing is not a mistake and that it would be futile trying to think that way. At this point the individual may become angry and express rage, and rightly so: their life has been interrupted; they cannot pursue happiness; they may have been put in

*The acceptance of death is a stage where no feelings
are shown—the dying patient has accepted fate
and now wants to be left alone.*

hospital and subjected to constant tests. These are constant reminders—
from the environment, other people, and perhaps their own body—that life
will end soon. Aware of what is at stake, this person often projects anger
toward hospital staff, family—even God. Realizing the inevitable, they
may begin trying to postpone death by bargaining. This is the beginning
of stage three.

STAGE THREE: Rather like a child being rewarded for "good behavior,"
the person now tries to negotiate for the relief of pain or discomfort and
even life extension. In dealing with conscience and spiritual beliefs, they
may promise to lead a life devoted to God or in service of others in return
for survival of a few more days, weeks, or months. When the patients know
that they can deny the illness no longer, when the anger has dissipated and
bargaining efforts have been spent, they enter a stage of depression.

STAGE FOUR: While in this stage of depression, a person may refuse vis-
itors, become very silent, or just spend time crying or grieving. Two types
of depression may occur in this stage. Reactive depression is one type, in
which the patient grieves over having to quit work or, perhaps, put the
children in a day-care facility because no one can be at home. It occurs with
regard to events in the recent past. The other type of depression is called
preparatory grief. Here, the person contemplates losses that will occur in
the near future. This process allows the patient to dissociate herself from
all love objects and facilitates entry to the "final" stage, which is the
acceptance of death.

STAGE FIVE: The acceptance of death should not be mistaken for
happiness or capitulation. Rather, it is a stage where no feelings are
shown—the dying patient has accepted fate and now wants to be left alone.

*Funerals help to separate one emotionally from the
deceased and to smooth the transition
of the bereaved back to an adjusted life.*

14.4.2 Grief and Mourning

For the survivors death will cause a psychological crisis. This suffering, called grief, is a mixture of loneliness, fear, and despair over the loss of a loved one. How grief affects the survivor depends on
• the specific relationship between survivor and the deceased,
• the meaning which the dead person had in one's own life,
• the functions of the dead person in the life of the survivor, and
• the nature of the changes in the survivor's life that result from the death.

The task of the mourner is to try to cope with the grief and get back to living. In adjusting to this stressful situation, the mourner usually passes through three distinct stages, similar to those which the dying person experienced. The time period denoted below for the duration of each stage merely illustrates the relationship among the stages of grief. They vary among individuals, and for some people, grief lasts for years.

ONE: In the first three days, there is shock, denial, weeping, and sometimes agitation;

TWO: In this stage, visual memories (painfully) come back, perhaps leading to depression, insomnia, and irritability. This occurs at about the first month and continues for two months or longer. There may even be attempts at bargaining to bring the person back, much like the dying person experiences in wishing to extend life.

THREE: In the third stage, grief has subsided, the mourner is able to continue or resume normal activities, and now may enjoy pleasant memories of the deceased. Usually within a year, the survivor has adjusted.

The process of grieving is facilitated by the funeral ritual, when the community eulogizes the unique qualities of the deceased. This is also the time when the bereaved sense their own mortality. Funerals help to separate one emotionally from the deceased (on an individual level) and to smooth the transition of the bereaved back to an adjusted life. Seeing the body of the deceased is said to lessen the "unconscious" threat to the body often experienced by the survivor and reassure him that, even when he dies, his body will be properly disposed of and life will continue. This theory of grief explains why, during the ritual, trying to deny or forget about the death would make it harder to overcome the associated pain and sadness.

14.4.3 Death in Our Society
The denial of death that exists in society is not completely new. Today, when someone dies, she is said to have "departed," "kicked the bucket," or "passed away." In the media, death is related to action and adventure. Ghost stories, mystery stories, wild west stories, and war stories give us violent images of death; but this vicarious experience is very different from the real, intense emotion felt between a dying person and a close friend or relative. In the nuclear family, children are separated from their grandparents and so are usually not around when they die. Because many adults and children have not seen death, it is difficult for them to understand that they, too, will die. It is not surprising then, if they grow up believing that they can live forever. The belief in medical technology as a panacea, once cancer and cardiovascular diseases are beaten, also is widely prevalent in our society. On the contrary, scientists believe that, even if all human ailments could be eradicated, only 20 years would be added to the currently established normal life expectancy of 70 at birth. In these various ways, modern urban life is organized to shield society from the reality of death.

14.4.4 Death in Other Cultures
One of the positive aspects of seeing how other cultures view death is that it reminds us that there are cultures, unlike our own, where death is not

feared. In fact, death is accepted by some, together with immortality of the soul or spirit. An example of this may be found in the Alaskan Indian culture. These people seem to know when they are going to die and prepare for it by being near family or friends. They may plan their own funeral and select who will participate. The village will know of the impending death and help prepare for it. After the burial, a feast is usually held. In this way, the person dies with a sense of dignity. Contrast this to the common scenario in our society, where the dying patient is in the hospital and attached to a life-saving device. Often a person is considered dead before his actual death!

The eastern religions of Hinduism and Buddhism have a number of similar beliefs concerning death. First of all, both religions believe in the inevitability of death and in reincarnation as another form of life. Death is not the ultimate goal; the goal is the liberation of the soul, both physically and spiritually, from the pattern of continuous time: life, rebirth, and redeath. The Hindus call this freedom "moska," while the Buddhists name it "nirvana," but both mean the same thing. Through life, death and rebirth, people of both religions believe they will eventually reach this high state, and so death is welcomed as part of the cycle.

14.4.5 Western Religious Views

The major western religions are Judaism and Christianity. The latter may be divided into Catholicism and Protestantism. They have different views of death and different rituals celebrating its occurrence (of course, the rituals mentioned below will vary from place to place).

The Roman Catholic religion regards death and the resurrection of Christ as symbolic conquests of death. A belief in life after death is characteristic: The soul, after death, is believed to be judged by God, and either punished, purged, or rewarded in the afterlife. There are many Roman Catholic rituals related to death, three of which will be described here. One ritual is called "extreme unction." This is known as the last rite and

*The eastern religions believe death is not the ultimate
goal; the goal is the liberation of the soul,
both physically and spiritually, from the pattern of
continuous time: life, rebirth, and redeath.*

involves anointing (the ceremonial application of oil) the dying person. Another ritual in some Roman Catholic countries is the "wake." This is a period of mourning held before the funeral. The body is laid out in an open casket (where possible) so that the family may pay their last respects. The funeral mass occurs in a church a few days after death. The casket is then taken to the cemetery, where the burial is conducted. The family and close friends congregate afterwards, at a particular place, to mourn the loss.

Protestant views on issues concerning death, such as immortality, and even Heaven and Hell, are more varied. The ceremonies also vary with regard to holding the funeral at the church, at the funeral parlor, or at the home. The casket may be open or closed, depending on the community. The church is supportive to the family, physically, emotionally, and spiritually.

The Jewish religion includes at least three theories on what occurs after death. These are known as the orthodox, reform, and conservative theories. A full description of these is too long to be included in this discussion. It is noteable, however, that in ancient writings, mention is made of the afterlife and resurrection. Transmigration is also mentioned. This is where the soul leaves one human body upon death and enters another one. In the mourning process, "keriah" is the wearing of a torn, black ribbon, and "shiva" is the seven day mourning period that follows death.

14.5 THE PROCESS OF DYING

14.5.1 The Where of Dying

HOSPITALS
In any given year, about 6% of the total population may be expected to die. Many years ago, the death of older people occurred at home. Even if it happened at another relative's home, the person's body was brought back to his house and the family was responsible for the funeral. (Funeral processions in the past normally started out from the home.) Most people

today die in institutions such as hospitals, resting homes, or nursing homes. Bureaucratization has lead to a depersonalization of the dying pro-cess. Institutions' attempts to insulate society from death and dying result in its occurrence being cast as somewhat routine and mechanical. Bodies in hospitals are not allowed to be moved during visiting hours, to reduce disruption and disturbance. When patients are obviously near death, they are immediately moved to another room to "protect" the other patients. The main factors that determine where a terminally ill patient spends their last days are financial status, emotional reactions of the family, the patient's wishes, and the patient's physical and emotional condition.

THE HOSPICE CONCEPT

An alternative to using the hospital as a facility for the dying is in the **hospice** approach. "Hospice" means a place of rest for tired travellers and implies a place where people can die with dignity. The hospice idea was first developed by Dr. Cicely Saunders, who opened St. Christopher's Hospice in England, in 1967. The hospice can be attached to a hospital or be a separate building altogether. The hospice movement represents a belief in letting the patient stay at home and be cared for there by relatives for as long as possible before terminal stages of illness. At home, family members are taught how to care for the dying person, allowing the patient to live as normally as possible. A support staff of doctors, nurses, psychologists, and social workers is available; they all have a background in the psychology of death and dying in order that they may help both patient and family cope with the patient's problems. Through facilities such as communal kitchens, dining rooms, and living areas, hospices try to recreate the home atmosphere. During visiting hours, family are encouraged to come and take part in hospice activities. Hospices generally are about one-third cheaper per day than hospitals.

A number of other self-help groups for the dying and their families have recently appeared. One is "Make Today Count," an organization founded

Make today count.

in 1974 to help people overcome the fear and isolation that terminally ill patients often experience. Some hospitals include nurses specifically trained in "death and dying" procedures. In California there is the Shanti (peace) project, which is a hot-line operated by volunteers (many of whom are terminally ill), that provides counselling to the dying, their family, and their friends. It is interesting to see that these organizations are formed by lay people, not by medical professionals.

14.5.2 The Afterlife and Near Death Experiences

Many researchers in **eschatology** (the study of life after death) have observed that a decrease in belief in the afterlife has increased the fear of death. Some regard the idea of life after death as foolish, while for others, the faith in life emerging (in some form) beyond the shroud of death eases the fear of death. Concepts of the afterlife vary greatly. They include
• survival of the soul,
• immortality of one's genes through reproduction,
• an ever-evolving purification and growth of the spirit,
• reunion with the Godhead,
• resurrection,
• the eternal existence of the soul in heaven or hell,
• transmigration,
• reincarnation,
• the unification of all minds, and many others.

Dr. Kubler-Ross became involved with this experience when one of her patients, who had apparently "died," was brought back to life and recounted her near-death experiences. She related how, when she was "dead" (i.e., had no vital signs such as breathing, blood pressure, and brain activity), she floated and hovered over her body for a period of three hours. She was able to describe in detail the medical procedures that the doctors performed to save her life.

*According to Daniel Grollman, the debate over
life after death is one which, in the end,
we will each be the final judge.*

As a result, Dr. Kubler-Ross and, independently, Dr. Raymond Moody investigated further cases of this phenomenon and recorded a number of common features in patients' accounts of their experience of "dying"
• being out-of-body,
• feelings of peace and quiet after the physical distress of dying,
• hearing noises such as loud buzzing sounds or ringing sounds,
• feelings of rapid movement through a dark space or tunnel,
• encountering very bright lights, often interpreted as beings of light, and
• coming back to one's self.

All of the evidence mentioned above is subjective, not proof that we can survive death. According to Daniel Grollman, the debate over life after death is one which, in the end, we will each be the final judge.

14.5.3 Euthanasia

Euthanasia is a term that is frequently interchanged with mercy killing, although they should be kept quite separate. Euthanasia (**eu**=good, **thanatos**=death) implies a death without prolonged suffering, an easy, painless, and happy death. Mercy killing, on the other hand, is killing the person to put him out of his misery. There are two types of euthanasia: direct (active) and indirect (passive). Direct euthanasia involves a deliberate action that would bring on the death of the dying individual. An example would be introducing a large dose of a substance, perhaps a depressant, through injection, that would result in death. Indirect euthanasia refers to withholding or omitting life-extending techniques, such as surgery, oxygen administration, or intravenous feeding, in the terminally-ill patient.

The legality of euthanasia is an issue hotly debated in medical, legal, and ethical circles. The "Hemlock Society" a grass roots American movement promotes "self-deliveration from life" to be legal. Convincing arguments for and against euthanasia exist. Some people argue that extreme suffering is degrading and inhumane to the individual. Opponents argue that the Bible prohibits killing and that euthanasia is an act of murder. This leads further to the question of who is responsible for controlling life or death, and what happens if that power is abused? At present, it is illegal to actively induce euthanasia, although a doctor, in consultation with the patient and the family, may withhold life-extending measures for the terminally ill.

14.6 SUMMARY

In this chapter aging, death, and dying have been discussed from various perspectives. From a social point of view, the ways in which longevity and life expectancy are determined, as demographic characteristics of a society, were explained. Then various theories of how physiological aging occurs were described. It should be noted that aging is still a mystery, and we still have no firm medical or scientific evidence favouring one theory over another.

Common problems of a financial, social, psychological, or physical nature, which are faced by the elderly, were discussed in the next section.

The latter part of the chapter dealt with dying. After considering different meanings which may be attached to death, the emotional impact of it was discussed. This was viewed from the perspectives of one who is dying and of those close to him or her. Meanings and rituals associated with death in other cultures and in various religions were presented, in order to illustrate the potential emotional impact that such differences might have. For instance, if death is seen as one step in a progression toward a further life, then its emotional impact will be lessened considerably.

Finally, some different processes for easing the transition from life to death or "this life to the next" were described.

14.7 REFERENCES

Adler, W.H. An Autoimmune theory of aging. In M. Rockstein, M. Sussman and J. Chesky (eds). **Theoretical Aspects of Aging,** 1974.

Aiken, L. **Later Life.** Stockton, California: W.B. Saunders and Co., 1978.

Bjorksten, J. Recent developments in protein. **Chemistry and Industry,** 48: 746, 1941.

Canada Year Book, 1980-81.

Carroll, C. and Miller, D. Health: **The Science of Human Adaption,** 3rd ed. Dubuque, Iowa: WCB Co., 1982.

Curtis, H.J. and Miller, K. Chromosome aberrations in liver cells of guinea pigs. **Journal of Gerontology,** 26: 292, 1971.

Diggory, J. and Rothman, D. Values destroyed by death. **Journal of Abnormal Social Psychology,** 30: 11, 1961.

Eisenberg, A. and Eisenberg, H. **Alive and Well: Decisions in Health.** New York: McGraw-Hill Co., 1979.

Fassbender, W. **You and Your Health,** 2nd ed. New York: John Wiley & Sons, 1980.

Haley, Alex. **Roots.** Toronto: Doubleday, 1977.

Harman, D. Aging: A theory based on free radical and radiation chemistry. **Journal of Gerontology,** 11: 298, 1956.

Hayflick, L. Cytogerontology. In M. Rockstein, M. Sussman and J. Chesky (eds.) **Theoretical Aspects of Aging.** New York: Academic Press, 1974.

Health of Nations, Open University, Health and Disease U205, Book 3, pages 15-16, Open University Press, 1985.

Insel, P.M. and Roth, W.T. **Health in a Changing Society,** 4th ed. Palo Alto, California: Mayfield Publishing Co., 1985.

Johnson, R.E. Some reflections on ageism. In S.M. Horvath and Yousef, M.K. **Environmental Physiology: Aging, Heat and Altitude.** New York: Elsevier/North-Holland, 1979.

Kart, C.S., Metress, E.S. and Metress, J.F., Aging, Health and Society. Boston, MA: Jones and Bartlett Publishers, 1988.

Kubler-Ross, E. **On Death and Dying.** New York: Macmillan, 1969.

Kubler-Ross, E. **Death: The Final Stage of Growth.** Englewood Cliffs, N.J.: Prentice Hall, 1975.

Moody, R. **Life After Life.** Toronto: Bantam Books, 1976.

Oken, D. What to tell cancer patients. **Journal of American Medical Association,** 175: 1120, 1961.

Rockstein, M. and Sussman, M. **Biology of Aging.** Belmont, California: Wadsworth Publishing Co., 1979.

Tappell, A.L. Will antioxidant nutrients slow aging processes? **Geriatrics,** 23: 97, 1968.

Walford, R.L. **The Immunological Theory of Aging.** Baltimore: Williams and Wilkins, 1969.

Statistics Canada. **Vital Statistics** (Vol. III, Deaths). Catalog Number: 84-206, 1977.

Statistics Canada. **Canada's Elderly.** Catalog Number: 98-800E, 1979.

14.8 STUDY QUESTIONS

1. Define the following terms in three or four
   sentences:

   a) aging   e) death
   b) longevity   f) thanatology
   c) life expectancy   g) grief and mourning
   d) retirement   h) euthanasia

2. Briefly outline the theories of aging.
3. Out of the nine or so theories discussed in this
   section, which one theory do you think will be
   more generally acceptable and why.
4. Summarize various attitudes towards death.
5. Describe the hospice movement and related
   organizations for the dying.

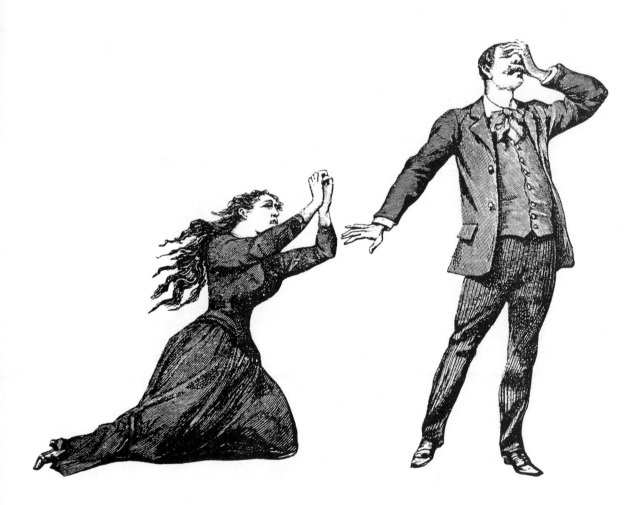

15

Family Violence

Both wife and child battering occur with astonishing frequency
and severity at all socio-economic levels.

OBJECTIVES

When you have completed this chapter you should be able to:
- **Define** the four forms of abuse experienced by women in intimate relationships.
- **Describe** the three phases in the cycle of violence typical of abusive partnerships.
- **Explain** why at least 6 beliefs commonly held by society with respect to wife abuse are untrue.
- **Discuss** the major factors, internal and external to the woman in an abusive relationship, that make it difficult for her to leave and not return.
- **List** and **describe** at least three lines of action that will help prevent wife assault from being perpetuated.
- **List** the common features shared by child abuse and wife assault.
- **Describe** a potentially abusive parent in terms of his/her background, current relationship and situation, and perceptions of the child.
- **List** at least 3 resources available to people needing more information about family violence.

KEY TERMS

atmosphere of violence	learned helplessness
blaming the victim	failure to thrive
cycle of violence	

15.0 INTRODUCTION

The issue of violence within the family unit is one which is only recently appreciated by society. Typically it is considered a problem of the **lower class** or **underprivileged**. However, both wife and child battering occur with astonishing frequency and severity at all socio-economic levels.

Region IV Council on Domestic Violence in the U.S. reports the nation's 700 shelters provided safety to more than 91,000 women and 131,000 children and were unable to provide to 264,000 more. There are 3,000 animal shelters but only 700 shelters for battered women .
*(From **In Transition**, Newsletter of the North Shore Crisis Services Society, Vancouver, B.C., Canada, December 1985).*

This chapter discusses wife assault and child abuse as separate examples of family violence (see reference note at the end of chapter). The frequency and severity of this problem, threatening as it does the physical and psychological well being of the victim(s) is an important contemporary health issue.

The high incidence of abuse reported in this chapter is only a conservative estimate since many cases are never reported. Society's response to the problem is usually to urge families to try to reconcile and stay together (regardless of past histories of brutality)—particularly when limited social agency funding makes provision of alternatives and counselling difficult. A serious consequence of this approach is the real and increasing danger facing the victims which is often underestimated, overlooked, or even denied. Ultimately many victims are permanently injured, both physically and emotionally; many die.

What solutions are there? Well, the first step is a recognition and understanding of the scope of the problem by society. This includes acceptance of the fact that family violence occurs at every social, economic, and vocational level (Ganley, 1981). It is not simply confined to families of alcoholics, the mentally ill, the poor, the immigrant, the uneducated, or other special groups. There is a good chance it is happening close to your own home.

15.1 BATTERED WOMEN

How serious and extensive is the problem of wife abuse? Consider the fact that approximately one in ten women in any crowd or gathering is being or has been physically assaulted by the man she is living with. This is a common estimate according to reports cited in Canada and the United States and does not include cases of psychological battering. The latter crime is often more painful and damaging to the victim than physical abuse (Walker, 1979).

The figures cited in the above quote are one indication of the extent of wife battering as a social problem. Consider the following statistics reported in British Columbia, Canada as further testimony to the pervasiveness and seriousness of this form of violence against women (B.C. Ministry of Labour, Women's Programs, and the Ministry of Attorney General, 1985, p.1). In the Vancouver metropolitan area alone, an estimated 4,000-5,000 women are beaten to the point of serious injury each year. Moreover, about 20% of homicide victims in Canada are murdered by their spouses, and most of these victims are women. Of the men, most are killed by their wives in self-defence during battering episodes.

Similarly, the following figures have been reported in the United States (O'Reilly, 1983). Nearly 6 million wives will be abused by their husbands in any one year. Some 2,000-4,000 women are beaten to death annually. The nation's police spend one-third of their time responding to domestic violence calls. Battery is the single major cause of injury to women, more significant than auto accidents, rapes, or muggings.

15.1.1 Defining Wife Abuse
PHYSICAL ABUSE
"Courts and social agencies use terms such as marital abuse and wife battering to describe serious or repeated injury by a person with whom the victim has a relationship involving cohabitation and sexual intimacy. Some 50% of the incidents involve persons no longer or never legally married." (O'Reilly, 1983, p. 19).

The injuries reported in cases of physical abuse include bruises, black eyes, strangulation, dislocated bones, fractures of fingers, arms, nose, jaw, collarbone, tailbone and ribs, internal hemorrhaging, knife wounds, burns, and even bullet wounds. Being punched or kicked in the stomach while pregnant is a frequent form of battery (McLeod, 1980; Carthy, 1982; Walker, 1979).

SEXUAL ABUSE

Closely linked to, and often part of physical abuse are incidents of sexual violence. This form of brutality is normally accompanied by real or threatened physical abuse for any non-compliance. One description puts the matter in a clear, if unpleasant light:

Some women report that their battering mates will force sexual activity after a beating, or require the performance of certain sexual practices while holding a loaded gun to their heads, or force certain unwanted sexual activities, or force sex with a third person. One woman said that her husband brought home pornographic magazines. He would beat her if she refused to do the sexual activity pictured in the magazine. Or, if she complied, he would beat her for going along with such "dirty sex".

Some cities and states recognize these sexual assaults as crimes and will prosecute offenders even if married to their victims. There are many other cities and states, which do not recognize rape within marriage as a crime (Ganley, 1981, p. 60).

PSYCHOLOGICAL ABUSE

The physical and sexual abuse described above is vivid, direct, and overtly violent. Psychological battery is much more difficult to define, however. It is nonetheless important that it is recognized and its severity in terms of impact on the victim not be underestimated. While this form of violence may often occur without accompanying physical injury, the reverse is not usually the case; physical abuse is nearly always accompanied by verbal and psychological battering. Even more important, as noted earlier, most women who report physical assault by their partners insist that such psychological abuse, concomitantly suffered, was often more long lasting and ultimately more harmful than any physical injury sustained (Walker, 1979).

Although various definitions of psychological abuse exist, one that makes a useful distinction is offered by Ganley (1981). She distin-

If a woman has reason to suspect she is being battered,
she probably is. If she errs in her judgement at all
it is in denying or minimizing the battering relationship.
Battered women rarely exaggerate (Walker, 1979).

guishes between psychological battering and emotional abuse according to whether or not physical violence has ever occured in the relationship. Although similar abusive behavior may occur in both situations, it is the accompanying **atmosphere of physical violence and fear** that makes psychological battering more serious and damaging to the victim than emotional abuse. The ever-present threat of real physical violence likens this type of psychological battering to the kind of abuse reportedly experienced by prisoners of war (POW's) in concentration camps of World War II (1939-45).

Abuse of women and POW's involve similar elements of victim isolation and increasing loss of control over their life. For example, the victim of spousal abuse usually has few outside contacts with whom to check perceptions of herself, her situation, and that of others, and thus retain some sense of reality. Both sets of victims experience degrading actions. Both are controlled by violence or the possibility of it. They live with the constant fear that the violence may return and with the belief that their captors are fully capable of carrying out any threat, since they have already demonstrated their abilities to be violent. Unlike the brainwashing of a POW, however, the psychological battering of women in our society is carried out by an **intimate**, one who at another time may be tender and loving. Such psychological battering is all the more disorienting to this victim because it is not clearly inflicted by one understood to be an enemy (Ganley, 1981, p. 60).

ABUSE OF PETS AND BELONGINGS
Another form of violence, often accompanying physical assault, is injury to a pet or personal property. In most cases property damage occurs to belongings or pets valued by the victim. Sometimes, however, the abuser destroys items given by him as gifts or items of common ownership, known to be precious to him. The woman is then blamed for "causing" the incident and any further violence that results from it.

15.1.2 Myths About Wife Battering

Even in modern times, violence against women is implicitly condoned by a society conditioned by erroneous, but commonly held beliefs. Some of these myths are accepted by both the man **and** woman locked in an abusive partnership. Several such myths and the accompanying reality are described below.

Myth 1: Wife battering occurs more often with poor, uneducated, and minority-group women than with middle-class, well-educated anglo women. As noted in the introduction to this chapter, it is erroneous to assume that battering occurs only within "disadvantaged" groups in society. Until recently it was mainly the disadvantaged women in any community who reported problems involving family violence, and thus it appeared most often that they were the ones experiencing abuse. Evidence now indicates that this is not the case (Ganley, 1981). Abusive men are represented in every occupation, race, religion, socioeconomic category, and size of community, as are the women they abuse. In fact, middle- and upper-class women who are battered are often more effectively silenced by the shame they feel, their concern for their husband's reputation, and by surrounding disbelief, than those of lower socio-economic levels. It may be their own families and friends who apply the most pressure on them to cover up and tolerate the brutality in their homes.

Myth 2: Women who are battered have done something to deserve the beating. It is a popular notion that battered women provoke beatings by being too bossy, too insulting, too obnoxious, too seductive in public, too "uppity, too sloppy, or too something else equally as vague. This myth, often referred to as "blaming the victim" (Ryan, 1971) effectively perpetuates the problem of violence by excusing the batterer for his crime. When victims continually receive the message from both an abuser and society, that somehow they caused their own abuse, battered women themselves even begin to believe their culpability (Stark, Fliteraft, and Frazier, 1979; Walker, 1979). A point to be emphasized here is that in law, assault of another person is an offence, regardless of any real or imagined provocation. An important point in understanding abusive behaviour is that reports by abused women commonly state that compliance with their partner's demands for their behavioural change did nothing to prevent further beatings. While in some cases women were able to postpone or partly control the timing of battering incidents, their submissiveness and generally nurturing behaviour was only a temporary restraint, at best, against further abuse. Batterers lose control not because of the woman's behaviour but rather due to their own self-direction (NiCarthy, 1982; Walker, 1979).

Myth 3: Battered women must be masochistic, that is they must enjoy being abused, otherwise they would not continue in a relationship with the abuser. This is an illogical observation. Women do not like being beaten, threatened, or to live in constant fear (Kuhl, 1984; Symonds, 1979). Such observations, if accepted, compound an already serious social problem. It may even alienate those in a position to help the victim. One reason why this myth is perpetuated is that many battered women fail to report the abuse they suffer, particularly in cases where they have tolerated it for several years.

Myth 4: Alcohol abuse causes wife abuse. Several studies on wife battering agree that men "drink to batter," but they do not batter **because** they drink, or **only** when they have been drinking. Some statistics indicate that in 50% of reported assault, the man has been drinking; in 20% of the cases the woman was drinking (McLeod, 1980). A recent research review presented contradictory evidence on the likelihood of alcohol (or other chemical substances) being a cause in cases of wife assault (Edleson, Eisikovits, and Guttman, 1985). These authors note

that convincing evidence establishing a cause-effect relationship between alcohol and wife abuse was singularly lacking.

The important thing to recognize is that an **association** of alcohol
with abusive behavior does not make it a **cause** of the brutality.
While alcohol may facilitate violent behaviour, in most cases where alcohol is reported as a precipitating factor, women report that beatings
frequently occur in the absence of drinking as well (Walker, 1979). It
appears that men often drink before a battering incident because it helps
justify the fact that they beat their wives. In addition, a woman may
use the fact that her partner had been drinking to rationalize his behaviour.

Myth 5: Batterers are psychopaths. In some ways, it is unfortunate that this statement is not true. If it were, an abusive, battering
type personality might become recognizable. As it is, however, few
men who beat their female partners are psychopathic. A current view is
that violent behaviour is socially learned and perpetuated. A corollary
is that is can be **unlearned**; of course this is only possible when the
batterer is willing to work toward change (Edleson *et al.*, 1985).

A parallel between the abusive man and the psychopath is the
"Jekyll and Hyde" personality of each. Walker (1979) reports that all of
the 120 women she interviewed in her work described their partners in
such terms. These men seemed able to extend an extraordinary charm
as a manipulative technique.

*A batterer can be either very, very good or very, very horrid. Further-
more, he can swing back and forth between the two characters with the
smoothness of a con artist. But unlike the psychopath, the batterer
feels a sense of guilt and shame at his uncontrollable actions. If he
were able to cease his violence, he would (Walker, 1979, p. 26).*

Myth 6: The batterer is not a loving partner.   Between interludes of coercion or violence the offender may be affectionate, considerate, even romantic and charming. This is one reason why women become trapped into believing that things may change, that abuse may stop permanently. The dream of their partner maintaining his loving behaviour consistently is a powerful incentive to believe his promises.

Myth 7: The high incidence of wife assault in recent years is due to the increasing liberalization of women and an accompanying real or perceived negative change in stature weakening masculine self-confidence.   This statement is historically inaccurate. It is based on a perception of family relationships which condones and supports male dominance, authority, and control over a female partner. This attitude, unquestioned prior to the women's rights movement, sanctioned wife beating even by law! Thus, it cannot legitimately be claimed that women's rights efforts and women's achieved equality are the cause of men's abusive behavior. Many battered women have chosen the more traditional role of "housewife and mother" over a career outside the home. These women, if they do decide to leave their partners, find it especially difficult to cope with the demands of the "working world." In such cases the batterer may be very successful in isolating and controlling his wife's movements; but this does not seem to prevent the pattern of beatings.

Myth 8: Economic hard times are a cause of wife battering. It is undeniable that economic hardship applies stress within families. However, domestic violence that appears to result from such pressure must be attributed to its rightful source. That is, the male's inability to cope effectively with stress, **regardless of the source of the stress**, is the reason why he batters. It is particularly crucial for the man in a violent relationship that the violence is not explained away by

blaming it on life's stresses and problems. By giving the man responsibility for his behavior he is given the opportunity to learn new ways
of handling the stresses and problems in his life. By excusing violence
as a "natural" result of such problems, the message given to the abuser
is that his reactions are controlled by his circumstances rather than his
own choice.

15.1.3 The Cycle of Abuse

It now seems clear that a definite cycle of abuse occurs. It is important
to understand the nature of this cycle for at least three reasons. First, it
increases the chance for effective outside intervention, so that the violence may be stopped. Second, it helps explain how women are trapped
into a continuing abusive relationship. Finally, it helps dispel erroneous beliefs leading to blame for the situation being ascribed to the
victim.

The three phases in the cycle of violence are the tension-building
phase, the actual battering incident, and a period of calm, loving, respite (Walker, 1979; 1983). The cycle is illustrated in Figure 15.1.
The length of time spent in any one phase, or the time taken for
completion of the whole cycle, varies greatly among couples and often
varies throughout a period in any one relationship. There is evidence
that particular circumstances effect the onset of a phase and that intervention may be more effective at certain points in the cycle than at
others (Walker, 1979).

PHASE I: TENSION-BUILDING

This phase may last anywhere from a few days to several years. It is
characterized by minor battering incidents, which gradually increase in
intensity as tension builds. Typically during this time a wife tries to
prevent the abuse from escalating by whatever form of behaviour seems
effective. She may become very nurturing, compliant, anxious to
please, and/or may simply try to stay out of the man's way. In her

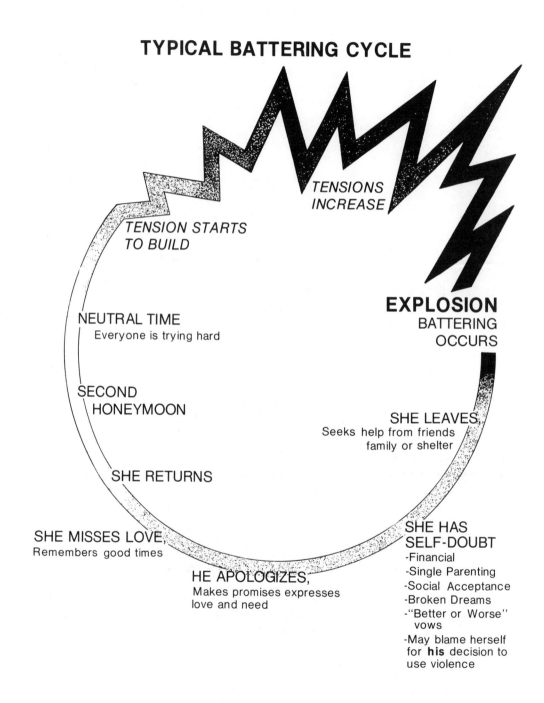

TYPICAL BATTERING CYCLE

TENSIONS INCREASE

TENSION STARTS TO BUILD

NEUTRAL TIME
Everyone is trying hard

SECOND HONEYMOON

SHE RETURNS

SHE MISSES LOVE,
Remembers good times

HE APOLOGIZES,
Makes promises expresses
love and need

EXPLOSION
BATTERING
OCCURS

SHE LEAVES
Seeks help from friends
family or shelter

SHE HAS
SELF-DOUBT
-Financial
-Single Parenting
-Social Acceptance
-Broken Dreams
-"Better or Worse"
 vows
-May blame herself
 for **his** decision to
 use violence

Figure 15.1 The three phases in the cycle of abuse.
Reproduced with permission from Walker, L.E., 1979.

attempts to avoid a beating, she is thus likely to overlook and accept the "minor" forms of abuse that take place. Unfortunately, as noted previously, these actions also communicate to the batterer that his abusive behaviour is acceptable.

If the woman is successful in avoiding a beating, she has done her job well. If a battering incident occurs, she is likely to blame herself for not behaving in the right way. The batterer's accusations claiming that she provoked or caused his explosion also reinforce her self-condemnation. The next time that Phase One occurs, the stage is effectively set for each to play out a similar role.

PHASE II: ACUTE BATTERING INCIDENT

As tension escalates between a couple it becomes more and more difficult for each to cope. The male behaviour becomes increasingly oppressive, hostile, and brutal; the female becomes unable to accommodate psychologically to the pain, anger, and fear she is experiencing. When both partners' control and coping mechanisms fail an acute battering incident inevitably occurs.

Occasionally, the woman will in fact provoke a battering incident at this point. She knows that a violent episode is imminent but has no way of knowing just when, where, or how it will occur. Often it becomes, not a matter of wishing to be beaten, but rather, wishing the suspense and the inevitable horror over with. From previous experience the woman knows that once the battering incident is over, the batterer moves into a phase in which a loving attitude is prominent (Walker, 1979).

Most of the time the woman is too ashamed, frightened, and depressed after a beating to report it immediately or to seek medical attention, if she can avoid it. Even when she does, this is the time when the batterer becomes the most loving, apologetic, and persuasive. Medical, counselling, and legal professionals alike are startled and horrified to watch a woman return some days later to the same man who recently brutalized her. However, Phase Three behavior is only one of the many reasons why women return. Other obstacles to her escape are discussed in section 15.1.4.

PHASE III: LOVE, KINDNESS, AND REMORSE

A batterer's actions during previous phases of the cycle are now reversed —he now will do **anything** in recompense (Walker, 1979). As noted earlier, batterers frequently possess and use great charm to manipulate a relationship. Part of the reason that they are so convincing at this phase is that they themselves believe that they will be able to change. They are convinced that now they can control themselves, and they are sincerely sorry for their former behaviour.

The woman, for her part, is not only relieved that the battering incident is over, but she now obtains a rare glimpse of the love and concern she has dreamed of receiving from the man. If she already has been through several battering cycles, the woman's awareness that she has traded her (and perhaps her children's) psychological and physical safety for temporary states of bliss only exacerbates her feelings of worthlessness and embarrassment.

15.1.4 Why Battered Women Stay

One of the questions asked most frequently about wife abuse is, "why does the woman not leave the man and, having once left, why does she return?" From the discussion so far, it should be apparent how the woman in an abusive relationship becomes psychologically trapped. However, there are also a multitude of other factors which work together to make it difficult for her to leave or stay away after she has left. Three major factors typically are:

1. Her own personal turmoil and state of mind;
2. Surrounding society pressures; and
3. Fear of the loneliness and struggle she faces if she leaves and remains separated.

A statement by a physician clearly
expressess the "value-free" approach
many doctors take to cases of
wife-batthering.

If a woman comes in with bruises, I ask about the
cause. If she says, "I fell down the stairs", I
accept her explanation. Upon examination, however, I may feel that she didn't sustain these
bruises by falling down the stairs. Somebody
may have hit her. I accept the patient's story....
We don't have the time or the background for the
reason of the assault.... It's a personal problem
between man and wife.

(Davidson, 1978, pp. 84-85).

THE WOMAN'S EXPERIENCE

Several personal factors affect a woman's position. In most women,
submissiveness and dependence as desirable traits are taught from an
early age. This is still largely true today for every social class of women, regardless of their educational or vocational status as adults. In
abusive situations, emotional dependence is fostered through continued
verbal abuse, which diminishes self-confidence, increased social
isolation, and, in many cases, a lack of any access to money.

A woman's first experience of abuse usually is in a relatively minor
series of incidents. When the first major battering incident occurs, she
is likely to experience shock, disbelief, and a considerable amount of
shame and guilt. It must be remembered that her partner has often been
telling her during more minor episodes that she is inadequate. She now
may blame herself for provoking the beating, and/or she may attribute
it to outside sources of stress on her mate. Her sense of shame will
usually prevent her from sharing the experience with outsiders. This
produces feelings of isolation in her, increasing the likelihood that she
will collude with her partner in denying the seriousness of the incident.
Moreover, most women report that first of all they believe the violence
just experienced will never be repeated, and they believe their partner's
avowal to reform (Dobash & Dobash, 1979; Langley and Levy, 1977).

In addition to these factors, an abused woman may feel obliged to
take care of her man, particularly when his remorse, emotional dependence, and desperation become apparent during Phase Three. She is likely to share in her partner's fear of being isolated and alone. To leave
him means she must resolve to face drastic changes in living habits at a
time when she feels inadequate, ashamed, helpless, and defeated.

Charles Baker, 42, was sentenced yesterday for kicking and punching his wife to death. Mr. Baker's 41-year old wife died on January 25, 1981, after a drunken quarrel between the couple. She had broken ribs, a ruptured pancreas and several bruises on her stomach, pelvis and legs. Mr. Baker had pleaded not guilty to a charge of second-degree murder, and a jury found him guilty of the lesser offence of manslaughter.

Crown lawyer Thomas Smith had asked that Mr. Baker receive a three-year to five-year term in a federal penitentiary. "Mr. Baker and his fists were a disaster waiting to happen and that is exactly what occurred on January 24," he told the judge prior to the sentencing. "Wife beating is always a concern because the victims cannot protect themselves," he said. "The sentence of this court must shout out that it's not going to be open season on wives who are victims..."

In sentencing Charles Baker the judge of the Ontario Supreme Court said the maximum sentence for manslaughter is life and the man probably deserved a penitentiary term. "However, I know what I do will not bring back to life Mrs. Baker." Instead, Mr. Baker was given two years less a day in a provincial reformatory. The judge recommended the man be sent to an institution where programs for alcoholics are available.

Standing Committee on Health, Welfare and Social Affairs, May 6, 1982.

SOCIETY'S PRESSURES

It was noted in section 15.1.2 that the woman in an abusive relationship will experience societal pressure to remain, particularly if she is married. Women are accustomed to taking responsibility for keeping marriage and family intact, and this sense of responsibility is encouraged by many of the people with whom the battered woman comes in contact. Often doctors, lawyers, judges, social workers, clergy, and even her friends and relatives urge a battered wife to return home to her husband, "where she belongs" (Hofeller, 1983). Her family and friends may not believe her claims of abuse, or they may even fear violence themselves from the man if they take steps to intervene.

THE REALITIES OF LEAVING

It cannot be denied that resolving to leave is difficult, especially if children are involved. The woman's fears for her own and her children's physical well-being when left suddenly alone and ill-prepared for self-sufficiency are real and justified. While the penalties for wife assault are more severe, and the powers of police to intervene and protect are now better defined, lack of effective, complete protection for victims is still an unfortunate reality. A recent report indicates that:

In the first half of 1979, police laid charges of assault in only 3% of all family violence cases, despite the fact that they advised 20% of the victims to seek medical treatment (Burris and Jaffe, 1985, p. 30).

In addition to physical danger, a woman often faces financial hardships, lack of employment opportunity (she may have few job skills), and lack of adequate housing for herself and her children. In many cases the community does not provide adequate support services such as daycare, job training, and counselling for such cases. For a woman who has been isolated socially and/or whose family and friends are not willing to support her actions actively, these obstacles may be insurmountable.

Table 15.1. Summary of assistance for battered women across Canada in the form of transition houses (Response, 1983)

Province	Number of Transition Houses	Average Length of Stay (days)	Provincial Legislation	Levels of Government Assistance
Newfoundland	1	3 days-3 months		Provincial
Prince Edward Island	1		Welfare Assist. Act	Provincial
Nova Scotia	2	21	Children Services Act	Provincial and Municipal
New Brunswick	7	14-28	Children and Family Services and Family Relations Act (Part II)	
Quebec	34	14-21		Provincial
Ontario	50	14-21	General Welfare Act	Provincial and Municipal
Manitoba	5	14-21	Community Services	Provincial and Municipal
Saskatchewan	6	45	Department of Social Service Act	Provincial and Municipal
Alberta	9	23	Dept. of Social Service & Community Health Act	Provincial
*British Columbia	30		Guaranteed Available Income for Need Act	Provincial

* Note: Due to recent changes in British Columbia's approach to social programmes, levels of assistance, and access, information presented may not be entirely accurate. Most assistance is provided by Winnipeg at the Municipal level in Manitoba.
Source: National Clearinghouse and Family Violence Survey "Women and Children in Transition" and interviewing with provincial authorities.

15.1.5 Assistance and Prevention

There are a number of things a woman in an abusive relationship can do to protect herself. Primarily, being able to flee a violent situation at a moment's notice is critical. Preparation includes such things as keeping hidden a spare set of car keys, extra money, and emergency telephone numbers. Emergency services now exist in most geographical areas, including emergency shelters for women (see Table 15.1), crisis lines, social service agencies, community mental health centres, and hospital emergency rooms.

Women who are being abused should be encouraged by friends or neighbours to talk to people who can lend support and guidance. As noted earlier, many women feel ashamed and reluctant to admit that they have been battered. It may be up to a family member or friend to come forward and make the woman aware of available support services.

Some communities now also offer counselling services and support groups for men who want to learn more acceptable ways of coping with their frustration and anger. As noted earlier, however, this can only be accomplished where the batterer accepts responsibility for his actions and recognizes that he, not others in his environment, must change. While it appears that abusive men can in fact learn new behaviour such as replacing aggression with assertiveness, it is unlikely that long-standing abusive relationships can change for the better. As explained by Walker (1979), "relationships that have been maintained by the man having power over the woman are stubbornly resistant to an equal power-sharing arrangement." Even with the help of skilled counsellors these relationships seldom become entirely resolved. "At best, violent assaults may be reduced in frequency and severity. Unassisted, they simply escalate to homicidal and suicidal proportions. The best hope for such couples is to terminate the relationship. There is a better chance that with another partner they can reorder the power structure and live as equals in a nonviolent relationship" (Walker, 1979, p.29).

Table 15.2. Directive from the Inspector of the Court Services Branch of the London City Police Force instructing officers to lay assault charges when they have reasonable and probable grounds to believe the assault took place.

Memo to: ALL RANKS   **From:** Inspector, Court Services Branch
Subject: Assault Complaints

1. Commencing immediately, charges are to be laid by our Force in all cases where there are reasonable and probable grounds revealed in the investigation. The practice of directing the victim to lay private informations is to cease.
2. Charges of common assault and assault causing bodily harm are to be laid in the Family Division of the Provincial Court only when the assault occurs between members living together in the same dwelling unit as a family.
3. All other assault charges are to be laid in the Criminal Division of the Provincial Court.
4. Wounding charges are to be laid in the Criminal Division of the Provincial Court.
5. The occurrence report and the charge sheets must indicate the relationship between the victim and the assailant.

(Source: Burris and Jaffe, p. 31, 1985)

Clearly, prevention of abuse in intimate relationships is a desirable goal, but one which is still a long way from being achieved. Attitudes toward violence and toward women must change if abuse is to stop. Until violence is rejected by our society and is condemned as a means of expressing anger or resolving conflict, some men will continue to see it as permissible at home. Men and women alike must understand that no one deserves to be beaten or physically threatened, regardless of the circumstances. There is a growing recognition by society that women cannot legitimately be expected to accept violence from their partners as a means of controlling them. This must also be reflected in law and law enforcement policies. The traditional response—or lack of it—by society's officials in cases of domestic violence is no longer acceptable; in many parts of North America the justice system is responding to this challenge. An example of this is the recently instituted policy of the London City Police Force in London, Ontario, Canada, described in Table 15.2.

15.2 CHILD ABUSE
Child and wife abuse patterns share several important features in terms of the interpersonal and psychological factors which characterize them. Specifically, these common features are as follows:
• Abuse results mainly from an inability on the batterer's part to handle stress—it has little or nothing to do with the behavior of the victim.
• Batterers and their victims are not only the poor, uneducated, psychotic, criminal, alcoholic, or otherwise abnormal element of society.
• Attacks are unpredictable and vary in frequency—this results in continued stress and fear on the part of the victim.
• The victim's self-esteem is eroded by repeated condemnation and criticism by his or her spouse/parent (i.e. the victim's most significant other).
• The batterer usually has had some experience of being abused.
• The batterer experiences low self-esteem, feelings of powerlessness

> **Said of the woman who has escaped and survived to begin a life without brutality:**
>
> She knows some of her own emotions have been killed, and she distrusts those who are infatuated with suffering—as if it were a source of life, not death. In her heart she is a mourner for those who have not survived. In her soul she is a warrior for those who are now as she was then. In her life she is both a celebrant and proof of women's capacity and will to survive, to become, to act, to change self and society. And each year she is stronger and there are more of her.
>
> Andrea Dworkin, 1985.

and frustration, and is fearful of true intimacy.

- The unpredictable nature of the abuse, and the frequent messages received by the victim that he or she is responsible for the beatings, leads the victim to try even harder to please, in order to avoid punishment.
- Consistent failure to succeed in pleasing, and thus in avoiding punishment, results in what is often referred to as "learned helplessness" (Walker, 1979). These are described next.

While some understanding of child abuse is facilitated by considering these common features, it also presents unique features.

15.2.1 Forms of Child Abuse

Child abuse generally is considered to include **physical abuse, emotional abuse**, physical and emotional **neglect**, and **sexual abuse** or exploitation. The first two are similar in character to the physical and emotional abuse experienced by women. Physical violence involves physically harmful action directed against the child, defined by any inflicted injury. Emotional abuse is defined as actively undermining a child's self-image, sense of worth, and self-confidence through consistent humiliation, rejection, or criticism. As with abused women, children who are physically battered nearly always experience emotional abuse also, but the reverse is not necessarily the case. Many children who are otherwise physically well cared for are abused or neglected emotionally, resulting in severe damage to the child's developing personality (Kempe and Kempe, 1978).

Neglect implies the failure to provide adequate nutrition, safety, health and medical care, attention and love, or other safeguards for the child's well-being (note that a distinction between physical neglect and willful injury, both of which can cause "accidental" harm, is often ill-defined). A common result of nutritional and medical neglect of infants and very young children is a condition known as **Failure to Thrive**. This is a life-threatening situation for a child, identified by such charac-

In 1982 official reports documented 1.3 million mal-treated children in the United States. Sixty-two percent suffered from a deprivation of necessities, 17% from minor physical injuries, 10% from emotional maltreatment, 7% from sexual abuse, and 2% from major physical injuries (American Humane Association, Highlights of Official Child Neglect and Abuse Reporting, 1982).

teristics as emaciation, seemingly frantic movement and expression, an inability to relax or respond to cuddling, and a voracious appetite once removed from the home (Kempe and Kempe, 1978).

Emotional neglect may be equally severe in terms of its effects on a child's development. As might be expected, this form of deprivation is much more difficult to document.

Sexual abuse as defined in a Canadian provincial government policy statement, is "Any sexual touching, sexual intercourse or sexual exploitation of a child and may include any sexual behaviour directed toward a child" (British Columbia, Canada, 1985). (A "child" under the Family and Child Service Act of British Columbia refers to a person under the age of 19).

15.2.2 Precipitating Factors

Not all potentially abusive parents abuse their children, nor do all parents, otherwise defined as adequate, treat their children fairly and appropriately all the time. If one were to chart the potential for abuse shown by all parents, the results would resemble the bell-shaped curve shown in Figure 15.2. However, it is important to consider the fact that circumstances, both past and present, play a large role in determining whether or not abuse or neglect actually occurs (Kempe and Kempe, 1978).

There are four factors which may be considered predisposing conditions likely to result in child abuse. The first involves the parents' background and problems. The second is the parents' perceptions of the child's physical and behavioural characteristics. The third and fourth factors relate to the immediate and ongoing stress in the lives of the parents. Specifically, child abuse is most likely to occur during moments of crisis and when there is no effective support system for a parent to rely on at such times.

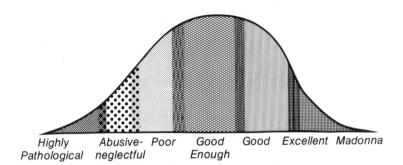

Highly Pathological   Abusive-neglectful   Poor   Good Enough   Good   Excellent   Madonna

Figure 15.2. The potential for abuse shown by all parents, represented on a bell-shaped curve. Reproduced with permission from Kempe, R.S. and Kempe, C.H., 1978.

PARENT'S BACKGROUND AND PROBLEMS

As noted above, the abusive parent is characterized as having very low self-esteem and feelings of powerlessness within his/her own life. A good description of the common pattern shown in the lives of potentially abusive parents was offered by Ackley (1977, p.22):

As children, potential abusers receive the message from their parents that they are inadequate and fundamentally disappointing. Potential abusers do not seriously question their parents' judgement on this point, but rather assume its accuracy. Thus, their first attempt at an intimate relationship, the one with their parents, fails to give them a belief in their own worth. Rather, the result is a daily parental message of disappointment and condemnation despite the child's desperate attempts to please.

A curious thing then occurs in adulthood. Potential abusers both seek and shun intimate relationships. On the one hand, they seek intimacy in order to obtain what was missing in the earlier parental relationship. This need leads them to define a close relationship as one in which, like the child, they can: (1) obtain emotional support and warmth without giving much in return, and (2) depend on their partner to solve the problems of living that adults are called upon to solve....

Alternatively, intimacy is shunned because the first childhood attempts were such failures.... The fear of disappointment keeps them from honestly trying but does not prevent the appearance of trying. The behavioral result of this complex set of feelings is that the potential abuser marries an individual who is less able than most to provide the emotional support sought. Such marriages are contracted, in part, because the basic feeling of worthlessness on the part of potential abusers precludes marriage to a truly giving individual. Furthermore, few mature people would be willing to accept a relationship on the terms set by the potential abuser. Potential abusers unsurprisingly find their marriages deeply disappointing.... The next step is to have children, the expectation being that they will finally have someone who truly loves them.

Such a parent, then, seeks to find the love and recognition that is lacking in his/her life, first in the marital partner, then in the child. The child is seen by the potential abuser as capable of satisfying adult needs, unrealistic as this may be. When this fulfillment does not materialize, the parent interprets this non-provision as intentional on the child's part. Parents see this child as "inadequate" in the same way that they, themselves were. The child then becomes a constant reminder of their own childhood feelings of inadequacy, anger, and bitterness which they still experience.

Often the parent sees physical punishment as an appropriate way to correct child behaviour. Given the distorted perceptions and expectations of the child that were reviewed above, it is but a short step for such correction to become abusive.

CHARACTERISTICS OF THE CHILD

As indicated above, the child is regarded as disappointing by a potentially abusive parent. While this partially results from the parent's own childish needs and unrealistic expectations, it also is often exaggerated by peculiarities within the child. This is seen in many cases where only one of several children in a family is abused. The abused child may have some type of physical or behavioural condition which puts him or her at greater risk than the other children. For example, a hyperkinetic child, who is difficult to manage under even ideal conditions, can easily become the target of abuse where the potential for it already exists in the character of the parent.

Apart from real physical or constitutional characteristics which make a certain child more trouble to a parent than another, some children have the misfortune of being simply "wrong" in the eyes of the parent. They may be the wrong sex, or have characteristics that remind the potentially abusive parent of a despised relative, or they may show features that are most hated by the parent within him or herself.

*Regardless of the form of abuse, deprivation, or
combination of effects which occur, an outstanding feature
of all seems to be the inability of the parent(s) to
recognize the child's needs and limitations.*

MOMENTS OF CRISIS

Child abuse situations usually occur in response to some crisis which "overloads" a parent's coping ability. The crisis itself may appear to an objective observer as a minor incident, but it is exaggerated out of proportion by a potentially abusive parent.

When such a crisis occurs, whether it be internal or external, the parent has few, if any, personal resources for dealing effectively with it. The childishness and inability to relate intimately to anyone, already described as characterizing the potentially abusive parent, now creates feelings of isolation, an inability to ask for help, impulsiveness, and poor problem solving skills.

LACK OF SUPPORT

The final factor that precipitates child abuse is that there is no effective support or "life-line" for the parent when needed. In many families this support is provided by one parent, who may take charge of the child in times of an emotional crisis or overload on the part of the other. Even if direct partner support is not actually present at a time of crisis, if emotional support is generally available to the parent, it often is possible for him/her to postpone an emotional outburst rather rather than becoming abusive.

15.2.3 Abuse versus Neglect

The relationship between abuse and neglect is not well understood. It is clear, however, that they result from similar factors, as described in section 15.2.2. Also, they may be expressed in both physical or emotional form. Regardless of the form of abuse, deprivation, or combination of effects which occur, an outstanding feature of all seems to be the inability of the parent(s) to **recognize the child's needs and limitations**.

In the case of physical or emotional battering, the parent's inaccurate perception of the child's or infant's behaviour as willfully defiant may be a cause for punishment (i.e., when the baby has a bowel movement at an "inconvenient" time or place). Neglect, on the other hand, often stems from the parent's fear that attention or care beyond that required for "survival" will spoil the child. In such a case, the needy and helpless child may become completely emaciated, and yet the neglectful mother perceives instead a monstrously greedy parasite who threatens to drain her of all reserves of food, affection, and energy. A typical example of the type of distortion found in perceptions of infantile behaviour by abusive parents is given by Kempe and Kempe (1978, p. 19):

Keith was seven months old and beginning to have activity which was increasingly irritating to his mother. Activity during diapering she found most unbearable and she said, "I had to whack him again and again to make him hold still". Keith was observed during diapering, lying completely immobile, intently watching his mother's hands with a serious expression on his face. Three months later, the mother complained that Keith had learned his lesson only too well. During diapering and dressing he now became quite limp, failing to hold up his hands to have his shirt put on. Mother said she would "have to show him he could only go so far before he got the flat of her hand again".

One other point about abuse and neglect is that parents who neglect their children generally have a high potential for indulging in physical battering as well. Thus, a parent who is found to have severely neglected a child (e.g., in cases where a child is hospitalized for Failure to Thrive) must have his/her own needs also considered in any form of intervention that takes place. Should this not occur, and instead only the responsibilities of parenting be reiterated and emphasized, there is a strong likelihood that this parent will become actively abusive toward the child (Kempe and Kempe, 1978).

> Most of us never tell. We learned, too early, to hide our fears, our confusions, and our anger about the sexual and personal violations which made our lives hell when we were only three or four or twelve years old. Our lonely and haunting manifestations of pain remain with us throughout our lives—shadows we can never escape.
>
> A Survivor of Incest (Vis-a-Vis, 1984)

15.2.4 Sexual Abuse

Statistics reported in the U.S.A. (Rush, 1980) show that:

- In a random sample of 4,000 women, 25% were found to have experienced a sexual encounter with an adult before age thirteen.
- In a study of college students, 19.2% of the 530 females and 8.6% of the 266 males sampled had been sexually victimized as children.
- Of 5,058 **reported** sex crimes in New York City in 1975, 27.2% of the victims were under age 14, and most of these (20%) were female.

A Committee on Sexual Offences Against Children and Youths (Department of Justice of Health and Welfare, Canada 1984) reported over 10,000 cases of sexual offence against children and youths.   They found that:

One in two females and one in three males were victims of unwanted sexual acts which include threats, exposures, sexual touchings and attempted or actual assaults. About four in five victims were under the age of 21 when the first offence was committed against them. The Committee found that virtually all offenders were male. One in four assailants was a family member or a person in a position of trust; half were friends or acquaintances; one in six was a stranger.

(Vis-a-Vis, Autumn, 1984)

These statistics are clearly disturbing. Perhaps even more important is the fact that most cases of child sexual abuse remain undisclosed. It has been estimated that, "Fifty to eighty percent of all such incidents go unreported" (Rush, 1980).

While sexual abuse may occur with children of any age (Rush [1980] notes that rape has been reported on children of six months or less), the most vulnerable are the most trusting (2-6 year olds) and those at the peak period of pubertal development (12-16 year olds). The physical and psychological effects of sexual abuse and exploitation on children are immense; psychological damage in particular may never be repaired (Miller & Porter, 1983; Mills, Rieker, and Carmen, 1984).

15.3 EFFECTING SOLUTIONS TO FAMILY VIOLENCE

Any comprehensive discussion of current approaches to intervention in family violence crises is beyond the scope of this chapter. Nevertheless, it is not enough to report the incidence of the problem without considering ways being studied to alleviate it. Public and social service agencies work at three different levels to modify and reduce the effect of all forms of family violence.

First, through public education and media publicity a major effort is being undertaken to increase public awareness and understanding of the dimensions and prevalence of domestic violence. Dissemination of such information and educational resources is considered the best possible means of prevention and eventual eradication of family violence. Clearly, legal, medical, and counselling intervention must be promoted also, but these latter measures are likely to be taken only after considerable damage to the victim has already occurred.

Real change is not possible until public awareness and consciousness has been raised enough to stop the violence from being tolerated on any level. Patriarchical attitudes prevalent in our society unfortunatey do not support this type of fundamental change; nonetheless, women's voices are forcing many such issues to the forefront of societal awareness. No longer can the magnitude of the problem be hidden or denied through enforced silence on the part of the victims. A wide array of books, films and self-help kits is now available for victims, parents, teachers, medical and mental health personnel, and any other person or group wishing to understand or cope better with family violence issues. Figure 15.3 shows one type of informational item now available.

Increasing pressure has been applied recently to the judicial systems, both in Canada and the United States, to take more effective action against the problem. It is not yet possible to guarantee physical and legal adequate protection against violent family members, but the

Streetproof your Children:
Helpful Rules to Keep Young People Safe

- Ten percent of Canadian families will be confronted by sexual abuse.
- One out of every three females will be sexually molested before age eighteen.
- One out of every ten boys will be sexually molested before age eighteen.
- More than 85% of abusers are known to the victim.

Most parents want to educate their children about sexual abuse, but they don't know how. These guidelines will help parents to teach their children how to keep safe. Remember, you can't tell a child too much; knowledge doesn't stimulate inappropriate behavior—ignorance does. Parents who talk openly with their children will be "askable" parents, and children will feel free to bring their worries and concerns to them in the future.

1. An unattended child is a child at risk. Arrange with your child an alternative place to wait if you are delayed, especially in the dark winter evenings. Suggest a well-lit store or inside an arena or school.

2. Always, where possible, have children walk in pairs or goups.

3. Children should always travel the same way home.

4. Use a secret family code. Children should never go with anyone, not even a close family friend, unless they are able to give the child the code. Once the code has been used, it should be changed.

5. Don't allow your young child to go to a public washroom unattended.

6. Check your babysitter's credentials thoroughly. In your absence, they are guardians of a priceless treasure.

7. Tell your child it is not rude to ignore an adult who is asking directions on the street. Another adult could be asked for more accurate directions.

8. Tackle the subject of sexual abuse prevention with the same honest, matter-of-fact manner you would attach to road safety. Remember, the only time a child will ask you about sexual abuse is after it has happened. Open the subject and your child will remember that you are askable.

9. Introduce your child to the "Hot and Cold" game. Describe a situation which is 'cool'—"imagine you are walking home from a friend's house"... then make it 'tepid'—"you hear footsteps and think someone is following you"... Request the child to make the situation 'cool' again and suggest that it would be appropriate to cross the street. Now make the situation warmer by indicating that the footsteps also have crossed the street. Suggest that the child cross back again, and explain that if the footsteps cross the street for a second time, then the situation is "hot". Ask for ways to "cool" down the situation. You might help with ideas such as going into a lighted store, going into a neighbour's house, looking quickly for a Block Parent, or because it is a "hot" situation, they might yell "fire" which will bring a quicker response than "help".

10. Discuss with your child the difference between fact and fancy, fact and fiction so that they may understand the nature of taking an oath. (This may be necessary for a court appearance).

11. If you suspect that an abuse has taken place:
- DO encourage the child to talk about it.
- DO establish in the child's mind that he/she is not to blame.
- DO NOT correct the child's story; listen to the original words, even those which are babyish or family words.
- DO NOT suggest or modify what the child is trying to say. Your ideas might confuse the truth.
- DO NOT show horror or anger; however if caught by surprise and unable to control your emotions, be clear that your anger is meant for the offender, not the child.

12. When you are aware of an incident of sexual abuse, call the police or the child welfare authorities immediately. Ensure that a social worker, a police officer and someone supportive to the child is present when the evidence is given.

From: **Vis-à-Vis 2(3)**: National Clearinghouse on Family Violence, Health and Welfare Canada.

Figure 15.3: Streetproof your children.

situation is improving, as evidenced by changes in policing instructions in many localities (e.g. see Table 15.2). Another way in which
various judiciaries have responded is to change policies for filing and
dropping charges relating to family violence. The main thrust of these
changes is to:

1. Require through state (U.S.A.) and provincial (Canada) law that
   all professionals report suspected cases of child abuse and neglect
   (Response, 1984).
2. Require any adult to report "reasonable grounds for believing that
   a child may be in need of protection." Note: The same legislation
   protects the reporting individual from legal action taken against
   him or her (i.e., in terms of breach of professional/client confiden-
   tiality or civil liability). In some areas, failure to report is considered an offence that may result in prosecution (e.g., Provinces
   of B.C. and Ontario, Canada).
3. Reduce the high rates of case attrition (i.e., instances where charges
   of assault against a family member have been dropped) by adopting policies that divest family victims of the burden of prosecution and assign it to the state or province. This may mean either
   (a) disallowing victims from unilaterally dropping charges against
   their abusers, once filed, or (b) specifying that the responsibility
   for actually filing charges lies with the state/province (the latter is
   preferable, as it is less likely to "backfire" on the victim).

A third form of action being taken is that of treatment intervention,
coordinated with improved laws and law enforcement. For example,
while transition houses and crisis services for battered women and their
children offer temporary shelter, they work closely with the police,
legal services, and counselling agencies who are able to offer appropriate assistance in their own area of responsibility. In cases where
police officers are the first to intervene, victims of family violence are
encouraged to seek emergency shelter and crisis counselling from local
services.

Schools are also taking a stronger role in detection, prevention, and assistance in cases of family violence. Increasingly school personnel have information on how to deal with children who may be in need of assistance (see Table 15.3). Joint programs with other community service agencies are being developed in many school districts. In some cases schools even offer special programs for children who have been in transition houses or some other form of family violence assistance program. For example:

A Toronto public school has provided a special program for children who come from four transition houses for battered women in the school area. A team composed of a teacher and child care worker assesses the child's needs on entry and designs an individual program based on each child's abilities and emotional state. With staff-to-child ratio of 1:4, the children are able to receive individual attention. It helps to know that other children in the same class are going through the same kind of painful experience.

(Vis-a-Vis, III(1), 1985).

In addition, counselling for the offender in areas of both wife assault and child abuse is now offered in many locales. The aim is to prevent further violence by helping abusive people learn more effective and less damaging ways of coping with their problems and stresses. One innovative program in Saskatoon, Saskatchewan (Canada) involves a comprehensive, community-wide network of educational and support services for families under stress.

Table 15.3. What Can School Personnel Do?

For Child Abuse and Neglect

- Know the indicators and the reporting laws for physical/emotional abuse and neglect.
- Plan a team approach with the principal, counsellor, nurse, and teachers.
- Report the abuse to the child welfare agency on the same day as you suspect it.
- Keep accurate records.
- Be sensitive to the child's social, physical, and emotional needs at school even after the child welfare agency becomes involved.

For Child Sexual Abuse

- Assume the child is telling the truth.
- Assure the child that he/she is not to blame.
- Contact the child welfare agency or the police immediately.
- After disclosure, do not feel that you must interview the child: that is the job of the child welfare workers or the police. However, remain responsive, supportive, and attentive if the child wishes to continue talking.
- If the report is intra-familial, do not contact the parents. Leave that task to the child welfare worker or to the police. If the report is extra-familial, contact the parents immediately.
- Remain with the child until the child welfare officials arrive to interview the child. The child must be protected from the alleged perpetrator.

For Wife Assault

- Be sensitive and aware. Acting-out at school is often a symptom of problems at home.
- Seek out helpful school and community resources which can offer public education and counselling.
- Keep in mind that children in families where there is wife assault also may be abused or neglected.
- Teach children that violence is not an acceptable problem-solver.
- Correct the imbalance in sex-role stereo-typing through the curriculum.

Domestic violence is condoned and/or perpetuated by ascribing blame or responsibility for the abuse to any source other than where it rightfully belongs.

Considered a pioneer in developing preventive and early intervention programs, the Saskatoon Society for the Protection of Children program includes:
1. Totline—a weekend crisis phone line;
2. A Parent-Aide Program—to assist inexperienced or high-risk parents to learn basic skills in coping with life stress and child management;
3. Parenting programs such as Stress Management Group and Parents Anonymous;
4. A Child Abuse Therapy Coordinator; and (perhaps the most innovative of all interventions)
5. The Crisis Nursery—short-term (up to 72 hours) housing for the children of families in crisis.

15.4 SUMMARY
Most of the myths identified here and in other literature on wife assault share a common theme. That is, domestic violence is condoned and/or perpetuated by ascribing blame or responsibility for the abuse to any source other than where it rightfully belongs. Variations on this theme are reflected in views that blame the woman (e.g., her problems, illness, behavior or inadequacies), alcohol, drugs, unemployment, financial hardship, lack of education, women's liberation, or psychopathic personality in the male. As noted in Myth 8, it is only by helping batterers to accept responsibility for their violent behavior that they can learn more adaptive responses to problems and stress.

15.5 RESOURCES/FURTHER READING

WIFE ABUSE
Getting Free: A Handbook for Women in Abusive Relationships. NiCarthy, G. Seattle, Washington: The Seal Press, 1982.

Learning to Live Without Violence: A Handbook for Men. Sonkin, David J. and Durphy, Michael, 1982. San Francisco: Volcano Press, Inc.

Men Who Batter ($7.50 U.S.). Similar to the Wife Abuse packet, this one contains information useful for those developing or working in programs for men who batter their wives. Available from the Centre for Women Policy Studies, see references.

Sheltering Battered Women: A National Study and Service Guide. Roberts, Albert R. New York: Springer Publishing Co., 1981.

Stopping the Violence: Canadian Programs for Assaultive Men. Browning, James, 1984. National Clearinghouse on Family Violence (see references).

Transition House: How to Establish a Refuge for Battered Women. MacLeod, Flora. Vancouver, B.C.: United Way of the Lower Mainland, 1982. Available from the National Clearinghouse on Family Violence, Health and Welfare Canada, Ottawa, K1A 1B5.

Understand Wife Assault: A Training Manual for Counsellors and Advocates. Sinclair, D., 1985. Available from Ontario Government Bookstore, Publications Services Section, 880 Bay St., Toronto, Ont., Canada, M7A 1N8.

Victimology: An International Journal, 2:(3/4), 1977/78. Special issue on spouse abuse and family violence.

Wife Abuse ($7.50 U.S.). A resource collection containing up-to-date information on all aspects of wife abuse. The packet also contains the CWPS 1984 Fact sheet on wife abuse and an annotated bibliography on the topic. Available from the Centre for Women Policy Studies, see references.

Wife Abuse in the Armed Forces. West, L., Turner, W.M. and Dunwoody, E. Washington, D.C.: Centre for Women Policy Studies, 1981. This report pulls together national and international information on the nature of wife abuse in the military community. See references.

CHILD ABUSE/NEGLECT
Self Help and the Treatment of Child Abuse. Borman, L.D. and Lieber, L.L. National Committee for Prevention of Child Abuse, 332 South Michigan Avenue, Suite 1250, Chicago, Illinois, 60604-4357, 1984.

Sigurdson, E. and Jones, K. The development of a rural team to deal with child abuse. **Canadian Family Physician, 28:** 1180-1184, 1982.

The Parenting Module. This education kit contains 16 units designed to inform junior and senior high school students about the parent-child relationship and to explore the function, needs, and future of the family. Available from: Red Deer Family Resource Team, Alberta Social Services and Community Health, 4920 51st Street, Red Deer, Alberta, Canada. T4N 6K8.

The Sexual Aggressor: Current Perspectives on Treatment. Greer, J.G. and Stuart, I.R. (eds). New York: Van Nostrand Reinhold Co., 1983.

15.6 REFERENCES

Ackley, D.C. A brief overview of child abuse. **Social Casework**, January, 21-24, 1977.

American Humane Association. **Highlights of Official Child Neglect and Abuse Reporting, 1982**. Denver, Colorado: American Humane Association, 1984.

British Columbia, Canada. **Inter-Ministry Child Abuse Handbook**. (Policy statement on child abuse for the province of B.C.) Victoria, B.C.: Queen's Printer for B.C., 1985.

British Columbia Ministry of Labour, Women's Programs, and the Ministry of Attorney General. **Information Relating to Wife Assault in British Columbia**, Victoria, B.C.: Queen's Printer for British Columbia, 1985.

Burris, C.A. and Jaffe, P. Wife abuse as a crime: The impact of police laying charges. In B.C. Ministry of Labour, Women's Programs, and the Ministry of Attorney General, **Information Relating to Wife Assault in British Columbia**. Victoria, B.C.: Queen's Printer for British Columbia, pp. 30-34, 1985.

Davidson, T. **Conjugal Crime**. New York: Hawthorn Books, 1978.

Dobash, R.E. and Dobash, R. **Violence Against Wives**. New York: The Free Press, Macmillan, 1979.

Dworkin, A. The bruise that doesn't heal. In B.C. Ministry of Labour, Women's Programs, and the Ministry of Attorney General, **Information Relating to Wife Assault in British Columbia**. Victoria, B.C.: Queen's Printer for British Columbia, pp. 11-13, 1985.

Edleson, J.L., Eisikovits, Z. and Guttman, E. Men who batter women: A critical review of the evidence. **Journal of Family Issues, 6**(2): 229-247, 1985.

Ganley, A.L. **Participant's Manual for Workshop to Train Mental Health Professionals to Counsel Court Mandated Batterers**. Washington, D.C.: Center for Women Policy Studies (reprinted in Information Relating to Wife Assault in British Columbia, 1985), 1981.

Hofeller, K. **Battered Women, Shattered Lives**. Palo Alto, Ca.: R. and E. Research Associates, Inc., 1983.

House of Commons, Canada. **Report on Violence in the Family: Wife Battering**. Standing Committee on Health, Welfare and Social Affairs, 1982.

Kempe, R.S. and Kempe, C.H. **Child Abuse**. Cambridge, Mass: Harvard University Press, 1978.

Kuhl, A.F. Personality traits of abused women: Masochism myth refuted. **Victimology, 9**(3-4): 450-463, 1984.

Langley, R. and Levy, R.C. **Wife Beating: The Silent Crisis**. New York: Pocket Books, 1977.

McLeod, L. **Wife Battering in Canada: The vicious circle**. Prepared for the Canadian Advisory Council on the Status of Women, 1980.

Miller, D. and Porter, C. Self-blame in victims of violence. **Journal of Social Issues, 39**(2): 139-152, 1983.

Mills, T., Rieker, P.P. and Carmen, E.H. Hospitalization experiences of victims of abuse. **Victimology, 9**(3-4): 436-449, 1984.

NiCarthy, G. **Getting Free: A handbook for women in abusive relationships**. Seattle: The Seal Press, 1982.

O'Reilly, J. Wife beating: The silent crime. **Time**, September

Response (to Violence in the Family and Sexual Assault). Newsletter of the Center for Women Policy Studies, 2000 p Street, N.W., Ste 508, Washington, D.C. 20036-5997.

Rush, F. The Best Kept Secret: Sexual Abuse of Children. Englewood Cliffs, N.J.: Prentice-Hall, 1980.
Ryan,W. Blaming the Victim. New York: Pantheon Books/Random House, 1971.

Standing Committee on Health, Welfare and Social Affairs. Third Report to the House: Wife Battering. Marcel Roy, Chairman. House of Commons, Issue No. 34, Thursday, May 6, 1982.

Stark, E., Flitcraft, A. and Frazier, W. Medicine and patriarchal violence: The social construction of a "private" event. International Journal of Health Services, 9(3): 461-490, 1979.

Symonds, A. Violence against women: The myth of masochism. American Journal of Psychotherapy, 33(2): 161-173, 1979.

Vis-a-Vis. Newsletter of the National Clearinghouse on Family Violence, Health and Welfare Canada, Ottawa, K1A 1B5.

Walker, L.E. The Battered Woman. New York: Harper and Row, 1979.

Walker, L.E. Victimology and the psychological perspectives of battered women. Victimology 8(1-2): 82-104, 1983.

15.7 STUDY QUESTIONS

1. Why is it important to place full responsibility for abusive behavior with the batterer and not blame it on uncontrollable or external causes?
2. Why do you think affluent women seldom use available emergency services such as crisis counselling and transition houses? Is it that they are not victims of abuse, that they have "their own" resources to rely on, or is it that shame and societal pressure cause them to suffer in silence?
3. What changes to law and law enforcement policies would you recommend in order to increase the safety of women and children from violent homes?

Note: Throughout this chapter the terms "wife assault" and "wife abuse" are used. It is important to note that marriage is not a prerequisite to battering, although it is reported most often by married women. Thus these terms are used in reference to the abuse of women by their male partners in a sexual relationship, whether married or not.

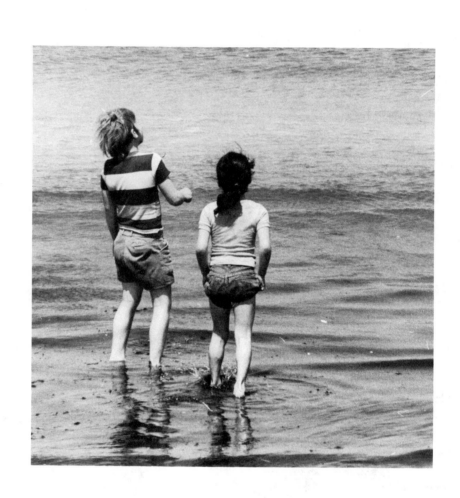

16

Summary

The doctor of the future will give no medicine but will interest his patients in the care of the human frame, in diet and in the cause and prevention of disease.

INTRODUCTION

In this book several contributors have reviewed contemporary health issues and practices and the comfort and happiness of people in various societies throughout the world. Of necessity in an introductory text like this, an in-depth study of every topic is impossible, if not undesirable, given the complexity of some of the subjects discussed. Even in the relatively short period of one year during which the original manuscript, after acceptance by the publisher, was readied for publication, significant changes in world events, international relations, and intra-governmental affairs closer to home in North America forced extensive rewriting of portions of the text. Even now, as you read it, some parts will already be out of date. The book itself is a significant departure from the conventional health text, because in it we have truly attempted to raise issues that bear upon the long term health and happiness of people, no matter how far removed these issues may seem from the immediate, pressing concerns of the moment. We have tried sometimes to raise the consciousness of the reader to global issues that may soon become national, community and quickly personal issues, which are currently, more often than not, of an undesirable nature. Undoubtedly to change the undesirable progress of events in the future, significant, even radical changes in thinking about how we live will be needed. In a relatively few years life has accelerated in the developed nations to such a pace that it allows no time, no space, no ability to live in consonance with it. In addition, unless people in developed countries are willing to contain their material desires, there is little hope for underdeveloped nations to improve their lot through their sharing more equitably in the resources of the world. Let us consider those areas where real concerns are beginning to stir action at inter-governmental levels.

The Environment:

Since the Industrial Revolution people in Western Nations have considerably advanced the comfort, stimulation, variety, and adventure in their

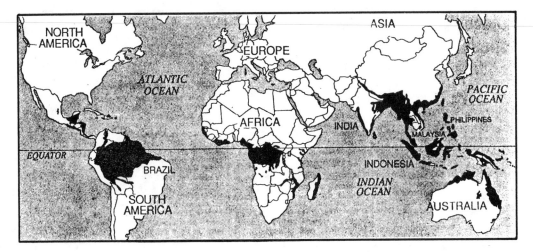

Figure 16.1. Within 50 years, most of the rainforests shown will have vanished; only those in the Amazon and Zaire basins will likely remain. Reproduced with permission from Bennell, B. **The Globe and Mail**, Jan. 25, 1986.

lives. During this progress little concern for the environment was shown. Why should it have been? The land, the sea, and the air were boundless; the complex interactions between events noted in Chapter 2 were unrealized; progress was limitless. In the forty years since the end of the Second World War, modern science accelerated the pace of environmental deterioration still more. Modern methods applied to every type of human activity bring a mixed blessing of surface progress and hidden menace.

Forest loss:
The rate of forest loss is catastrophic. 100 years ago 15 million sq. kilometers of forest covered the earth. Now only 9 million remain and these are eroding at a rate of 200,000 sq. kilometers a year. Consider the significance of this; recent progress made in feeding the world is directly due to the forest's wild plant strains of cereal crops. Many modern crop varieties contain genetic material from these wild forms, making them resistant to disease or suitable for multiple cropping. A central component of the Green revolution package, improving Mexico's, India's, and China's wheat production several fold was a wheat bred from wild Mexican strains in the 60s. Many medicines and potent drugs are manufactured first from plant life before their eventual chemical synthesis. In the next 30 years 250,000 wild plant species will disappear with the vanishing forests together with hundreds of millions of years of evolution.

Within 50 years, at this current rate of depletion, most of the rain forests shown in Figure 16.1 will have vanished. Concomitantly, as forests are burned they add two billion tons of carbon products (CO_2) per year to the atmosphere, rather than removing carbon dioxide from the atmosphere to produce oxygen by photosynthesis.

Global Temperature Changes:
Carbon dioxide, however, accumulates far more from our burning of fossil fuels (oil, gas, coal) than from destruction of the tropical forests. There is

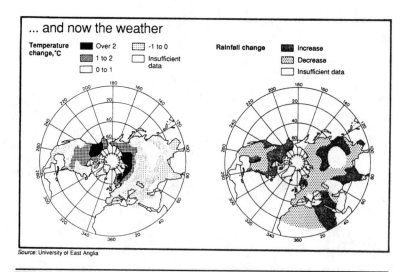

Figure 16.2. Estimates of world temperature and rainfall changes accompanying a warming of the globe. Reproduced with permission from Science and Technology. **The Economist,** Nov. 29, 1986.

a possibility that by the year 2100 the concentration of CO_2 in the atmosphere will have doubled from present levels, warming the globe by between 1.5 to 4.5°C over its surface due to the green house effect noted in Chapter 4. Estimates of world temperature and rainfall changes accompanying this rise in temperature are shown in Figure 16.2. The long term effects of such changes are not yet understood, but probably relate to natural calamities of flood, agricultural disasters, desertification, etc. One solution would be to close down fossil-fueled power stations in favour of nuclear power but nuclear power presents its own attendant health risks.

Nuclear Power:
To rely exclusively on nuclear fission for power is to court health disasters similar to the one at Chernobyl (Russia) on April 26th, 1986. The health care legacies of such disasters are extraordinary. It has been estimated that, as a result of radiation released by the accident, 40,000 extra deaths from cancer will occur in the next 70 years among the 75 million people living in the Western Soviet Union. Already, in 1987, blood samples from victims exposed to radiation show a link between the degree of radiation exposure and the number of mutated cells in the blood system. Western nuclear experts doubt Russian plans to fix flaws in similar reactors in the rest of the country which would ensure their safety.

A yet unresolved problem still being researched is the safe disposal of nuclear waste. In Canada by the year 2010, thirty years of research by Atomic Energy of Canada at Lac du Bonnet in Manitoba, some of it carried out jointly with the U.S.A., will have preceded the first commitment of spent high level radioactive fuel cells to permanent container facilities deep underground. It will linger there forever, some elements of the fuel remaining radioactive for tens of thousands of years. Meanwhile, accumulating waste lies in limbo in deep tanks of water at reactor sites around the country; waiting until the research on safe disposal is completed and a decision on appropriate sites is made. The health risks inherent in such disposal seem increasingly remote, but so did the risk of meltdowns at Chernobyl, Russia in 1986, and before that at Three Mile Island near Harrisburg, Pennsylvania in 1979, and before that, of a reactor fire in 1976 at Sellafield, North of Liverpool and, in the same year, of a nuclear waste tank explosion at Kasli, in Russia.

Spent fuel is not the only reactive waste produced. Uranium mine tailings in Canada have accumulated to 160 million tons. Protective clothing, materials from hospitals, universities, laboratories, and so forth are lower level wastes, but still hazardous if carelessly treated.

How continuously vigilant are the operators of commercial Nuclear Power Plants around the world? In the U.S.A. it seems, not very. The Nuclear Regulatory Commission (Del Vecchio, 1987) recently observed that California's Diablo Canyon Nuclear Power Plant's management had faltered from its previously high level safety and maintenance record since the second of the plant's two reactors was licensed. At the other end of the country, only a few miles from Three Mile Island, the Commission has closed the Peach Bottom Atomic Power Station because of operator violations of safety procedures. It seems accepted in the Industry that plants are infinitely better designed and safer than was the case previously, but now human fallibility is the danger. Human error arising from the monotony and boredom of increasingly invariant, vigilant tasks is responsible for all nuclear accidents so far. Another major problem is how to ensure responsibility of nation states to share, unselfishly and promptly, information on their acute catastrophies as well as their chronic, more insidious, environmental problems in order to safeguard the health of neighboring countries. The nature and extent of the Russian nuclear disaster, which obviously could not be contained within national boundaries, was not communicated to the West until many hours after it occurred and after pollution of neighbors' space, land, and food supply took place. Similarly the disastrous chemical fire at the Sandox factory in Basle in 1986, which polluted the Rhine for many miles through several neighboring countries, was not

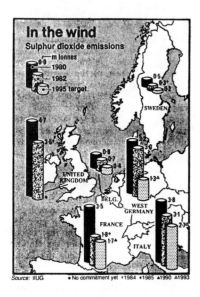

Figure 16.3. Europe's commitments to lower the health hazard of 18 million tons of sulphur dioxide annually polluting European skies. Reproduced with permission from Villages Correspondent, **The Economist**, Mar. 14, 1987.

immediately reported by Switzerland. Even within the single principal community of nations existing at this time, the European Economic Community, each member of the group still tends to protect its own interests. 1987, however, is the European Year of the Environment. Figure 16.3 shows Europe's commitments to lower the health hazard of 18 million tons of sulphur dioxide annually polluting European skies.

Pollution of the air with sulphur dioxide, nitrogen oxides and ozone is suspected of being the chief cause of lake sterilization and deforestation of central Europe, where for the past 6 years trees have been getting sick and dying in 15 European countries. The German's call it Waldsterben - Forest Death. Similar inexplicable declines in North American forests are taking place. This adds further deforestation to the planned razing of the forests, noted earlier, to provide arable land. The critical time scale of the search for solution and eradication of the problem can be no more than a decade before irreparable damage is done but no concensus of when to start has yet been achieved. Figure 16.4 compares the immediate environmental quality of the forest in North America just a century apart. Yet eighty-two metropolitan areas in the USA, containing 1/3 of the population, continued to violate key federal air pollution standards in 1986, particularly with regard to safe ozone levels.

Only recently did the U.S.A. commit $2.5 billion (to be matched by industrial contributions) to help solve a similar air pollution problem shared with neighboring Canada. It is estimated that failure to limit toxic gas emissions from coal-fueled furnaces of the American mid-west will destroy many of the lakes and forests in central and eastern Canada in the next 30 years, to say nothing of the untold damage to property and health close to the sites of such emissions. The ill-resolve of central government to act previously on this problem in the USA has prompted six U.S. states (Pennsylvania, Maine, Rhode Island, Virginia, New York, and Minnesota), to join forces to promote acid-rain control legislation at the state level.

The solid residues of modern living that threaten our health are more

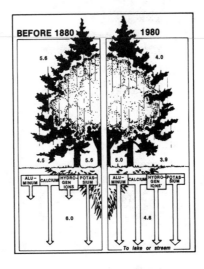

Figure 16.4. Compares the immediate environmental quality of the forest in North America just a century apart. Reproduced with permission from Cross, M., **South China Post**, Dec. 8, 1986.

obvious accretions than the gaseous, which escape into the surrounding air. Burgeoning new homes in suburban areas often threaten to overcome waste treatment and sewage systems. Chapter 4 indicated that sewage systems of many major cities even in developed countries rely only upon primary rather than the secondary and tertiary treatment of household effluents that are really needed. More hazardous still are the toxic wastes of industry. Technological development of incineration temperatures of up to 17,000°C will dispose of a good part of organic waste in the future. Biodegradation is increasingly able to deal with even the most troublesome of the chemicals previously dumped in landfills for lack of incineration capacity. These landfills now are so diluted with dirt that they cannot be incinerated properly. In the USA a "Superfund" was set up in 1981 to clear up the toxic waste dumps, but the reappropriation of funds to it is fraught with industrial lobbying and political irresolution on who should pay. Thus, currently, nearly 1,000 of the most hazardous waste sites nation-wide continue to spill into the environment. Most notable of these is that from the West Contra Costa County sanitary landfill in Richmond, California, which has leaked into San Francisco Bay wetlands. At its current level of funding the Environmental Protection Agency indicates that the timetable of closure for these sites begun in 1984 will have to extend into the 1990s. There remain a further 18,000 abandoned and uncontrolled hazardous waste sites not covered by Superfund and 93,000 municipal and industrial landfills with such a long history of uncontrolled dumping into them before regulation, that no one knows what is in them. Then there are 180,000 miniature industrial lakes of waste across the country, 2.3 million underground fuel tanks, 84% of which are made of bare steel unable to resist corrosion—now 5 to 10% of them are leaking. In addition, there still are 20 million septic tanks periodically cleaned out with toxic chemicals. Similar kinds of pollutant sources exist to greater or lesser degrees throughout all modern industrialized societies and it is essential that they be reduced by simultaneous efforts to decrease or destroy them at their point of origin

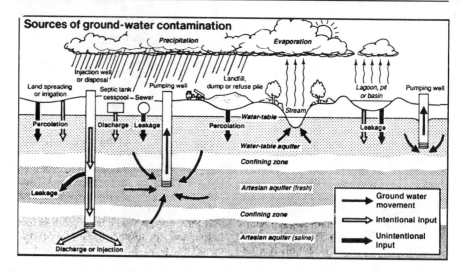

Sources of ground-water contamination

Figure 16.5. Shows the sources of ground-water contamination. Reproduced with permission from Feature Article, **The Economist**, Oct. 4, 1986.

and to continue to clean up existing areas of serious ground pollution which threaten the most vital of all human resources....water.

Water:

Where ground water is an important source of a country's water supply, ground pollution is an acute problem. Eight percent of all water used and 40% of that used for irrigation in the U.S.A. lies in underground reservoirs called aquifers, located in tiny pockets or in huge deposits like the Ogallala aquifier underlying parts of eight states from South Dakota to Texas. Figure 16.5 shows the vulnerability of these underground supplies to pollutants. Even this vast continuously renewable resource is now being depleted in the West, where withdrawals have increased from 35 to 90 billion gallons a day in just 30 years. Each year Arizona uses 2.5 million acre-feet more than can be replenished by nature. Aquifers replenish slowly at a rate of 5-50 feet annually. When the aquifer in a region becomes exhausted, desert returns. This is the case in some parts of Texas where the Ogallala has been depleted. Half of America's population rely upon groundwater for drinking supplies. Thus, to have it contaminated by leaks from storage sites, fuel tanks, septic tanks, agricultural run off (pesticides, herbicides, fertilizers) is potentially catastrophic. Already 40 polluted public water supplies contain more than the acceptable limit of nitrate. The Office of Technological Assessment (see reference in Chapter 2) has observed that "the consumption of ground water contaminated with chemicals can result in acute, subchronic and chronic health impacts".

These converging, interacting effects from diverse sectors of modern living (recall Chapter 2 feedback effects) illustrate the complex management task facing humanity in order to recover and maintain the natural balance pre-existing our intrusion.

Figure 16.6 illustrates a typical problem together with some existing and planned solutions. Water in the west is becoming scarce. Large diversion schemes previously funded mainly by Federal funds (e.g., the Los

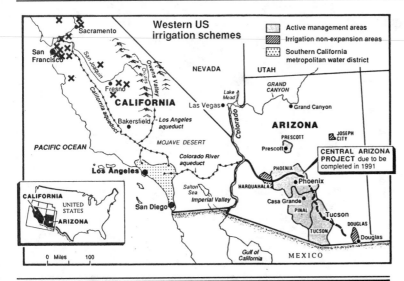

Figure 16.6. Western U.S. irrigation schemes. Major toxic waste sites in California are shown marked by an X. Reproduced with permission from Feature Article, **The Economist**, Oct. 4, 1986.

Angeles aqueduct, the Colorado river aqueduct, and the Central Arizona Project) will in the future have to be funded by the State in a major way and thus are unlikely to be implemented. Toxic hazard waste sites have sprung up throughout the area (59 in California alone, some of which are shown in Figure 16.6). Water consumption is burgeoning.

Solutions undertaken include:
- Cleaning up the toxic waste sites
- Active state management of water, as in Arizona, by:
  1. legislating limits on water use by householders, farmers and industry; discouraging profligate use.
  2. Controlling the use to which land may be put (e.g., for new agricultural projects).
  3. Retiring agricultural land from irrigation.

In active management areas, larger urban populations in Arizona have the objective that, by 2025, withdrawals from ground water aquifers will not exceed their natural recharge by:
- Considering water as a marginally available (and therefore costly) commodity for trade; marketing it as such ($400-$500 per acre-foot), thereby decreasing the excessiveness and improving the effectiveness, of its use.
- Considering the addition of treated water (e.g., run-off from heavily fertilized marginal land) estimated to cost $400-$500 per acre-foot, to the trade in water from regions with surplus to those without.

Such procedures accord with the U.S. Agricultural Department's scheme to reduce sediment run-off into streams from highly erodable farmland by 23% and reduce pesticide use by 11% by paying the farmer to withdraw such land from use.

Nineteen and a half million acres towards a planned holding of 40 million acres have already been withdrawn. This level of reduction, besides being environmentally desirable, will also reduce crop surpluses by 6-8%. In Britain, excessive crop surpluses in the European Economic Community (EEC) are a primary motive to practice the same type of land withholding scheme. Potential environmental benefits are the same. It is interesting that different, originally stated objectives in resource management, one to conserve a scarce commodity, the other to eliminate a surplus, are achieved by a common action.

The resources and environment of the world support the people, in fact all living things, but the people of the world have to control their profusion if a balance between resource use and renewal is to be achieved, thus safeguarding the future. Food is another major commodity.

Hope for the Starving:
The remarkable success of the Green Revolution technology applied to the growth of high-yielding new varieties of wheat, rice and maize has the potential to provide 2/3 of the total daily per capita calorie intake needed in West Asia, South and South-East Asia, and China, where previously 70% of the World's malnourished lived (Timmer, 1977). China, having embraced the technological packet of the Green Revolution.... new crop varieties, intensive planting, pesticide and fertilizer application, backed by intensive irrigation, has now seemingly achieved nutritional self sufficiency. The real secret of China's success, however, seems to have been a political leadership which has ensured distribution of the increased food supply equitably among all the people without urban bias by disallowing commercial exploitation of the product by larger commercially-minded farmers or land owners (i.e. by selling it outside a region where it is grown).

No solution is ever complete, however. Secondary effects erode production successes. One effect is that any new domestic cereal production discourages imports in order to improve trade balance, so that no real growth in the food supply is felt. Another effect shifts agricultural emphasis to cereals away from nutritionally higher quality protein crops such as legumes. In addition, outside centrally planned economies (e.g., China and Cuba), that have succeeded remarkably in feeding their people, market forces direct maldistribution of the product. The poor still may remain malnourished, as what might have been grain for them, is purchased by the more affluent to feed to livestock for their own beef consumption.

Important steps to be taken by any government to ensure maximum effects of the new technology are:
- to assist in purchase of the original inputs (i.e. fertilizer, seed, pesticide, water, etc.),
- to enact land redistribution reform if necessary to give access to farming land to a majority of people, and
- to anticipate the downstream effects that might threaten the primary goal of sufficiency for all, such as a growing differential in purchasing power leading to displacement of poorer people from land and their direct access to a food supply and earnings (Timmer, 1977). Norman Borlang, the Nobel Laureate who discovered the dwarf wheat which launched the Green Revolution in India and China, is having similar success with a package prepared for African States. In the Sudan, 420 trial plantings have increased per-hectare sorghum yield six-fold and doubled yields in Ghana (**The Economist**, May 17, 1987).

Hope for the Unemployed:
It is ironic that many developed nations of the west, toward whose standard of living Third World nations aspire, and from whom they frequently seek aid, are themselves, facing crisis. The very speed of scientific discovery and its technological implementation has left many gasping in economic distress. The pace of adjustment from conventional occupations to new types of hi-tech jobs ranging from office automation to the robotization of manufacturing is being forced into a single decade. In the process many conventional jobs are disappearing and the need for flexibility and innovation, both in creating and adjusting to new jobs, is putting a tremendous

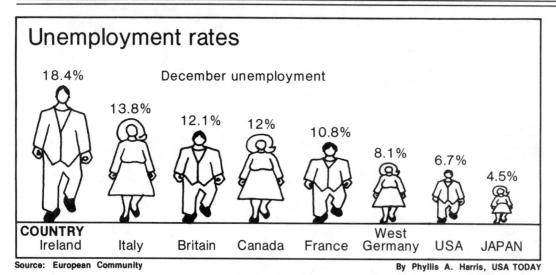

Unemployment rates

December unemployment

18.4%

13.8%

12.1%

12%

10.8%

8.1%

6.7%

4.5%

| COUNTRY | | | | | | | |
| Ireland | Italy | Britain | Canada | France | West Germany | USA | JAPAN |

Source: European Community

By Phyllis A. Harris, USA TODAY

Figure 16.7. European unemployment rates 1987, compared with Japan and North America. Modified and reproduced with permission from **USA Today**, Feb. 9, 1987.

stress upon people in many countries. Thus, temporarily, maybe permanently, many people are unemployed. Figure 16.7 shows jobless rates in some European countries, Japan, Canada, and the USA. Compounding the stress and difficulties of transition is the rise in manufacturing strength of nations with cheaper labor pools in North and South Korea, Taiwan, Hong Kong and other nations of the Pacific Rim, so that, not only is the manner of manufacturing changing to one that needs fewer people, but the products from those labor intensive processes still surviving are being manufactured off-shore. The countries creating jobs are those with flexible, efficient work forces, initially well-trained and then, continuously retrained in developing new technology... an informational technology (IT) from which everything new will be spawned.

New designs for cars, bridges, trains, and so forth, from computer aided design (CAD); new manufacturing sequences and processes, new efficiency, e.g. robotics and just-in-time delivery of parts, saving inventory space, from computer integrated manufacturing (CIM); improved medical treatment from computer aided medical diagnosis and treatment (CAMDT); and not least new communication systems spanning the globe; all these represent but a small fraction of the infinite possibilities stemming from the collection, storage, and manipulation of information and processes by computers.

There is an ironic parallel between the IT revolution sweeping across the economies of affluent nations and the displacement of the small farmer from the land and thus his living, in Third World countries. For the increasing number of unemployed in the former countries the result is also similar i.e. displacement of a reasonably affluent middle class from a job and a standard of living which can no longer be maintained. An alarming schism is thus in danger of developing in these societies between an affluent minority and a majority of poor. Even in the USA, a country with one of the most impressive records of providing 1.9% more new jobs each year throughout the last decade, a Congressional report in 1984 indicated that

Table 16.1. Distribution of enrolments in university education 1983-1984 (%).

	Under 20	Age† Range 20-24	25-29	over 30
Australia	27.1	31.6	14.9	26.3
Austria*	12.5	49.8	24.7	12.9
Britain (2)	34.7	45.7	8.6	11.0
Canada	14.1	42.3	16.5	25.2
Denmark	4.1	42.1	28.4	24.7
Finland	4.8	45.6	29.4	20.3
France (1)	21.3	44.7	19.3	14.7
Greece (2)	30.3	52.7	9.4	4.1
Holland	13.3	47.6	24.6	14.5
Ireland	45.3	45.5	5.3	3.9
New Zealand*	33.3	42.6	10.1	13.9
Norway (2)	5.0	50.9	25.2	18.9
Portugal*(1)	12.3	55.5	17.6	14.5
Spain (2)	25.4	47.9	11.1	7.5
Sweden*(3)	15.6	36.5	22.6	24.4
Switzerland	15.5	50.3	21.8	12.4
United States (2)	24.1	40.8	14.5	20.6
West Germany	3.9	52.1	31.2	12.8

Source: OECD (1) 1982; (2) 1983; (3) 1975; *all higher education; † excluding unknowns. Reproduced with premission from the Feature Article. Training for Work. **The Economist**, December 20, 1986.

the wealthiest 40% of families received 67.3% of the available income while the poorest 40% received only 15.7%. A recent US Census Bureau Report (**American Demographics**, March 1987) indicates that the poorest 42.5% of households earned less than $20,000 per annum and only 14.7% of households earned more than $50,000, although median household income was continuing to rise. In Chapters 1 and 3 we indicated that the degree of health and happiness of a people depended importantly upon the degree of care and leadership provided by their society. Unless these economic ills of developed societies begin to be solved, fewer people without jobs will be able to afford the cost of personal health care, a cost formerly shared by an employer. Historically, such a major dichotomy, in both earnings and access to social services between significant segments of a society, has been accompanied by an increasing desperation and lawlessness, ultimately characterized by violence and crime. The evidence, from nations most successfully accommodating to modern economic forces, is that the flexible skills required by future generations are produced by societies providing greatest accessibility to education at every level and age, including manpower training (apprenticeships and vocational). Figure 16.8 and Table 16.1 show comparable "density of education" statistics in several developed countries.

Social Malaise:

The evolution of modern complex societies has not been accomplished without the attendant growth of social ills, many of which have received scant attention in competition with the primary goal of material growth. In pursuit of this latter goal we have not always made people safer, happier, or healthier. In fact, the 20th century, which has witnessed the greatest increase in material wealth of developed nations, has also witnessed continuing global strife and emerging inter- and intra-national "have" and "have not" sub-societies. Paradoxically, the two often exist in close proximity to each other.

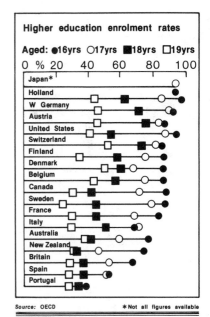

Figure 16.8. Higher education enrollment rates. Reproduced with permission from **The Economist**, Feature Article, Training for Work, December 20, 1986.

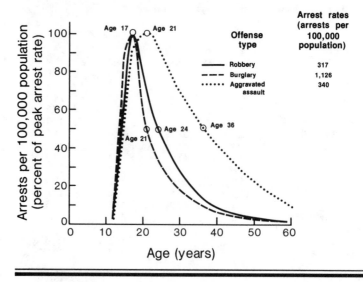

Figure 16.9. Crime and youth: age-specific arrest rates show the ages at which burglary, robbery, and aggravated assault decline to half their peak rates. (Source: Federal Bureau of Investigation, 1984). Reproduced with permission from News and Comment, **Science**, 233: Sept., 1986).

Strife, stress, and conflict in society affects species, ages, genders, ethnic groups, and material classes, often without distinction. In Chapter 4 we read how humans have altered the environment profoundly, acutely affecting the lives of all living things and now, in full circle, are seeing these effects threaten their own very existence.

Crime and Violence:

More threatening to security in the short term than the ever present threat of nuclear warfare is the increasing crime rate in the majority of societies.

Tougher arrest and parole laws in the United States have compounded a problem of prison overcrowding, a common problem in many other countries too. The USA incarcerates 300 people per 100,000 of its population for criminal offenses, a level matched only by the Soviet Union and South Africa. In the early months of 1987 prisons in Texas overflowed to such an extent that prisoners were being released early, almost on a daily basis, in order to accept newly-sentenced arrivals. Texas already has 40,000 parolees—more than its whole inmate population. A recent report to the Academy of Criminal Justice Sciences predicted that by 1999 economic and racial strife could produce urban unrest, disorder, and violence of a magnitude only previously seen in the civil disorders of the 1960s.

The increasing criminal activity of the last 20 years in the USA and other countries (Table 16.2) may be partly attributed to the coming of "criminal" age, of those born in the "baby boom" years following the second World War (1945-1964). A Federal Bureau of Investigation Report (1984) indicates that the prime ages for criminal activity are between 16 and 25 years (Fig. 16.9). Additionally, the relationship between high frequency criminal activity and drug abuse is unmistakable. Young urban males are chief offenders. The increasing desire of people to have criminals restrained will cost billions of dollars (in buildings, supervision, etc.) to the American economy well into the twenty-first century. Depending on

Table 16.2.
General statistics on crime from several countries reported for 1985.

Britain	Australia	Canada	USA
Highest crime rate in Europe	1.25 million (M) serious crime victims in 1985	2.2 M serious crimes in 1985. 1 M more than reported in 1970 and overall a 65% growth in all crime in 15 years.	22 M households affected 12 M serious crimes Burglary every 10 sec Motor vehicle loss every 30 sec Assault every 44 sec Robbery every 60 sec Rape every 6 min Murder every 28 min

how well we succeed in reducing through positive social changes, the developing sense of alienation on the part of many, and begin to understand the genesis of criminal behavior, it may well extend for a considerably longer period.

Violation of the Elderly:

Chapter 15 on Family Violence, focused on violence of a different sort from "street" violence, but one no less harsh and life threatening. Police in 78 cities across the USA now arrest violent domestic abusers more than 5 times as much as in 1984. The principal concern in Chapter 15 was with wife and child safety. Now elder-abuse has emerged as a public issue of the 80s, a natural successor to acknowledgement of child abuse in the 60s and wife battering in the 70s.

There seems to be a continuation of marital disputes into old age. One USA study found that 58% of reported abuses were between spouses. The Canadian Federal Government's National Clearinghouse on Family Violence estimated that 100,000 Canadians (2-4% of Senior Citizens) are victims of elder-abuse. A similar figure (3.2%) was found in the U.S.A. in a smaller sample population of 2,020 persons over 65 in the Boston area (**Globe and Mail**, Jan. 2, 1987). The problems of increasing infirmity and dementia in the elderly has prompted some legislation to institutionalize those neglecting themselves, but abuse appears to be just as likely in institutions as with family. Reports in the USA indicate that elders have also been abused by their children after being taken in, during the de-institutionalization of public mental hospitals. The latter decreased institutional care from 550,000 patients in the 1950s to 130,000 in the 80s. While many hazards to the elderly, living alone, with family, or in institutions have been identified, not many solutions to the multifaceted problem have been suggested.

Recall from Chapter 14, on aging, that the elderly are an increasingly larger proportion of the population in developed countries. By 2050, 5% of the United States' population will be 85+ years old. Figure 16.10 shows

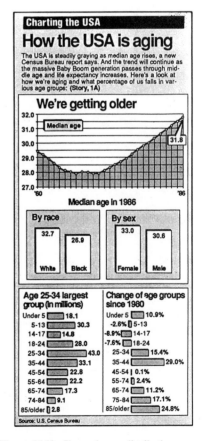

Figure 16.10. Shows the age distribution of the American population in 1986. Reproduced with permission Dunn, W. from **USA Today**, March, 1987.

the distribution of the population in the USA in 1986. In many countries, the baby boomers from the post World War II period (1945-64) are now having children. This is causing a secondary increase in the population currently under 5 years old. An aging population implies several potentially disturbing consequences to the stability of the social system. Not the least of these is the question of who works the economy and who takes care of the aged.

Health Care for All:
Several systems of health care delivery were outlined in Chapter 3. Many of those of underdeveloped countries are rudimentary and represent a great challenge for concerned nations to improve. Among developed nations, most systems rely on massive government funding for providing adequate "sick" care. Their continuance at their current burgeoning cost must remain conjectural as governments attempt to reduce debt load. America claims the highest standards of health care from a system with a substantial element of free enterprise in it. However, its system remains inaccessible to many. An estimated 35 million out of a population of 241 million (some 14.5%) are uninsured or underinsured. These people are swamping large city public hospitals and isolated rural hospitals with unpaid bills which have climbed to $7.4 Billion (B) in 1985 from $3.5 B in 1980. It is estimated that as many as 600 of the nation's 2700 rural hospitals will close by 1990, at the present rate of debt accumulation.

A principal source of funding for many health care systems are social security contributions from those still working. Such funds are in jeopardy in developed countries achieving zero population growth. As their populations age, the much greater proportion of those working and paying into benefit schemes to those receiving benefits eventually reverses and quickly exhausts reserves. It is estimated that Medicare in the USA, which insures hospital and medical care for the aged, will become exhausted by 2002 without either reduction in Medicare coverage or a 15% increase in

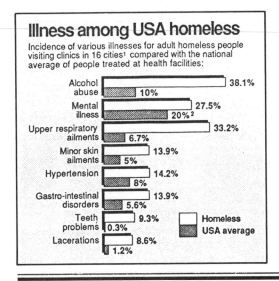

Illness among USA homeless

Incidence of various illnesses for adult homeless people visiting clinics in 16 cities[1] compared with the national average of people treated at health facilities:

Alcohol abuse — 38.1% / 10%
Mental illness — 27.5% / 20%[2]
Upper respiratory ailments — 33.2% / 6.7%
Minor skin ailments — 13.9% / 5%
Hypertension — 14.2% / 8%
Gastro-intestinal disorders — 13.9% / 5.6%
Teeth problems — 9.3% / 0.3%
Lacerations — 8.6% / 1.2%

☐ Homeless
▨ USA average

1 - Clinics were in Albuquerque, N.M.; Baltimore; Birmingham, Ala.; Boston; Chicago; Denver; Detroit; Milwaukee; Newark, N.J.; Nashville, Tenn.; New York City; Philadelphia; San Antonio, Texas; Seattle; San Francisco; and Washington, D.C. The survey was of 11,886 people visiting clinics more than once.

2 - Percentage of people National Institutes of Health says needs mental care.

Source: Health Care for the Homeless Program; National Institutes of Health; USA TODAY research

Figure 16.11. Shows the distribution of illness among the homeless compared with the national USA average. Reproduced with permission from Moss, D., **USA Today,** March, 1987.

contributions. A Medicare Bill introduced into Congress, more generous than one recently proposed by President Reagan (1987), would in fact take such a course by increasing contributions from the more affluent elderly, while simultaneously extending coverage extensively, and capping the maximum amount payable per year for hospital care at $520 and physician care to $1,043. This does not address the problem of medicaid for the poor, homeless, and mentally ill (many of whom are now homeless from the deinstitutionalization carried on from 1950 onwards). Between 1/4 million and 2.5 million homeless now crowd the shelters and steam grates across the country and they have serious health problems. Figure 16.11 shows the distribution of illness among the homeless compared with the national USA average.

The enormous cost of health care practice in its present form is increasingly being called into question. The situation is aptly summarized by the comment of former Colorado governor R.D. Lamm that, not more spending is needed, but just smarter spending (**USA Today,** Feb., 1987).

Valuable contributions to alleviating overall morbidity and mortality statistics from preventive tactics such as education, occupational safety, accident prevention, education, and lifestyle factors generally, are frequently underestimated and receive little recognition in competition for health care funding. Few would now argue however, that it is the contribution of modern medicine alone, with its rather limited capacity for treatment (surgery, diagnostic procedures, etc.), rather than the significant changes in lifestyle effected by a large segment of society, that has reduced such illnesses as cardiovascular disease up to 30% during the last three decades in Canada and the USA.

Similarly, the direct medical costs of smoking in 1984 have been estimated at $23 Billion in the USA with an additional $30.7 B estimated for wage loss due to premature death, disability and sick days (**San Francisco Chronicle,** March 21, 1987). These costs would be totally eliminated without any intervention from conventional medicine if no one smoked. With the immense social and legislative pressure building against the habit, such a result may well happen in the not-so-distant future.

Table 16.3. Health hazards of alcohol abuse.

Health Hazard	Result
Motor Vehicle Accidents (MVA's)	• 1/3 drivers dying in MVA's have higher than permissible blood alcohol • 1/9 have more than 2 times the limit
Other accidents	• 1/4 of home accident victims had been drinking • 15% of job accidents are alcohol related
Mental illness	• in England rise in admission rate to mental hospitals from alcohol abuse rose from 11,500 to 17,200 between 1973 and 1983
'sick' absenteeism	• in England 8 million (m) to 14 m days per year
premature death (PD) and illness (I)	• in Britain 4th major cause (PD) in USA 3rd major cause (I)
Violence injury	• in Britain 43% of wounding and assaults offences committed by persons whom victims claimed had been drinking

Drug and Alcohol Dependency:

Alcohol is a paradox. It may be enjoyed equally in the quiet intimacy of a dinner date, the noisy comraderie of a bar after strenuous activity, or relaxedly with peanuts in front of a TV football game. Most of us have grown up tolerating, even enjoying its availability. It is difficult for some to conceive that it may ever be the pariah that the cigarette has become. Yet it is a decidedly insidious enemy to many individuals, to their families, and to the wider community in which they work (see Chapter 10). Consider that approximately 2.5% or more of any developed country's population is alcoholic.... 600,000 Canadians, 5 million (M) Americans, probably 7-8 M Russians, 1M Britons, 1.8M Japanese. Seven in 100 Americans in a 1985 survey by the Centers for Disease Control considered they were heavy drinkers (2 or more drinks per day) but British experts' opinions of what constitutes a safe drinking level ranged from 7 pints (beer) to 31 pints a week (1-4 drinks per day).

Thus, how much, and how frequently, is too much remains quite unclear. In many degenerative disease states (liver damage, neurological damage, heart disease), all potentially developing from alcohol ingestion, it is difficult to relate the course of their development to the size of the risk factor, producing them, in this case alcohol. The dangerous relation between dose and response is not clearly drawn for many and permits a "personal exclusion from consequences" syndrome to prevail, allowing denial and continuing indulgence. The range of damage produced by alcohol impairment is extensive (Table 16.3) and dollar costs are considerable (Table 16.4).

Awareness of risk and moderation of habit by the general public is currently absent. Any impartial attitude on the part of government to attempt to reduce alcohol consumption is handicapped by their obvious interest in tax receipts from alcohol sales, although this return cannot possibly equal the reciprocal spending needed on health and societal-related consequences of excess alcohol consumption (Table 16.4). Worldwide, esti-

Table 16.4. Health care and economic costs of alcohol abuse (Canada, 1981).

Item	$ Cost
Health care	2 billion (B)
Job productivity	1.2 B
Social welfare cost	increased by 1.4 B
Law enforcement	0.65 B
Ratio Alcohol: Revenuse/costs	0.42 B

Table 16.5. Legacies of doubt in Adult Children of an Alcoholic.

- They guess at what normality is
- Have difficulty completing projects
- Lie when it would be just as easy to tell the truth
- Rigidly attach themselves to the truth no matter the cost
- Judge themselves unmercifully. Have self-doubt and
  low self-esteem
- Have difficulty with intimacy
- Are afraid of changes and become anxious about changes
  over which they have no control
- Constantly seek affirmation from others
- Can be extremely responsible—or irresponsible
- Are extremely loyal even if misguidedly so
- Are impulsive

mates of these costs total $100 Billion annually. In the USA there are presently 22 million adult children of Alcoholics (ACoA) who share some common traits (Table 16.5). Some legacies from the operating conditions of their childhood: Don't feel—you won't get hurt, Don't trust—you won't ever be disappointed, and, Don't tell anyone that someone in your house drinks (Benati, 1987). Some suggestions to limit abuse and encourage sensible drinking habits have been proposed (Table 16.6) . Their implementation and the continuance of society's support groups, such as Alcoholics Anonymous (AA), which has 40,000 groups throughout the world, and ACoA groups, of which 400 operate throughout the USA, are both short and long term solutions to alcoholism. However, they currently operate in the absence of a social sentiment against excess which would come close to that voiced against smoking.

It is estimated that 67% of all Americans have drunk alcohol at least once, and that 50% currently drink regularly, even if only small amounts. These figures on prevalence reflect its present social acceptance. Abuse of substances such as tobacco, alcohol, heroin, marijuana, or cocaine, to name the few most widely abused, may be considered a self-induced affliction (contrary to the general concept of a disease as one involuntarily contracted from an infectious agent. This distinction has not prevented serious study of drug abuse by classical epidemiological methods in the USA (Kozel & Adams, 1986). Descriptive epidemiology of drug abuse characterizing prevalence (use) in the US population draws information from two surveys sponsored by the National Institute for Drug Abuse (NIDA). These are the National Household Survey on Drug Abuse, and the High School Senior Survey. Additional information is gained from two hospital based data systems—The Drug Abuse Warning Network (DAWN), and the Client Oriented Data Acquisition Process (CODAP). The standardized procedures and measurements made regularly on large sample populations during several years in these surveys and data systems enables significant trends to be noted, as well as analysis of a variety of

Table 16.6. Possible methods inducing sensible drinking habits. Reproduced with permission from Kozel, N.J. and Adams, E.H. **Science**, 234:970, 1986. Copyright © by the AAAS.

Method	Possible Success Rate
Education	Little relationship has been found between the severity of habit and individual understanding of the health hazards of alcohol excess.
Laws	Many exist but are weakly or erratically enforced.
Product price elevation	Good deterrent to youthful drinkers who have less money.
Changing social character of drinking establishments	Combining food service with alcohol service reduces alcohol ingested but retains profit margin and increases women clientel, further reducing per capita drinking but maintaining gross sales.
Mandatory health warnings on alcohol products	Has had success in anti-smoking campaigns.
Societal support for AA and ACoA agencies	Less tolerance for people drinking and driving or behaving even mildly reprehensibly under the influence of alcohol is clearly being seen and felt.
True social pressure for change against heavy drinking	This will lead to observance of the law by the majority's example and unwillingness to tolerate individual exceptions to the rules.

Table 16.7. Trend in estimated prevalence of marijuana use among three age groups, 1972-1985 in the U.S.A. Reproduced with permission from Kozel, N.J. and Adams, E.H. **Science**, 234:970, 1986. Copyright © by the AAAS.

Prevalence	Population using marijuana (%)						
	1972	1974	1976	1977	1979	1982	1985
12- to 17-year olds							
Ever used	14.0	23.0	22.4	28.0	30.9	26.7	23.7
Used in past year		18.5	18.4	22.3	24.1	20.6	20.0
Used in past month	7.0	12.0	12.3	16.6	16.7	11.5	12.3
Sample size	880	952	986	1,272	2,165	1,581	2,287
18- to 25-year olds							
Ever used	47.9	52.7	52.9	59.9	68.2	64.1	60.5
Used in past year		34.2	35.0	38.7	46.9	40.4	37.0
Used in past month	27.8	25.2	25.0	27.4	35.4	27.4	21.9
Sample size	772	849	882	1,500	2,044	1,283	1,804
26 years and older							
Ever used	7.4	9.9	12.9	15.3	19.6	23.0	27.2
Used in past year		3.8	5.4	6.4	9.0	10.6	9.5
Used in past month	2.5	2.0	3.5	3.3	6.0	6.6	6.2
Sample size	1,613	2,221	1,708	1,822	3,015	2,760	3,947

Table 16.8. Trend in estimated prevelence of marijuana use among high school senior classes, 1975-1985 in the U.S.A. Reproduced with permission from Kozel, N.J. and Adams, E.H. **Science**, 234:970, 1986. Copyright © by the AAAS.

| | High school seniors using marijuana (%) | | | | | | | | | | |
Prevalence	1975	1976	1977	1978	1979	1980	1981	1982	1983	1984	1985
Ever used	47.3	52.8	56.4	59.2	60.4	60.3	59.5	58.7	57.0	54.9	54.2
Used in past year	40.0	44.5	47.6	50.2	50.8	48.8	46.1	44.3	42.3	40.0	40.6
Used in past month	27.1	32.2	35.4	37.1	36.5	33.7	31.6	28.5	27.0	25.2	25.7
Used daily in past month	6.0	8.2	9.1	10.7	10.3	9.1	7.0	6.3	5.5	5.0	4.9
Sample size	9,400	15,400	17,100	17,800	15.500	15,900	17,500	17,700	16,300	15,900	16,000

questions on interrelated problems of drug abuse. These include induction of habit in one drug from previous habit in another, and identification of particular age groups or ethnic groups at risk from specific drugs or routes of administration.

Data reported on heroin, marijuana, and cocaine prevalence in the last several years are shown in Figure 16.12 and Tables 16.7, 16.8 and 16.9 respectively. The established methods of analytical epidemiology represent an interactive system, feasible for modeling future developments (see Chapter 2), thus anticipating events so that preventive measures may be taken. A singular disturbing effect noted in these data is the sharp increase in DAWN-reported cocaine emergencies. In the period from 1981 to 1985, these rose from slightly more than 3,000 to almost 10,000, with cocaine related deaths showing a similar 3-fold increase. Treatment admission (CODAP) for primary cocaine abuse climbed from 1.8% of the total in 1977 to 5.8% in 1981 and to 14% in 1985. If secondary cocaine abuse were included, almost 29% of admissions were cocaine related. Truly, a river of cocaine rises in Columbia, Bolivia, and Peru (Figure 16.13) to flood into the U.S.A. It costs $2.50 to collect 25lbs. of coca leaf in Columbia and 550 leaves produce a pound of cocaine. Thus, the approximate production cost of cocaine is $55 per lb. or $123,200 per ton ($23 per kilogram). Since the current average selling price is approximately $21,000 per kg. this is a massively inflationary figure (x 170). Figure 16.14 shows the rise in the drugs illegally imported into the U.S.A. and federal costs spent in policing actions. Illegal drug exports contribute to an "underground" economy in these Third World Countries (Fig. 16.15). The approximate production costs of 130 tons of cocaine, some $16 M become worth $33 Billion (130 x $25 M) almost 66% of all drug sales in the U.S.A. in 1985.

The distribution of cocaine in a freebase, smokable form called "crack", selling in small affordable quantities for $10, ominously enhances its chances for distribution among younger age groups in the future.

A new technique for attacking the distribution of drugs, which seems unable to be stemmed at national borders, has been instituted by police

Table 16.9. Trend in annual prevalence of cocaine use among follow-up populations,1 to 4 years after high school, 1980-1985 in the U.S.A. Reproduced with permission from Kozel, N. and Adams, E.H. **Science**, 234:970, 1986. Copyright © by the AAAS.

| | Used cocaine in past 12 months (%) | | | | | |
Sample	1980	1981	1982	1983	1984	1985
Total	18.0	18.1	19.2	17.5	17.5	17.2
Full-time college students	16.9	15.9	17.2	17.2	16.4	17.3
Sample size	2,855	2,862	2,861	2,821	2,790	2,690

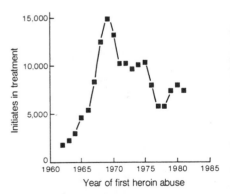

Figure 16.12. Incidence of heroin abuse in the U.S.A. Data are based on admissions to a panel of federally funded treatment programs. Epidemic proportions of use may be observed in the late 60s, early 70s and again between the late 70s and early 80s. Reproduced with permission from Kozel, N. and Adams, E.H. **Science**, 234: 970, 1986. Copyright © by the AAAS.

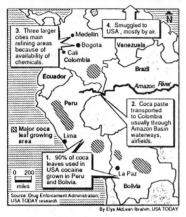

Figure 16.13. Showing possible channels of coca refinement and illegal shipment to the U.S.A. Reproduced with permission from **USA Today**, Beissert, Feb. 6, 1987.

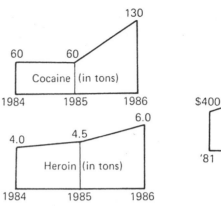

Figure 16.14. Showing continuing growth of illegal cocaine and heroin imports into the U.S.A. despite rising Federal spending on drug enforcement. Reproduced with permission from **USA Today**, Beissert, Feb. 6, 1987.

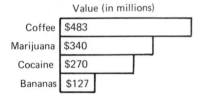

Value (in millions)	
Coffee	$483
Marijuana	$340
Cocaine	$270
Bananas	$127

Figure 16.15. Value of legal and illegal exports contributing to Columbia's legal and undertground economy. Reproduced with permission from **USA Today**, Beissert, Feb. 6, 1987.

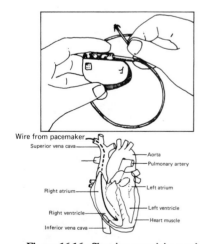

Figure 16.16. Showing an activity sensitive pacemaker. The wire inserted into the right ventricle carries a small electrical signal generated from the activity sensor to excite and pace the heart's contractions at the right pace. Reproduced with permission from Science/Medicine, **Globe and Mail**, Jan. 3, 1987.

departments in New York, Washington, Baltimore, South Florida and Los Angeles. The technique is to destroy major drug rings at street level, thus continuously disrupting deals, making arrests, and precipitating a snowballing attrition in selling. It is hoped that some new users will thus be dissuaded and current users may enter drug treatment schemes in frustration from an inability to satisfy the habit.

The long term impact of such methods are, of course, not yet studied. An undesirable result of this arrest policy however is its exacerbating effect on the already overcrowded prison system in the U.S.A.

Modern Medicine:

In the future we may expect continuing remarkable technological advances in organ transplants, implanted monitoring or regulating devices, limb replacement, and surgical techniques similar to those described in Chapter 11. Recent developments, for instance, include an activity-sensitive heart pacemaker device (Figure 16.16) which adjusts the heart rate appropriately to the activity level of the recipient instead of relying on fixed rate pacing. Another example is a bionic prosthesis relying on amplified natural muscle electrical signals to effect movement in a naturally acting cosmetic human limb (Figure 16.17). The adaptation of laser beams carried by a fiberoptic strand to perform precise, contained, bloodless surgery in cases previously cured by much grosser surgical procedures (e.g., partial or total hysterectomy for recurrent uterine bleeding) is a third instance. Significant discoveries are taking place into the causes of diseases of the brain, such as Alzheimer's disease, characterized by brain deterioration, memory impairment and senility, Parkinsonism, causing tremor and rigidity, and mental illness such as manic-depression, producing alternating periods of abnormal excitement and deep depression. Within the last year, a drug tetrahydroaminoacridine (THA) has been used to improve, interimly, the responses of Alzheimer patients suffering dementia. Up to now, Alzheimer's disease has been confirmed, only at autopsy, from

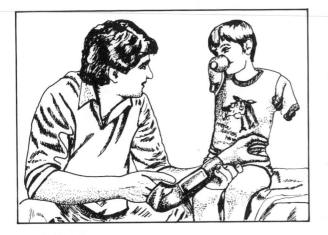

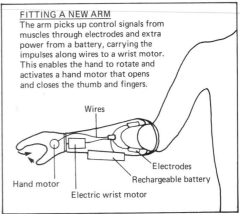

FITTING A NEW ARM
The arm picks up control signals from muscles through electrodes and extra power from a battery, carrying the impulses along wires to a wrist motor. This enables the hand to rotate and activates a hand motor that opens and closes the thumb and fingers.

Wires

Hand motor

Electric wrist motor

Electrodes

Rechargeable battery

Figure 16.17. Showing a new bionic arm for Enofel Zharkoff, working naturally from nerve signals arising in muscles normally functioning in the arm. The new arm is fashioned by prosthetist Mr. T. Chaffin of the Shriners' Hospital for crippled children in Portland. Reproduced with permission from Crick, **The Oregonian,** Aug. 28, 1986.

collections of tangled fibers (neurofibrillary tangles) and dead cells in certain areas of the brain. However, chemical protein found in the brain and spinal fluid of Alzheimer patients may eventually be used to distinguish Alzheimer's sufferers earlier from those with disorders such as depression, anxiety, alcoholism, and malnutrition which show similar symptoms. Another chemical, a neurotoxin MPTP, recently found accidently to produce the same symptoms as Parkinsonism in drug users, enabled an animal model of Parkinsonism to be simulated in various age groups, so that investigations exploring methods for regenerating the damaged brain regions have been facilitated.

Shortly after these discoveries were made surgeons were able to make autografts (tissue from a person's own body), in this case from the adrenal gland, into the brain of patients with Parkinson's disease (first in Sweden, then Mexico, and most recently in the USA). In the American procedure, a portion of the adrenal medulla, which normally secretes neurochemicals similar to the active chemical messengers deficient in the area of the brain producing Parkinson's symptoms, was grafted on to a female patient's brain near this region. It was adequately bathed in cerebrospinal fluid (the brain's internal circulating system), and the hope was that the cells would modify and take on the character of nerve cells secreting the correct neurotransmitter controlling Parkinsonism. Seven days later the same dramatic improvement of tremor noted previously by Mexican surgeons in their patients but not by the Swedes, were observed in the woman. Long term results remain to be evaluated. The short term effect could be due to a placebo effect or to the adrenal tissue's unmodified neurotransmitters themselves exerting a positive effect.

In theory, fetal brain tissue should perform even better, since one step of the process, i.e. differentiation of the transplant into brain tissue (if indeed this occurs), would not be needed. In addition, young cells are in a rapid stage of growth and differentiation. They are thus marvelously plastic and transformable. The needed neurotransmitter, dopamine, would also be a normal secretory product of the transplanted tissue. The transplant material would come from aborted fetus or accident victim tissue. In anticipation of such surgical procedures, an expert medico-ethical-legal panel, convened in March, 1987 at the Centre for Biomedical Ethics at Case Western Reserve University School of Medicine, proposed a set of ethical guidelines, for governing human brain tissue transplants (**Science,** 1987).

Even such radically new procedures whose very mechanism of action is as yet poorly understood pales beside the potential scope of another procedure already upon the surgical horizon: that of genetically engineering a cure for a wide variety of neurological deficiencies. Recently the results of a 10-year study of manic-depression in three generations of an Old Order Amish family in Pennsylvania linked the illness to an aberrant gene on chromosome 11 (see Chapter 11). Another study of five large families in Jerusalem implicated a gene on the X chromosome, confirming the influence of heredity on mental illness. Recently, people with an hereditary form of Alzheimer's disease have been found to carry an abnormal number of a gene on chromosome 21. Down's syndrome patients suffer a brain disorder similar to Alzheimer's disease carry an extra chromosome 21, and thus an extra number of the gene also. The gene governs production of a protein called beta-amyloid, thought to cause the disease. Increasingly, genetic markers for other diseases, such as cystic fibrosis and atherosclerosis, are being found. Possibly the time will come when such aberrant conditions in the germ cell may be corrected. In a recent decision which has a future bearing on this issue, the USA became the first country to allow the patenting of new forms of animal life. This is an issue with broad moral and ethical implications. In the personal opinion of Dr. J.C. Fletcher, chief of the bioethics program at the National Institutes of Health, the new patent policy is the reluctant recognition that, "human beings have discovered how to deliberately change and alter biological evolution".

This is a proposal which many people will find difficult to accept, particularly at the pace with which new scientific discoveries bound to moral questions are now presented to the public. The divisiveness of the issues is illustrated by just a small sample of initial reactions to the new policy (Schneider, 1987):

- "If you look down the road you're looking at men having the tools to make animals."
- "It paves the way for industrialization of this technology." (This refers to the marketing of gene-altered organisms, such as two bacteria now awaiting field tests. One of these inhibits frost bite in crops and the other produces its own natural pesticide to protect crops).
- "Years of animal breeding by farmers will become the raw material for biotechnology companies who will tinker, obtain their patents, and sell their new breeds at high prices."
- "We're going to make animals that nature never made."
- "This policy (i.e., the new patent policy) has little to do with the needs of agriculture and a lot to do with the needs of a few corporations."
- "If you invest the time and money in developing products, whether animal or chemical or whatever, then you want to have protection. This (i.e., the patent policy) is going to lead to developments we haven't even considered before."
- "It's a staggering decision. It removes one more barrier to the protection of human life." (Patents applications involving human life will not be considered under the present policy).
- "Good God, once you start patenting life forms, there is no stopping it."
- "There's going to be a major political battle in this country, starting today, between corporations and people concerned about the ethics of this policy."

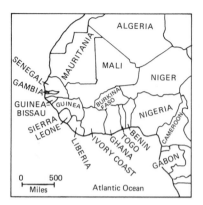

Figure 16.18. Showing populous countries of the sub-Sahara where the Human Immunodeficiency Virus HIV, is now spreading. Brooke, J. Copyright © 1987 by **The New York Times Company**. Reprinted by permission.

Overearching and dominating health, education, social habits, religion, and politics on both national and international levels in the immediate years ahead however, will be the HIV, or AIDS problem, which was extensively discussed in Chapter 12. The inexorable progress of this infection around the world continues. Central Africa's AIDS problem is now spreading to the populous west coast of Africa (Fig. 16.18), whose countries to this point had previously taken little direct preventive action against the spread of the virus. This spread appears to be due to heterosexual contacts, often through foreign travel, and an increasing degree of prostitution, causing diffusion at home in modern African cities. It is feared that general education of the populace on the characteristics of the disease and its control will not be effected in time to avoid a widespread epidemic in West Africa.

Cuba, which has more than 300,000 troops returned from African countries, besides medical teams, construction workers, and teachers on assignments there, recently reviewed the status of AIDS in its country, noting that 103 of 667,000 people tested had the AIDS virus. They have been quarantined. One hundred and seven of 20,000 foreigners tested who proved positive were sent home. Three cases had died. Precautions reportedly taken by the Cuban government have been to:

- accept no blood donations from Cubans who have lived abroad for an extended period;
- accept no blood donations from people with previous histories of repeated sexually transmitted disease;
- include information on these events on National Identity Cards;
- require mandatory tests of all Cubans returning from abroad with 6-month follow-ups;
- examine anyone with known AIDS contact every 3 months;
- outlaw and eliminate prostitution; and
- eliminate drug addiction.

Some of these "ideal" solutions presently seem unattainable in democratic societies and probably in any kind of modern society too, no matter what its political character. However, they reflect a political will and personal discipline human beings may have to exert in order to contain and eradicate this modern scourge. Bavaria also recently introduced similar drastic preventive measures against AIDS in spite of much less stringent control policy widely adopted by European Common Market countries as a whole.

On a hopeful note, genetic information from the HIV-I virus necessary to produce reverse transcriptase, the enzyme essential for the virus's reproduction (see Chapter 12), has been spliced into a common bacterium, ensuring its safer production and handling than in the virus itself. The enzyme is in high demand, since it is the focus of research to produce methods designed to inhibit its action in enabling the virus to replicate as DNA (Farmerie et al., 1987). Inhibition or destruction of reverse transcriptase would act at a point previous to that of the presently licensed antiviral drug, AZT. The latter confuses replication of the virus ordered by the enzyme (Figure 16.19). In the USA, between \$0.6-1.6 Billion will be spent on AIDS research in 1988 and \$120 Million on education about it in the schools, media, and television. In the absence of a cure or a vaccine against the virus, prevention seems the only presently viable strategy.

It has been said that the AIDS issue in the next decade will force people to question what principles are important in their society, what values and trusts should be shared, and what is the degree of an individual's responsibility to others (Stark, 1987).

The single, greatest, ever present, threat to global health, however, is the danger of nuclear warfare between nations. By the end of the century it is estimated that 40 nations will have nuclear capability. Thus, an East-West agreement in itself will no longer suffice and global accord, policies, and strategies will need to supervene. In the words of Pope John Paul, (1980), undoubtedly there is "A fundamental dimension which is capable

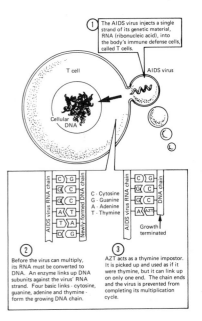

Figure 16.19. Showing how the antiviral drug AZT effects a slowing in the progress of AIDS. Reproduced with permission from Petit, **San Francisco Chronicle**, March 21, 1987.

of shaking to their very foundations the systems on which the whole of humanity is built and of liberating human existence both individual and collective, from the dangers that threaten it. The fundamental dimension is man in his wholeness, man who lives at one and the same time in the sphere of material values and in that of spiritual values."

If indeed our salvation lies within us, there are sufficient, significant issues in the near and long term, that bear upon national and global health and happiness to inspire emergence of the highest leadership and dedication to the task. Increasingly and somewhat hopefully, political, economic, and literary commentary is accentuating co-operative, national and global policies (Etchison, 1987; Obasanjo International Report, 1987; Wainright Capitol Hill, 1987; Peccei, 1981) so that, after all, our course toward the twenty-first Century may be more purposeful than was once imagined.

REFERENCES

Abelson, P.H. (ed.). Treatment of hazardous waste. **Science, 233:** Aug. 1, 1986.

Across State Lines. Study: Seven in 100 are heavy drinkers. **USA Today,** Feb. 13, 1987.

Across State Lines. 176 cities surveyed on policing violence. **USA Today,** Feb. 18, 1987.

AIDS vaccine tests are nearing. **USA Today,** March 27, 1987.

Alber, J.L. and McLean-Ibrahim, E. NATO and Warsaw Pact forces in Europe. **USA Today,** March 5, 1987.

Altman, L.K. AIDS: cooperation vs competition. **New York Times,** April 14, 1987.

American Survey. Toxic wastes: super fund—super bungle. **The Economist,** Feb. 22, 1986.

Associated Press. Bacteria production process could speed AIDS research. **New York Times,** April 18, 1987.

Associated Press. Brain graft gives patient new hope. **New York Times,** April 17, 1987.

Associated Press. Experts support transplant plan. **New York Times,** Mar. 13, 1987.

Associated Press. Genetic research praised as a lifesaver of the future. **Chicago Tribune,** April 21, 1987.

Associated Press. Injections cut sclerosis cases. **New York Times,** April 11, 1987.

Associated Press. Parkinson's victim is first in U.S. to undergo transplant in brain. **New York Times,** April 10, 1987.

Associated Press. Public hospitals ask congress for help with medical aid for the poor. **New York Times,** Mar. 13, 1987.

Associated Press. Waste: northern California hazardous waste sites. **The San Francisco Examiner,** March 16, 1987.

Barnes, D. News and Comments. Grim projections for AIDS epidemic. **Science, 232:** 1589-1590, 1986.

Barnes, D. Research News. Defect in Alzheimer's is on chromosome 21. **Science, 235:** 846-847, Feb. 20, 1987.

Barron, J. Youth suicides: are their lives harder to live? **New York Times,** April 15, 1987.

Beissert, W. Drug cartel rich in cash and power. **USA Today,** Feb. 6, 1987.

Benanti, M. Close-up. Grown children of alcoholics. **USA Today,** Feb. 1987.

Benedetto, R. Tobacco becomes a burning state issue. **USA Today,** Feb. 3, 1987.

Benedetto, R. Welfare reformers on a roll. **USA Today,** Feb. 28, 1987.

Bennell, B. Demise kill off of life. **Globe and Mail,** Jan. 25, 1986.

Berkow, I. Lloyd and Wiggins of Rickets banned for drug use. **New York Times,** Jan. 14, 1987.

Blakeslee, S. Genetic discoveries raise painful questions. **New York Times,** April 21, 1987.

Bollag, B. The AIDS-tainted blood drug: Hemophiliacs pre-1985 use shows up in U.S., Europe's figures. **San Francisco Chronicle,** March 20, 1987.

Book and arts. The death of wage slavery. **The Economist, 95,** May 10, 1986.

Britain, One round too many. **The Economist,** Sept. 13, 1986.

Britain, The environment, a green face for farming. **The Econo-mist,** Dec. 13, 1986.

Brody, J.E. Laser lessens the trauma of surgery in uterus. **New York Times.** April 14, 1987.

Brooke, J. AIDS cases spreading in populous West Africa. **New York Times,** April 15, 1987.

Brooks, A. Real estate: sewer line pacts aid developers. **New York Times.** April 3, 1987.

Canadian Press. Six U.S. states unite to push acid-rain laws. **The Globe and Mail,** Jan. 25, 1986.

Capitol Hill. Enlisting the young in public service. **New York Times,** April 12, 1987.

Carroll, J. The fate of the rain forests. 11, **San Francisco Chronicle,** March 17, 1987.

Champion, D. Acid rain in national parks causing 'Havoc'. **San Francisco Chronicle,** July 22, 1987.

Charting the U.S.A. Dirty air could choke cities federal funding. USA Today, Jan. 23, 1987.

Charting the U.S.A. Aging vetrans top topic at convention. **USA Today,** Feb. 9, 1987.

Chien, C.A. Family violence arrests on rise. **USA Today,** Feb. 18, 1987.

Cocaine: in at the kill. **The Economist,** Oct. 11, 1986.

Cohen, A. Demand increasing for more regulation of toxic wastes. Financial Post, Nov. 16, 1985.

Crack use by kids: serious but exaggerated. **USA Today,** March, 1987.

Crack use reported rising in New York. **New York Times,** April, 1987.

Crick, R.J. Science: bionic arm to give boy more normal life. **The Oregonian,** Aug. 28, 1986.

Cross, M. Science/Nature National Geographic. "Waldsterben" is alarming scientists. **South China Post.** Dec. 8, 1986.

Cross, M. National Geographic Service. Time running out on desert spread UNEP head says. **The Globe and Mail.** Dec. 24, 1986.

Cummings, J. Doctors, fighting the war on AIDS find they are among the casualties. **New York Times,** April 11, 1987.

Dequine. Florida battles bulge of prisoners. **USA Today,** Feb. 3, 1987.

Delvecchio, R. Nuclear agency's critical look at Diablo Canyon. **San Francisco Chronicle,** March 20, 1987.

Diamond, S. Soviet reactor fixes fall short, meet told. **The Oregonian,** Aug. 28, 1986.

Drug interception failing, study says. **San Francisco Chronicle,** Mar. 18, 1987.

Dunn, W. On alert for earth: biologist sounds another warning. **USA Today,** Feb., 1987.

Dunn, W. U.S.A. aging: new median age 31.8. **USA Today,** Mar. 7, 1987.

Eaton, W.J. Soviet lab tests for AIDS. **USA Today,** March, 1987.

Ellis, T. Teaching about sex endagers children. **USA Today,** March 16, 1987.

Environment. A green face for farming. **The Economist**, Dec. 13, 1986.

Etchison, D. Pursuing a North American Accord. **New York Times**, April 15, 1987.

Europe. How green is my continent. **The Economist**, March 14, 1987.

Farmerie, W., Swanstrom, R., Loeb, D., Casavant, Cl, Hutchison, C. and Edgell, M. **Science**, 234: April, 1987.

Farrington, D.P., Ohlin, L.E. and Wilson, J.Q. **Understanding and Controlling Crime: Toward a New Research Strategy**. New York: Springer-Verlag, 1986.

Feature article. Abuse of the elderly. **The Globe and Mail**. Jan. 3, 1987.

Feature article. Water in America. **The Economist**, Oct. 4, 1986.

Feature article. Training for work. **The Economist**, 93-101, Dec. 20, 1986.

Feature article. The anatomy of cities. **The Economist**, 73-81, Dec. 20, 1986.

Feature page. Alcohol, a global binge. **The Globe and Mail**, March 14, 1986.

Findlay, S. A breakthrough in Alzheimer's. **USA Today**, Feb. 5, 1987.

Findlay, S. Is the government doing enough? **USA Today**, April 2, 1987.

Findlay, S. More proof Alzheimer's is genetic. **USA Today**, Feb. 3, 1987.

Findlay, S. Scientists predict health in 2000. **USA Today**, Mar. 5, 1987.

Fisher, M. Dispute brews at waste site. **The Globe and Mail**, March, 1986.

Flattan, E. Population control and China's stability. **Chicago Tribune**, April 25, 1987.

Foster, O. Don't compound the sex education failure. Black Americans for Family Values. **USA Today**, March 16, 1987.

Gaylin, W. On AIDS and moral duty. **New York Times**, 1987.

Gerson, G. Waste disposal management: special report. The **Financial Post**. Nov. 16, 1985.

Gibb-Clark, M. Nuclear waste a pressing problem awaits solution. **The Globe and Mail**, Aug. 16, 1986.

Glass, R.I. new prospects for epidemiologic investigations. **Science**, 254: 951-963, 1986.

Goldgaber, D., Lerman, M.I., McBride, O.W., Saffiotti, U. and Gajdusek, C. Reports. Characterization and chromosomal localization of a cDNA encoding brain amyloid of Alzheimer's disease. **Science**, 235: 877-880, Feb. 20, 1987.

Gordon, B. AIDS educators hope their frank approach will pay off. **San Francisco Chronicle**, March 17, 1987.

Gruson, L. AIDS toll in children is termed a deadly crisis. New **York Times**, April 9, 1987.

Gruson, L. Reactor closing shows industry's people problem. New **York Times**, April 2, 1986.

Halloran, R. Drug use in military drops: pervasive testing credited. **New York Times**, April 23, 1987.

Health and behavior. How to get the facts for discussing AIDS. **USA Today**, March 15, 1987.

Health and behavior. Testing for AIDS: needing to know: facing the answer. **USA Today**, Feb. 25, 1987.

Hellmich, N. Health and Behavior. Tackling the tough topic of condoms. **USA Today**, Feb. 9, 1987.

Holden, C. News and Comment. A revisionist look at population and growth. **Science, 231:** 1493, Mar. 28, 1983.

Holden, C. News and Comment. Growing focus on criminal careers. **Science, 233:** 1377-1378, 1986.

Holden, C. World model for the joint chiefs. **Science**, Nov. 11, 1983.

Idso, S.B. Carbon dioxide and climate. Letters, **Science, 210:** Oct. 30, 1980.

Involuntary smokers face health risks. **Science, 234:** 1066, 1986.

Iuculano, R.P. Fairness to all requires knowledge of risks. American Council of Life Insurance. **USA Today**, Feb. 24, 1987.

Johnson, D. Fear of AIDS stirs new attacks on homosexuals. **New York Times**, Mar. 24, 1987.

Kay, J. Dumps miss deadline to shut down. **San Francisco Examiner**, March 16, 1987.

Keating, M. Where there's smoke: polluters beware. **The Globe and Mail**, Aug. 9, 1986.

Kellog, J. It's wrong for insurers to use these tests at all. Lambda Legal Defense and Education Fund. **USA Today**, Feb. 24, 1987.

Kerr, P. Police shift focus in war on drugs to street deals. **New York Times**, April, 1987.

Kerr, R.A. Research News. Carbon dioxide and a changing climate. **Science**, Nov. 1983.

Kerr, R.A. Research News. Climate since the ice began to melt. **Science, 226:** Oct. 19, 1985.

Klare, A. Cameroon-type volcanic blast called highly unlikely in Northwest. **The Oregonian**, Aug. 28, 1986.

Kozel, N.J. and Adams, E.H. Epidemiology of drug abuse: an overview. **Science, 234:** 970-974, 1986.

Krawiec, R. Is anybody out there listening. **USA Today**, March 20, 1987.

Kristof, N.D. China's birth rate on rise again as official sanctions are ignored. **New York Times**, April 21, 1987.

Lemon, C. Be scared but not to death. **USA Today**, March, 1987.

Leovy, C.B. Carbon dioxide and climate. Letters, **Science, 210:** Oct. 30, 1980.

Letters. Singer, S.; Mathhews, A.; Holdren, J.P., Ehrlich, P.R., Ehrlich, A.H.; Bodoia, R.; Street, J.M., Fuller, G.A., Currey, B.; Sanderson, W., Johnston, B.F.; Davis, W.H., Gowgill, G.L.; Simon, J.L. Bad news is it true? **Science, 210:** 1431-1437, Dec. 19, 1980.

Lewin, R. Research News. Age factors loom in Parkinsonian research. **Science, 234:** 1200-1201, Dec. 5, 1986.

Los Angeles Times Special. Doctor tests AIDS vaccine on himself. **San Francisco Examiner**, March 19, 1987.

Makin, K. Cynicism undermining parole principle. **The Globe and Mail**, Jan. 3, 1987.

Mandatory recycling of garbage is signed into law in New Jersey. **New York Times**, April 21, 1987.

Maranto, G. Special Report. Are we close to the roads end? **Discover**, 28-38, Jan., 1986.

Marshall, E. News and Comment. The lessons of Chernobyl. **Science, 233:** Sept. 19, 1986.

Mayfield, M. Adults are avoiding vaccinations. **USA Today**, Feb. 27, 1987.

McLaren, C. Looking back at a dying planet: the world in year 2010. **Globe and Mail**, Dec. 24, 1985.

McQuay, T. Texas prisons bar new inmates. **USA Today**, Feb. 18, 1987.

Meddis, S. Crime study projections: U.S.A. crisis. **USA Today**, Mar. 1987.

Meddis, S. Drug war termed a sad state of affairs. **USA Today**, Feb. 6, 1987.

Meddis, S. Push to ban tobacco ads moves to congress. **USA Today**, Feb. 6, 1987.

Meddis, S. Study: future holds more crime, violence. **USA Today**, Mar. 17, 1987.

Mental illness linked to genetic defects. **San Francisco Chronicle**, Mar. 21, 1987.

Moore, P. How to fight AIDS: bipartisanship. **New York Times**, April 16, 1987.

Morris, J. Texas prisons, an open and shut case. **USA Today**, Mar. 13, 1987.

Moss, D. Study details health problems of homeless. **USA Today**, March 2, 1987.

Neuman, J. Regan flies to Canada to talk trade. **USA Today**, March, 1987.

New York Times. Reagan seeks more acid rain funds. **The San Francisco Chronicle**, March 20, 1987.

New York Times Report. Cancer caused by N-accident expected to kill 24,000 Soviets. **Seattle Post Intelligencer**, 1986.

News and Comments. Chernobyl: errors and design flows. Science, **233:** Sept. 5, 1986.

News Report. Number of gas victims tops 1,500. **Seattle Post Intelligencer**, Aug. 27, 1986.

Nordheimer, J. AIDS specter for women: the bisexual man. New **York Times**, April 2, 1987.

Obasanjo, O. Debt and drugs in the third world. **New York Times**, April 15, 1987.

One road too many. **The Economist**, Sept. 13, 1986.

Opinion. Teaching about sex protects children. **USA Today**, March 16, 1987.

Opinion. The debate: drugs and travel, random drug tests ensure public safety. **USA Today**, Feb. 3, 1987.

Opinion. The debate: fighting despair. **USA Today**, March 20, 1987.

Opinion. The debate: street people don't warehouse those who need help. **USA Today**, Mar. 5, 1987.

Overhauling welfare is good investment. **USA Today**, Feb. 26, 1987.

Parker, S. Warning signals. **USA Today**, March 12, 1987.

Peccei, A. One hundred pages for the future. New York. **Mentor**, p. 187, 1982.

Petit, C. How AZT drug confuses AIDS virus inside cells. San **Francisco Chronicle**, March 21, 1987.

Pointer, V. Year 2050: 5% of us will be 85+. **USA Today**, Mar. 4, 1987.

Pollack, A. Judge allows field test of man-made organism. New **York Times**, April 24, 1987.

Population Institute Study Report. Family planning advocated to stem population growth. **New York Times**, April 20, 1987.

Push to ban tobacco ads moves to congress. **USA Today**, Feb. 17, 1987.

Raymond, B.B. and Johnson, J. Keep adolescent pressure from crisis point. **USA Today**, March 12, 1987.

Researchers tests a herpes vaccine. **New York Times**, April 23, 1987.

Reuters. New findings on AIDS existence. **New York Times**, April 15, 1987.

Roberts, S. Urban Journal. Victim poses a dilemma for system. **New York Times**, April 30, 1987.

Robbins, W. Farming program on erosion gain. **New York Times**, March 14, 1987.

Ross, M. Lab find offers clue to Alzheimer's. **Globe and Mail**, Oct. 4, 1986.

Schneck, H.M. New infection may activate AIDS viruses, study finds. **New York Times**, April 15, 1987.

Schneider, K. New animal forms will be patented. **New York Times**, April 18, 1987.

Schneider, K. Patenting life. **New York Times**, April 18, 1987.

Schneider, S.H., Kellogg, W.W., Ramanathan, V. Carbon Dioxide and Climate. Letters, **Science, 210:** Oct. 30, 1980.

Science/medicine. Keeping pace: device slows, speeds heart. **Globe and Mail**, Jan. 3, 1987.

Science and Technology. Chernobyl: asking the unanswered question. **The Economist**, May 17, 1986.

Science and Technology. Not in my backyard. **The Economist**, Mar. 8, 1986.

Science and Technology. Russian roulette at Chernobyl. **The Economist**, Aug. 30, 1986.

Science and Technology. Counting cancers: Chernobyl. **The Economist**, Sept. 6, 1986.

Science and Technology. Acid rain: don't rain on Gro's parade. **The Economist**, Sept. 13, 1986.

Science and Technology. When decision makers turn to the experts. **The Economist**, 95, Sept. 13, 1986.

Science and Technology. Grass saves India's soil, where banks do not. **The Economist**, 97, Sept. 20, 1986.

Science and Technology. Good news from Arcadia for the old. **The Economist**, Nov. 29, 1986.

Science and Technology. Living in a global greenhouse. **The Economist**, 91, Nov. 22, 1986.

Science and Technology. Giving India's trees to the people. **The Economist**, 101, Dec. 6, 1986.

Science and Technology. Why some people get AIDS and others don't. **The Economist**, 101, May 23, 1987.

Selkoe, D.J., Bell, D.S., Podlisny, M.B., Price, D.L. and Cork, L.C. Reports. Conservation of brain amyloid proteins in aged mammals and humans with Alzheimer's disease. **Science**, 235: 873-876, Feb. 20, 1987.

Shabecoff, P., E.P.A. acting to halt leaks in underground fuel tanks. **New York Times**, April 2, 1987.

Sheldon, M. (ed.). The rain that kills. University of California, Berkley, **The Wellness Letter**, August, 1987.

Sherlock, J. AIDS medical costs to soar. **USA Today**, April 1, 1987.

Shriver, J. Teen suicide problem is growing. **USA Today**, March 12, 1987.

Simon, J.L. Resources, population environment: an oversupply of false bad news. **Science, 208:** June 27, 1980.

Special report. Of 1.2 million robberies a year, a third of the victims are injured. **New York Times**, Apr. 20, 1987.

St. George-hyslop, P.H., Tanzi, R.E., Polinsky, R.J., Haines, J.L., Nee, L. et.al. Reports. The genetic defect causing familial Alzheimer's disease maps on chromosome 21. **Science**, 235: 885-890, Feb. 20, 1987.

Stark, S.D. AIDS will transform the '88 campaign. **New York Times**, April 11, 1987.

Steed, J. Features. The middle class is under pressure. The rich get richer and the poor more numerous. **The Globe and Mail**, Oct. 4, 1986.

Sullivan, W. Parkinson's surgery faces U.S. use. **New York Times**, April 15, 1987.

Survey high technology. Getting smart. **The Economist**, 13-18, Aug. 23, 1986.
Tobacco becoming a burning issue. **USA Today**, Feb. 3, 1987.

Treaster, J.B. Cuba cites 3 AIDS deaths and new isolation unit. **New York Times**, April 18, 1987.

Tyson, R. At summit, focus is acid rain. **USA Today**, March, 1987.

Unemploymen Rates in America. **USA Today**, Feb. 9, 1987.

United Nations. More aid to Africa is urged. **New York Times**, April 13, 1987.

Villages Correspondent. The greening of the dark continent. The **Economist**, 42, Mar. 14, 1987.

Wainwright. Third world debt: a global solution. **New York Times**, April 14, 1987.

Waite, J.J. Soviet arms shift wins raves in Europe. USA Today, March 2, 1987.

Welfare reformers on a roll. **USA Today**, Feb. 28, 1987.

Wells, T. A river of cocaine rises in Colombia. **Seattle Post Intelligencer.** Aug. 27, 1986.

What smoking costs Americans. **San Francisco Examiner**, Mar. 20, 1987.

Whitaker, B. Alcohol a global binge. **The Globe and Mail**, March 14, 1987.

Whitaker, B. **The global connection: the crisis of drug addiction.** New York. Jonathan Cape, 1987.

Woller, B. Study shows mental illness can be inherited. USA **Today**, Feb. 26, 1987.

World Business. The cloud over Russian crops and energy. **The Economist**, May 10, 1986.

Yarrow, A. NY Times News Service. Early marital break-ups on the increase. Champaign, Urbana. **News Gazette**, Jan. 13, 1987.

Index

RA
425
.C774
1988

RA
425
.C774

1988

$33.85